POSITIVE APPROACHES TO HEALTH

POSITIVE APPROACHES TO HEALTH

CLAIRE DUMONT
AND
GARY KIELHOFNER
EDITORS

Nova Science Publishers, Inc.
New York

Copyright © 2007 by Nova Science Publishers, Inc.

All rights reserved. No part of this book may be reproduced, stored in a retrieval system or transmitted in any form or by any means: electronic, electrostatic, magnetic, tape, mechanical photocopying, recording or otherwise without the written permission of the Publisher.

For permission to use material from this book please contact us:
Telephone 631-231-7269; Fax 631-231-8175
Web Site: http://www.novapublishers.com

NOTICE TO THE READER

The Publisher has taken reasonable care in the preparation of this book, but makes no expressed or implied warranty of any kind and assumes no responsibility for any errors or omissions. No liability is assumed for incidental or consequential damages in connection with or arising out of information contained in this book. The Publisher shall not be liable for any special, consequential, or exemplary damages resulting, in whole or in part, from the readers' use of, or reliance upon, this material.

Independent verification should be sought for any data, advice or recommendations contained in this book. In addition, no responsibility is assumed by the publisher for any injury and/or damage to persons or property arising from any methods, products, instructions, ideas or otherwise contained in this publication.

This publication is designed to provide accurate and authoritative information with regard to the subject matter covered herein. It is sold with the clear understanding that the Publisher is not engaged in rendering legal or any other professional services. If legal or any other expert assistance is required, the services of a competent person should be sought. FROM A DECLARATION OF PARTICIPANTS JOINTLY ADOPTED BY A COMMITTEE OF THE AMERICAN BAR ASSOCIATION AND A COMMITTEE OF PUBLISHERS.

LIBRARY OF CONGRESS CATALOGING-IN-PUBLICATION DATA
Positive approaches to health / Claire Dumont and Gary Kielhofner (editor).
    p. ; cm.
  Includes bibliographical references and index.
  ISBN-13: 978-1-60021-800-2 (hardcover)
  ISBN-10: 1-60021-800-8 (hardcover)
 1. Medicine and psychology. 2. Health attitudes. I. Dumont, Claire, 1954- II. Kielhofner, Gary, 1949-
  [DNLM: 1. Attitude to Health. 2. Behavioral Medicine--methods. W 85 P855 2008]
R726.5.P67 2008
613--dc22
                        2007030902

Published by Nova Science Publishers, Inc. ✤ New York

Contents

Preface		vii
Chapter 1	Cognitive Functions as Adaptation Factors and Resilience in Neglected Children *Pierre Nolin, Frédéric Banville and Bernard Michallet*	1
Chapter 2	Volition: The Motivational Dimension of Health, Illness and Impairment *Gary Kielhofner and Renee R. Taylor*	23
Chapter 3	Possibility Spaces in Everyday Life: On Creative Potentials in Interventions for Persons with Life-Threatening Incurable Illness *Staffan Josephsson, Karen LaCour and Hans Jonsson*	37
Chapter 4	Theorization of Spirituality in Health Care: An Illustration through Occupational Therapy *Étienne Pouliot*	47
Chapter 5	Ecological Approaches to Health: Interactions between Humans and Their Environment *Claire Dumont*	65
Chapter 6	Positive Psychology and Health *Renee R. Taylor and Gary Kielhofner*	141
Chapter 7	Empowerment Approaches to Identifying and Addressing Health Concerns among Minorities with Disabilities *Yolanda Suarez-Balcazar and Fabricio Balcazar*	153
Chapter 8	Intersectoral Action and Empowerment: Keys to Ensuring Community Competence and Improving Public Health *William A. Ninacs and Richard Leroux*	169
Chapter 9	Literature and Medicine: Possible Amalgam? *Jean Désy*	187
Index		203

Preface

Our aim, in bringing together the chapters of this text, was to offer the reader a number of different perspectives on health-related interventions. This text seeks to go beyond the dominant biomedical perspectives that emphasis disease, diagnosis, cure or management of symptoms/impairments. While this biomedical perspective has been highly successful in managing disease and some of its sequelae, there are many dimensions of human experience that are not effectively touched by this approach. Moreover, the biomedical perspective tends to rely on normative view that sees disease and impairment as an aberration.

The perspectives offered in this book are highly diverse, but they have one thing in common. They each discuss a positive approach that aims to enhance health and well being. Moreover, they look beyond the lacks or dysfunctions associated with disease and impairment and emphasize instead people's strength, abilities, and potentials to harness inner motivation, stories, spirit, and hope as well as to be lifted up by creative contexts, literature and other resources of the environment.

It is not our intention here to offer a single unified thesis. Rather, we have needed to add new themes to the discussion of what should be done in the face of illness and impairment. We also gave the contributors of each chapter the freedom to approach their topic as they saw best. Some chapters, therefore, are empirically grounded, others are more theoretical and speculative, still others focus more on issues of practical application. Our intention, in letting each of the themes of this book to be presented in its own way, was to give the reader a look at this particular way of thinking from someone who was deeply embedded in the topic at hand. As a result some chapters will be read as a discussion of possibilities (e.g., a chapter on narrative) while others are more cautionary (e.g, the chapter on spirituality) and yet others are practical (e.g, the chapter on volition). Each of the chapters does provide a rich survey of the territory of the perspective so that the reader can gain an appreciation and also know where to look for more resources.

The themes (chapters) in this book are as follows:

- Resilience
- Volition
- Narrative
- Spirituality
- Ecological perspectives
- Positive psychology

- Empowerment of disadvantaged persons
- Community empowerment
- Literature

Each represents a different way of thinking about such issues of health, illness, impairment, healing, care, and rehabilitation. In the following sections, we offer a brief overview of the chapters.

The first chapter is about resilience. It explores the topic of resilience through presenting the results of a study. The study had three aims: a) to investigate whether neglect is associated with cognitive deficits as measured by a neuropsychological assessment; b) to determine whether socioeconomic status influences performance on neuropsychological tests; and c) to determine whether some neglected children manage to obtain a neuropsychological profile similar to control children, indicating their ability to adapt or their resilience. A neglected group of children were compared with a control group of children matched for age, gender and socioeconomic status and with a second control group matched for age and gender but from middle to high socioeconomic status. Neuropsychological assessment focused on attention, visual-motor integration, memory and learning, language, and frontal/executive functions. The neglected children showed a significantly poorer performance than the children in the two control groups on complex tests measuring attention and visual-motor abilities. Surprisingly, verbal learning and planning abilities were significantly better for the neglected children and mid/high socioeconomic status children than for the low socioeconomic status children. The results of this study point to the heterogeneity of cognitive profiles in children based on socioeconomic status and neglect. A promising conclusion is that the study showed that some neglected children do manage to develop good cognitive functions, viewed as an individual protective factor in terms of their ability to adapt in times of adversity. Protective and adaptation factors have been recognized as components of the more global concept of resilience. The chapter ends with a discussion of resilience and its potential as a resource.

The second chapter concerns the concept of volition which refers to the human drive to act and the associated thoughts and feeling that humans have about themselves as actors in the world. Volition, based upon theories of motivation that stress the human desire for exploration, mastery, competence and achievement. Volition is seen as a powerful force in the face of illness and disability. When a person's volition is negatively influenced by illness or impairments, the process of coping and living is compromised. On the other hand, strong volition can lead to willful, conscious decisions that can lead an individual to a positive life even in the face of illness and impairment. The chapter discusses volition in relation to health, illness, and impairment. It also characterizes stages or levels of volition. Strategies for evaluating difficulties with volition using clinical assessments are discussed. Finally the chapter overview approaches to restoring and capitalizing upon volition to enhance quality of life and functioning for individuals with disabilities. Examples within clinical practice situations are provided to illustrate the importance of volition-related concepts, measures, and interventions.

The third chapter concerns narrative approaches to meaning in the midst of illness and disability. The authors discuss how narrative understanding is a human process of meaning-making involving the process of emplotment of life events and circumstances. The chapter elaborates on how narrative approaches and understanding can be used to create meaning, forge connections to life and imagine a possible future. The chapter illustrates the potential of narrative by examining a workshop of creative activities for elderly persons with life-threatening illnesses. Life-threatening illness is experienced as a disruption of life and it requires a process of meaning-making. The authors argue that involvement in creative activities provides not only a platform for enjoyment and competence but also opportunities to connect to life both in a more abstract existential way symbolized through the concrete process of creation. These will be co-construction of disrupted narratives between client and therapist.

The fourth chapter discusses the idea of integrating spirituality in health care. Spirituality has become a major interest in many health care professions. The author discusses one profession, occupational therapy and its attempt to incorporate spirituality into a model for practice. The author illustrates how spirituality is made into a domain of knowledge in the field. The process of how professions tend to make spirituality into an object, professionally defined is revealed as a misconstruction of spirituality and its presence in the context of illness and health services. The author offers a different approach in which spirituality is understood in a horizon of practice. The necessity and nature of a change of paradigm in how spirituality is conceived in relationship to professional health practice is discussed.

The fifth chapter discusses and analyses how ecological models and approaches could contribute to improve human health. In the first section of the chapter, the evolution of human thought is redrawn, from ancient conceptions of the world up to the most recent ecological models. The second section presents a review of ecological theories, models, and approaches relevant to the field of health. In the third section, common characteristics of ecological theories, models and approaches are described. The fourth section deepens the concepts of environment and interactions, since these concepts were to date less defined in previous publications. New theoretical referents are proposed for these two elements. The fifth section presents the results of numerous studies with the aim of providing scientific evidence in support of ecological models and approaches. These studies are grouped according to the targeted components of ecological models, which are the person, environment or occupation, as well as the interactions between these components. Finally, the sixth section brings a different perspective. Some fundamental ecological mechanisms of interaction are analyzed according to human health and to the current context. Many research questions are proposed to improve knowledge in the field of human ecology in this section. Concrete suggestions for people involved in the field of health are also identified in order to improve population health.

The sixth chapter is about positive psychology. A question that has been raised with respect to all models of psychotherapy is whether they might overemphasize pathology and underemphasize the importance of recognizing, cultivating, and sustaining positive aspects of thinking and experience. In response to this question, the field of positive psychology was introduced. Positive psychology involves the study of positive emotions, such as confidence, hope and trust, positive traits, such as strengths, virtues and abilities, and positive institutions. Other valued emotions, or subjective experiences, include well-being, contentment, and satisfaction with the past, hope and optimism for the future and flow and happiness in the present. Valued individual traits include the capacity for love and work, courage, interpersonal aptitude, spirituality, wisdom, high talent aesthetic sensibility, perseverance, forgiveness, originality, and future mindedness. The need for a positive psychological approach to psychotherapy may be more pronounced when treating individuals with chronic medical conditions. Some clients may perceive cognitive therapy strategies, such as Socratic questioning, elicitation of automatic thoughts, and frequent summaries of presenting problems, as overly negativistic, pessimistic, frightening, or otherwise threatening - irrespective of whether alternative approaches to thinking and behaving are introduced. Some clients will have a strong need for reassurance and may request a more optimistic approach on the part of their therapists. In these circumstances, positive psychology approaches to cognitive therapy that emphasize hope and optimism are recommended.

The seventh chapter discusses personal empowerment and disability as participatory approaches to health promotion. Participatory approaches to empowering people with disabilities to increase control over decisions that affect their lives have been suggested in the literature in a variety of disciplines. However, little is known about participatory strategies to promote personal empowerment as it relates to health promotion. This chapter will suggest a contextual framework for participatory and empowerment strategies for health promotion among individuals with disabilities with emphasis on minorities with disabilities. The suggested framework includes the interaction between environmental and person-related variables that can assist individuals in removing barriers to health promotion and strengthening support systems. Examples will be provided to illustrate different empowering strategies. For instance, person-related strategies include peer mentoring. An example of peer mentoring include a peer mentoring approach developed to promote health and prevent secondary conditions among low-income minority individuals with violence-induced spinal cord injuries (VASCI) transitioning in the community after hospital discharge and pursue community integration while maintaining their health and preventing infections or pressure sores. Examples of environmental strategies include advocating for accessible exercise facilities in the community. The implications of empowering approaches to health promotion and the prevention of secondary individuals with disabilities will be discussed.

The eighth chapter is about intersectoral action, individual and community empowerment as keys ensuring community competency in public health. A community is competent when it provides access for its members to the resources required to ensure their health and well-being and when its members use the accessible resources to their advantage. Intersectoral action is a key to succeeding on the first level while empowerment is a prerequisite to achieving the second. Successful intersectoral action depends on an understanding of the role that each sector plays with regards to a community's diverse functions. The public and private sectors are generally instrumental while the non-profit sector includes an existential component. Concerted action between the sectors can thus result in a broader perspective of health promotion and more comprehensive, partnership-based service delivery. Enabling factors include a win-win approach and realizing that the process takes time and resources. Obstacles include lack of flexibility, especially in government institutions, hidden agendas and unrealistic expectations. There are at least two simultaneous empowerment processes required for a community to be competent and there exists a dialectical relationship between the two. The individual empowerment process is comprised of four components (participation, technical ability, self-esteem, critical consciousness), each of which evolves along a continuum of its own. Empowerment stems from the interweaving of the four, with each component simultaneously building on and strengthening the others, and thus intervention is needed on all four levels at the same time. The community empowerment process also has four interwoven components: participation, knowledge and ability, communication, and community capital. Intersectoral participation is influenced by the essential interaction of each process' components, since the two processes build upon and strengthen each other. An organisation can be an empowering environment since it is a functional community. The role of organisations in intersectoral participation is thus central. Since the majority of community-based organisations operate in the health arena, either by offering social support to specific — and often at risk — population groups or by providing crisis or specialized interventions on problems such as homelessness, poverty, suicide prevention, prostitution, mental health, food security and nutrition, substance abuse, HIV/aids and domestic violence, ensuring that these organisations support individual and community empowerment can be considered to be a vital public health issue. Finally, an organisation is an entity unto itself and, within the larger community that it is part of, it evolves through an empowerment process similar to that of an individual, but with recognition replacing self-esteem. Intersectoral strategies must take this process into consideration in order to be successful.

The ninth chapter is a special contribution. It closes the book with a more literary and poetic text. Certain masterpieces of the literature offer powerful parables to understand the mazes of the human soul. This chapter proposes different reflections on being a health practitioner from various literary works. The author states a possible fusion between the knowledge of the medical field and those of the literary field. This fusion can only enrich a more positive and wider vision of the health. At this particular moment of the human History, it is required to retie the world of the arts (and of the literature) with the world of the sciences. There is only one real representation of the human life in its totality, found in certain particular texts, which can lead to a certain resolution of the new problems in which the humanity is confronted. The biggest challenges in biology cannot remain sensible and relevant if the artistic point of view does not make counterweight to the scientific point of view. The arts, as the literature, intervene when the science can nothing more, in front of the problem of suicide and death in particular. Without being able to answer the question: does the literature make us better, the author nevertheless asserts that the literature, very often, makes us more lucid.

We hope that these complementary positive perspectives about positive approaches to health will help readers to develop better professional practices, with the aim of improving population health.

The authors in this text are as varied as its topics.

Fabricio E. Balcazar, Ph.D., is a Professor in the Department of Disability and Human Development at the University of Illinois at Chicago. Dr. Balcazar has conducted research over the past 23 years on the development of systematic approaches for promoting the empowerment of minorities and under-served populations, including Latinos with disabilities and their families. His research has included the development and evaluation of approaches for promoting empowerment approaches to vocational rehabilitation service delivery, school-to-work transition, dropout prevention, the promotion of the ADA in Latino neighbourhoods, and career development leading to employment opportunities for minority youth with disabilities. Dr. Balcazar is the director of the Center for Capacity Building on Minorities with Disabilities Research and has been actively engaged in the development and dissemination of cultural competence trainings for researchers and service providers. Dr. Balcazar is a fellow of the American Psychological Association.

Frédéric Banville has a Master in psychology and is doctoral candidate at the *Université du Québec à Trois-Rivières*. He is program evaluator since 2004 in the domain of physical rehabilitation. He is also member of the *Groupe de Recherche en Développement de l'Enfant et de la Famille* (GREDEF). He practices neuropsychology since 1996 at the *Centre de réadaptation en déficience physique Le Bouclier* in the province of Quebec, and in a private clinic. His research interests are about evaluation and neuropsychological intervention for executive dysfunctions using virtual reality, intervention following mild traumatic brain injury, and analysis of the process of certain interventions in the fields of neurotraumatology and language impairment.

Karenla Cour, is a lecturer at University College South in Naestved, Denmark and a doctoral candidate at the Division of Occupational Therapy at Karolinska Institutet, Stockholm, Sweden. Her doctoral studies focus on creativity and engagement of people with advanced cancer from an occupational perspective. Her research emphasizes a critical gaze on creativity as a resource enabling people in dealing with and creating connections to everyday life when dealing with life-threatening illness.

Jean Désy is physician and practices medicine in the Great North of the province of Quebec mainly for Inuits. He teaches as associated Professor at the Faculty of Medicine of Laval University. He also obtained a PhD in Literature at Laval University, with the aim of meaning-making of the suffering he meets every day. He wrote many books and obtained many literature prizes in the province of Quebec.

Claire Dumont obtained her PhD in public health in 2003. She is occupational therapist and works in the field of rehabilitation since more than 20 years at the *Institut de réadaptation en déficience physique de Québec*, a rehabilitation centre affiliated to Laval University and recognized as University Institute. She is associated professor at the Rehabilitation Department of the Faculty of medicine at Laval University. Her main interests in research are social participation of people with disabilities, interaction between personal and environmental factors and new technology. She published many articles, and she currently is a member of a team working in program evaluation at the *Institut de réadaptation en déficience physique de Québec*.

Hans Jonsson, is Associate Professor at the Division of Occupational Therapy at Karolinska Institutet in Stockholm, Sweden. He conducts research in the field of Occupational Science and Occupational Therapy with a focus on occupational transitions and occupational balance and patterns of daily life. He has contributed to theoretical articles and book-chapters about narrative theory and methodology.

Staffan Josephsson, is Assistant Professor at the Division of Occupational Therapy at Karolinska Institutet in Stockholm, Sweden and affiliated as researcher at the Sør-Trøndelag University College in Trondheim, Norway. He has used narrative theory in a number of studies regarding conditions for creativity and agency for persons with disability. He has published within the field of narrative methodology and in the borderland of art and health.

Gary Kielhofner is currently Professor and Wade/Meyer Chair, Department of Occupational Therapy, College of Health and Human Development Sciences. He obtained a classical bachelors degree in psychology and philosophy from St. Louis University, a Masters of Arts in occupational therapy from the University of Southern California, and a Doctorate in Public Health from the University of Southern California. Dr Kielhofner's research has focused on how persons with disabilities cope and manage everyday life. He is the co-author/editor of 16 books and has published over 125 articles. He is recipient of 3 honorary Doctoral Degrees, two of which were awarded from European Universities. He was named by the University of Illinois as a University Scholar.

Richard Leroux has a Master in sociology and a Certificate in pedagogy. He teaches at the *Cégep de Victoriaville* since 1978. He was the coordinator of the Department of Mathematics and Human sciences, educational adviser, individual educational assistant, and main researcher in different studies in pedagogy and in program evaluation. Mastering the concepts and the tools of the quantitative and qualitative research, he also realized several studies, researches and evaluations in the province of Quebec. He notably published the didactic volume "The quantitative methods, from the application to the concept". Involved in the community environment of the Bois-Francs region since 1978, he participated in the implementation and the management of numerous community organizations. He develops a particular expertise in evaluation, program elaboration, education, and in social and community intervention in a perspective of empowerment.

Bernard Michallet obtained a PhD in speech therapy at the University of Montreal. He is program evaluator at the *Centre de réadaptation en déficience physique Le Bouclier* in the province of Quebec. He is also speech therapist since many years, and he mainly worked with children having language impairments and their families. He is member of the *Centre de recherche interdisciplinaire en réadaptation* (CRIR) and of the *Groupe inter-réseaux de recherche sur l'adaptation des familles et de leur environnement* (GIRAFE). His research has focused mainly on needs identification of family having a child with dysphasia, and clients' empowerment during and after rehabilitation.

William A. « Bill » Ninacs, is consultant, researcher and professor in the fields of social and community intervention focusing on empowerment, economical development, and social economy at the *Coopérative de consultation en développement LA CLÉ à Victoriaville (Québec)*, from which he is the president. M. Ninacs obtained his Ph.D. in social services at Laval University. He is associated Professor at Laval University. He was the coordinator of the first community development cooperative in the province of Quebec. He is co-director of the Canadian Network in social community development. He does research in this field and has published many books and articles in French and in English. He taught at the School of Community Economic Development of Southern New Hampshire University and at Concordia University (Montreal).

Pierre Nolin obtained his PhD in neuropsychology at the Quebec University at Montreal. He is tenure Professor and researcher at the Quebec University at Trois-Rivieres, since 1989. He is member of the *Groupe de Recherche en Développement de l'Enfant et de la Famille* (GREDEF) and the *Groupe de Recherche et d'Intervention en Négligence* (GRIN). His current research interests are neuropsychological assessment, virtual reality in neuropsychology, neuropsychological effects of neglect, memory, learning for people with traumatic brain injury and other. He got a teaching prize at the Quebec University at Trois-Rivieres in 2003 and the professional prize of the Quebec Psychologist Board in 2005.

Étienne Pouliot, is professor and research professional at the Faculty of Theology and Religious Sciences of Laval University (Quebec). He is also a member of the ethic unity of the research centre affiliated to Laval University Robert-Giffard (CRULRG). He obtained a PhD in theology with a specialization in spirituality oriented on ethics in 2003. He has completed a formation in clinical pastoral and has been practicing in this field in mental health. Because of his double interest in spirituality and ethics, his researches focus on epistemology and language philosophy. They are also centred on hermeneutics, and more particularly on semiotic (post-structuralism).

Yolanda Suarez-Balcazar, Ph.D., is a Professor and Head of the Department of Occupational Therapy at the University of Illinois at Chicago (UIC). She obtained her PhD from the University of Kansas, and came to UIC from Loyola University Chicago, where she was an Associate Professor in the Department of Psychology. She has two related areas of scholarship. Her research examines the impact of community health programs designed for ethnic minorities and for minorities with disabilities. Additionally, she seeks to build service providers' capacity for providing evidence-based, culturally competent services. Dr. Suarez-Balcazar is currently the Associate Director of the Center for Capacity Building for Minorities with Disabilities Research, and Co-Chair of the Community Action Research Centers. She is a member of the American Occupational Therapy Association, the American Evaluation Association, the Society for Community Research and Action and a Fellow of the American Psychological Association.

Renée Taylor is an internationally-known researcher on the psychobiological aspects of post-infectious fatigue and chronic fatigue syndrome. She is an associate professor of occupational therapy and psychology at the University of Illinois at Chicago and practices psychotherapy part-time. In 1995 and 1997, Taylor received her M.A. and Ph.D. in clinical-community psychology from DePaul University (Chicago, Illinois, USA). She completed post-doctoral training in child and adolescent psychology at Ravenswood Hospital in Chicago in 1998. She then served two additional post-doctoral years as project director for a widely-cited, large-scale National Institute of Health funded epidemiological study of chronic fatigue syndrome. Since that time, Taylor has received as a principal investigator over $3,000,000 in U.S. federal research grants. Currently, she is completing a National Institute of Health-funded, prospective study of post-infectious fatigue following acute Epstein-Barr infection in adolescents. Recently, she has also initiated collaboration with Dr. Brigitte Huber at Tufts University in Massachusetts to explore genetic polymorphisms that may be associated with post-infectious fatigue. Taylor also participated in three by-invitation international workgroup meetings hosted by the U.S. Centers for Disease Control and Prevention at Cold Spring Harbour Laboratory in New York. Taylor has published over 60 articles on fatiguing conditions and four books.

Chapter 1

COGNITIVE FUNCTIONS AS ADAPTATION FACTORS AND RESILIENCE IN NEGLECTED CHILDREN

Pierre Nolin[*,1]*, Frédéric Banville*[2] *and Bernard Michallet*[2]

[1]Department of Psychology, University of Québec at Trois-Rivières
Groupe de recherche en développement de l'enfant et de la famille
[2]Centre de réadaptation en déficience physique Le Bouclier

ABSTRACT

Objective: The aim of the present study was threefold: first to investigate whether neglect is associated with cognitive deficits as measured by a neuropsychological assessment; second, to determine whether socioeconomic status (SES) influences performance on neuropsychological tests; and third, to determine whether some neglected children manage to obtain a neuropsychological profile similar to control children, indicating their ability to adapt or their resilience.

Methodology: Twenty-seven children aged 6 to 12 years and currently receiving Child Protection Services because of neglect (Group 1) were compared with a control group of 27 children matched for age, gender and SES (Group 2) and with a second control group of 27 children matched for age and gender but from middle to high SES families (Group 3). Neuropsychological assessment focused on attention, visual-motor integration, memory and learning, language, and frontal/executive functions.

Results: Cognitive profiles were obtained for each group. The neglected children showed a significantly poorer performance than the children in the two control groups on complex tests measuring attention and visual-motor abilities. The neglected children and low SES control children obtained lower scores than the mid/high SES control children for attention and language functions. Surprisingly, verbal learning and planning abilities were significantly better for the neglected children and mid/high SES children than for the low SES children.

Conclusion: The present study underscores the relevance of neuropsychology to neglect research. The results support the heterogeneity of cognitive profiles in children

---

[*] Correspondence should be addressed to: Pierre Nolin, Department of Psychology, University of Quebec at Trois-Rivières, P.O. Box 500, Trois-Rivières, Quebec, Canada, G9A 5H7. Email: Pierre.Nolin@uqtr.ca. Telephone: (819) 376-5085, ext. 3544. Fax: (819) 376-5195.

based on SES and neglect. A promising conclusion is that the study showed that some neglected children do manage to develop good cognitive functions, viewed as an individual protective factor in terms of their ability to adapt in times of adversity. Protective and adaptation factors have been recognized as components of the more global concept of resilience.

Keywords: child neglect, maltreatment, neuropsychology, cognitive functions, socioeconomic status, resilience.

INTRODUCTION

According to the Third National Incidence Study of Child Abuse and Neglect (NIS-3) (Sedlak and Broadhurst, 1996) and to the Canadian Incidence Study of Reported Child Abuse and Neglect (Trocme et al., 2001), the primary reason for investigation is neglect. Nevertheless, co-occurrence of different types of maltreatment for the same child is frequent (Trocme et al., 2001).

Neglect is defined as the chronic failure of parents to respond to their child's health, hygiene, protection, education or emotional needs. Neglect is thus the absence of beneficial parental behaviors rather than the presence of detrimental behaviors (Éthier Lacharité and Gagnier, 1994).

The Canadian Incidence Study of Reported Child Abuse and Neglect (Trocme et al., 2001) suggests a rate of 21.52 cases for every 1,000 children. However, this rate includes three types of cases: cases that were corroborated upon an investigation of the family (9.71 cases for every 1,000 children) as opposed to cases that were not corroborated (7.09 cases for every 1,000 children) or remained presumed (4.71 cases for every 1,000 children). Of these, neglect was the primary reason for 40% of all reported cases.

Maltreatment and Cognitive Performance

Studies on cognitive deficits observed in neglected children have for the most part confined their investigation to intelligence and language. Furthermore, many of the studies examined a combination of children who were experiencing various forms of maltreatment. Below is a summary review of the scientific literature on the topic, which then leads up to the rationale and description of this research, which took a neuropsychological approach.

On the *intellectual* level, Erikson Egeland, and Pianta (1989) reported lower intellectual performance in physically abused and neglected children who had been administered the WPPSI. Diminished intellectual performance was also demonstrated by Barahal Watermen, and Martin (1981). Hoffman-Plotkin and Twentyman (1984) compared the performance of maltreated children to control children and found a lower IQ in a group of maltreated children aged 3 to 9 years. Other authors have found significantly lower results for maltreated children on some verbal and non-verbal sub-tests of the IQ test (Oates and Peacock, 1984). The findings of Palacio-Quintin and Jourdan-Ionescu (1994) are along the same lines. Using a group of 38 maltreated children and a control group, they showed clearly lower intellectual development in the maltreated group, and particularly for verbal performance. Poorer intellectual performance in maltreated children has therefore been documented.

Maltreatment sequelae have also been reported in terms of *language*. Receptive vocabulary proved to be deficient in physically abused children 2 to 12 years of age (Perry, Doran and Wells, 1983) assessed using the Peabody Picture Vocabulary Test. Expressive language problems have also been noted (Coster and Cicchetti, 1993). Other authors have documented problems in more than one language sphere (Culp *et al.*, 1991).

There is relatively strong support for cognitive delays and dysfunctions in maltreated children for certain domains, but in terms of the vast field of neuropsychology, such support is fragmented. In fact, very few maltreatment studies have adopted a neuropsychological approach. Neuropsychology focuses mainly on brain/behavior relationships. Not only do neuropsychological assessment instruments enable clinicians to confirm the presence of brain damage, they can provide a neurofunctional profile of an individual. The first objective of this chapter is to investigate whether neglect is associated with cognitive deficits as measured by a neuropsychological assessment.

Neglect and Socioeconomic Status (SES)

One of the difficulties encountered in neglect studies is the fact that neglectful families are very often also low income families. Poverty is not a rare occurrence in North America (McLoyd, 1998). Many studies have shown that disadvantaged socio-economic status (SES) is a significant risk factor for intellectual development (Palacio-Quintin, 1997). This has been demonstrated for various components of cognition, including creativity (Forman, 1979), perception (Willis and Pishkin, 1974), graphic expression (Gauthier and Richer, 1977), preoperational logical-mathematical thought (Palacio-Quintin, 1992), intelligence and language (Duncan, Brooks-Gunn and Klebanov, 1994; Smith, Brooks-Gunn and Klebanov, 1997; Zill, Moore, Smith, Stief and Coiro, 1995). A good number of studies that controlled for maternal IQ, level of education, age and behavior during pregnancy have found significantly negative effects on children's cognitive and verbal skills (Korenman, Miller and Sjaastad, 1995; Liaw and Brooks-Gunn, 1994; Smith, Brooks-Gunn and Klebanov, 1997). For example, Duncan Brooks-Gunn, and Klebanov (1994) used a longitudinal study to show that family income and poverty significantly predicted IQ in five-year-old children, even after controlling for maternal level of education, family structure, ethnic origin and other factors.

The combined information gained from the studies cited above support a link between SES and children's performance on tests measuring intelligence and cognitive functions. The second objective of this chapter is to determine whether socioeconomic status (SES) influences performance on neuropsychological tests.

Adaptation and Resilience in Maltreated Children

Resilience is a complex and abstract concept and there is no consensus in the clinical and scientific communities as to its definition. It is generally seen as a dynamic process resulting in the continuation of positive development in spite of adversity (Vanistandael and Lecompte, 2000). The development of an aptitude for resilience has often been described in the literature with respect to children who have undergone a serious psychological trauma. For some authors, an abrupt rupture in an individual's development is necessarily involved. The Mother-Child Project approached resilience as a process that situates a person from an ecosystemic and developmental perspective. In that context, resilience refers to a person's ability to succeed and master a specific stage in his/her development (Egeland, Carlson and Sroufe, 1993).

The two factors most often linked statistically to resilience are locus of control and hardiness. Locus of control is the extent to which the person feels they have control over events in their environment (Chorpita and Barlow, 1998). In a study by Robin et al., (1996) (cited in Hart, Hofmann, Edelstein and Keller, 1997), resilience is viewed as the capacity to have the right degree of control. Resilient children do better in school. They have fewer concentration problems, move more rapidly towards a so-called internal locus of control, develop better comprehension of friendship and have better social relations. The concept of hardiness was introduced by Kobasa (1979) in order to compare different responses to daily stressors. For him, locus of control is encompassed in the concept of hardiness. A person demonstrates hardiness when she or he is able to experience a high degree of stress in their daily life without manifesting any psychosomatic disorders. Individuals who display hardiness have three main personal traits: they believe in their ability to control and influence events in their life (i.e. internal locus of control), they are deeply committed to (or involved in) their daily activities, and they perceive change as exciting, challenging, or as a chance to grow and learn. For Callahan (2000), the concept of hardiness is a personal trait that enables an individual to resist life's stressors. So, when control is possible in a given situation, environmental challenges and the psychological stress potentially associated with these challenges may facilitate the adaptive functioning of the person over time.

Resilience may be viewed as a personal, social or cultural trait leading to positive adjustment in a difficult life context. Thus resilience is not just a set of individual characteristics or personality traits. As it is not acquired for life (Cyrulnik, 1999, 2003; Masten, 2001; Rutter, 1998), the protective factors a person develops at a particular time do not make them "invincible" to subsequent ordeals. Indeed, for Larose (2003), the person becomes resilient to something in a specific context. It is therefore logical to assume that transference of resilience competencies from one situation to another does not always occur. Paradoxically, it appears that having overcome significant challenges in the past acts as a protective element. Indeed, when a person credits themselves with successful adjustment, they remember their "control capacity" in an adverse situation. As a result, emotional stability at a specific point in their life may have a major impact on their capacity to use and express their "acquired adaptive competencies". In some cases, accumulation of adverse situations may strengthen the person; in other cases it makes them more vulnerable. According to Chorpita and Barlow (1998), certain individuals may benefit from a steeling effect: some stressors may enable a certain individual and psychological "immunity" to be actualized. In other words, the ordeal may be a learning experience as a result of which the individual develops new adjustment reflexes in adverse situations.

Dyer and McGuiness (1996) examined the concept of resilience to understand the variations between individuals in crisis situations. They found that some people react symptomatically to an objectively minor event, whereas others experience no distress when faced with trauma even though they objectively assess it as significant. It would appear that a weakening of a person's adaptation systems before or after an ordeal increases his/her risk of developing adaptive problems, particularly when the situation persists (Masten, 2001). Chorpita and Barlow (1998) reported that early incidences of loss of control in life experiences create a learning process where children expect to suffer negative repercussions in everyday events. This leads them to continue feeling anxious when life events occur, interpreting them as being more serious than they are in reality.

Neglect is clearly a condition in life that jeopardizes children and their development. De Bellis (2005) states that neglect can be experienced by children as a trauma, the stressor being their inability to reach a state of trust in their parent (Schore, 2001). According to that perspective, neglect can mobilize the children's capacity for resilience. Along the same lines, Moran and Eckenrode (1992) show that maltreated children under the age of 11 years who display low self-esteem and an external locus of control are more likely to suffer from depression. This implies that an internal locus of control acts as a protective factor that is vital to resilience, an idea supported by Robin et al. (1996) (cited in Hart, Hofmann, Edelstein and Keller, 1997). For that reason, the third objective of the current study is to determine whether some neglected children manage to obtain a neuropsychological profile similar to control children, indicating their ability to adapt or their resilience. This would lead us to believe that good cognitive abilities constitute a protective factor. Lastly, as mentioned previously, resilience is a complex abstract multifactorial concept. For the purposes of this chapter and given the results of our study, resilience will be examined from an individual psychological perspective. This means that the main aspects of resilience will be discussed almost exclusively in terms of their link to cognitive and psychological protective factors.

Aim of the Study

The aim of this chapter is to determine whether it is possible to cognitively differentiate low SES neglected children from their non-neglected peers from low and mid/high SES families, and whether some of the neglected children manage to develop good cognitive abilities in spite of the detrimental effect of their surroundings. If so, the fact that they develop good cognitive abilities could be interpreted as a protective or resilience factor.

METHOD

The neglected children in the current study had been targeted by the Province of Quebec's Child Protection Services (CPS) whose legal mandate is to identify cases of child maltreatment. This agency is not part of a hospital setting. The children were identified as being exposed to neglect. All the neglected children came from families where child protection intervention involved legal action and were under CPS care.

Participants

Group 1, referred to as the Neglect group, was composed of twenty-seven child victims of neglect. The mean age for this group was 8.7 years (SD = 1.9 year) and it consisted of 15 boys and 12 girls. Group 2, the first comparison group, was made up of twenty-seven children from low SES families and is referred to as the Low SES Control group. The mean age for this group was 8.8 years (SD = 1.8 year) and it consisted of 16 boys and 11 girls. Group 3, the second comparison group, was composed of twenty-seven children and will be referred to as the Mid/high SES Control group. The mean age for this group was 9.00 years (SD = 1.8 year) and it consisted of 17 boys and 10 girls from mid/high SES families. There were no differences between the three groups in terms of age [$F(2, 79) = 1,19$, $p > .05$] and gender [$X^2 = 0.6$, $p > .05$]. The families of the Neglect children and Low SES Control children earned $29,000 (Cdn.) or less annually. The children in the Mid/high SES Control group came from families earning an annual income over $30,000 (Cdn). Significant differences were noted between Group 3 and Group 1 [$X^2 = 88.03$, $p < .05$] and between Group 3 and Group 2 [$X^2 = 87.72$, $p < .05$], according to their SES.

Assignment to Group 1: Neglect

To form the Neglect group, the children's CPS files were consulted. Standard CPS procedure requires that the type of maltreatment be determined through a detailed study conducted by agency case workers. Child protection procedure involves a number of steps before child neglect or maltreatment is officially confirmed. First, reports of neglect and/or abuse are investigated. A case worker conducts an investigation of the family, which may include a visit to the family home, and may also call upon health professionals, such as a doctor, for help in coming to a decision. The case worker is equipped with a computer program in the form of a decision tree that examines certain aspects in greater detail, depending on each situation. As quickly as possible, and within a maximum of 24-48 hours following the report of child neglect and/or abuse, the case worker must determine if there are sufficient indications to refer the case to the second step in the investigation. If this leads to the conclusion that CPS intervention is necessary, a second, more thorough, assessment is conducted. At this stage, the case worker has a maximum of 12 days (ideally less) to clearly document the situation and the type of maltreatment involved (neglect, physical abuse, sexual abuse, etc.). Meetings are set up with the child, the child's parents and other persons deemed important in the case, such as the child's teacher. At this point, the parents are confronted with the facts and possible legal consequences of the investigation. A decision is made based on: 1) objectified facts, 2) the child's vulnerability from a health and developmental standpoint and 3) the quality of parenting skills involved. The decision takes the form of legal action, where care for the child becomes the responsibility of Quebec's CPS. Voluntary measures may then be proposed to the parents (for example, beginning a six-month intervention program for members of the family) or legal action may be taken (for example, placing the child in foster care without the approval of the biological family). The children and parents who agreed to participate in the research project were then referred to the team of researchers.

A research professional met with the children's parents for a six-hour assessment. At that time, the type of maltreatment was re-evaluated with a number of questionnaires. *The Family Life Information Questionnaire* was developed by the research team (Ethier, Lacharité, Desaulniers and Couture, 2002) and provides information on the couple and their relationship with the children. The first question deals with changes in the couple's status. Questions 2 and 3 address the quality of the relationship between the spouses and each of the children in the family. The fourth question concerns foster care placements of the children since birth. The *Information on the Primary Environment of the Target Child (0 to 12 years of age) Questionnaire* was also developed by the research team (St-Laurent, Nolin and Desaulniers, 2003). Four questions address the mother's physical and psychological health as well as any prenatal drug or alcohol use. Nine questions deal with the perinatal period and the child's present and past state of health. Lastly, the questionnaire contains 30 questions concerning life events that may have occurred in the immediate family since the child's birth.

Exclusion Criteria

Children who were physically or sexually abused, who showed mental retardation or whose birth had been difficult (premature infant, umbilical cord around the neck, prenatal alcohol or drug use by the mother), or children who had been diagnosed as having brain damage (traumatic brain injury, epilepsy, concussion, anoxia, meningitis, encephalitis) were excluded from the current study.

Comparison Groups

Children in the same class at school as the neglected children brought home letters requesting their participation in a study on child cognitive development. Children who most closely matched the characteristics of the children in the neglected groups were then selected, based on the data of the 148 children assessed with their parents' consent. The children were put in group 2 (low SES) or group 3 (middle to high SES).

The children in the study were French-speaking and came from the same geographical area – in or near a mid-sized city (population: 150,000) in Quebec, Canada. The children's parents (or the foster parents of children who were in foster care at the time of the assessment) all signed a consent form. Children who were ten years old or older also signed a consent form and children under the age of ten gave their consent verbally; this was recommended by the university's ethics committee. The research project was approved by the ethics committee of University of Quebec at Trois-Rivières.

Instruments

The selected battery of tests covered five neuropsychological domains: attention, memory and learning, visual-motor integration, language, frontal/executive functions. All these tests are currently used in both clinical neuropsychology and research (see Baron, 2004; Lesak, 2004).

1. Attention

The *Digit Span Forward* subtest assesses the child's ability to repeat increasingly longer series of digits. This subtest is scored for accuracy and the result is the number of digits in the longest series repeated by the child. This subtest has good psychometric properties for its validity and reliability (see Wechsler, 1991).

The *Visual Attention* subtest of the French-Canadian form of the *NEPSY* (Korkman, Kirk and Kemp, 1998) assesses attention, speed and the accuracy with which a child can visually scan a set of elements and locate a targeted element. The child observes the images and crosses out the targets as quickly and accurately as possible. This subtest is scored for speed and accuracy. Raw scores were converted to age-corrected standard scores. The scale is from 1 to 20 (M= 10, SD = 3). This subtest has good psychometric properties for its validity and reliability (see Korkman, Kirk and Kemp, 2003).

The *Auditory Attention and Response Set* subtest of the French-Canadian form of the *NEPSY* (Korkman, Kirk and Kemp, 1998) assesses the children's capacity for vigilance and maintaining selective attention, as well as their ability to modify their pattern of response. The children must place different colored foam squares into a box by following audio-taped instructions. This subtest is scored for speed and accuracy. The raw scores were converted to age-corrected standard scores. The scale is from 1 to 20 (M= 10, SD = 3). This test has good psychometric properties for its validity and reliability (see Korkman, Kirk and Kemp, 2003).

2. Visual-Motor Integration

The *Beery-Buktenica Developmental Test of Visual-Motor Integration* (VMI) (Beery, 1997) is an un-timed test used to assess visual integration, visual motor skills, spatial organization and visual-perceptive ability. The design-copying portion of the test consists of a developmental sequence of 24 geometric shapes. Normative data are provided in the form of standard scores (M = 100; SD = 15). This test is scored for accuracy and it has good psychometric properties for its validity and reliability (see Beery, 1997).

3. Memory and Learning

French-Canadian norms (Lussier, 1996), of the *California Verbal Learning Test for Children* (CVLT-C; Delis, Kramer, Kaplan and Ober, 1994) which evaluates memory and verbal learning, were used in this study. The CVLT-C consists of a list of 15 words (List A) in three semantic clusters. The list is read five times to the child, who has to recall as many words as possible each time. An interference list of 15 words is then presented (List B). This is followed by immediate free recall of the words on List A, and then cued recall. Twenty minutes later, free and cued recalls are performed to assess retention of information over time. Finally, the child performs a recognition task, which involves identifying the 15 List A words among distractors. This test is scored for accuracy. The score used in the study was the total number of words recalled during the five learning trials. This test has good psychometric properties for its validity and reliability (see Delis, Kramer, Kaplan and Ober, 1994).

4. Language

The *Comprehension of Instructions* subtest of the French-Canadian form of the *NEPSY* (Korkman, Kirk and Kemp, 1998) assesses ability to process and respond to verbal instructions of increasingly complex syntax. The first items require the children to point to rabbits of different colors, sizes and facial expressions in order to test their receptive language. The last items require the children to respond to verbal instructions by pointing to targeted shapes according to their color, their position and their relationship with other shapes. This subtest is scored for speed and accuracy. Raw scores were converted to age-corrected standard scores. The scale is from 1 to 20 (M= 10, SD = 3). This subtest has good psychometric properties for its validity and reliability (see Korkman, Kirk and Kemp, 2003).

5. Frontal/Executive Functions

The *Verbal Fluency* subtest of the French-Canadian form of the *NEPSY* (Korkman, Kirk and Kemp, 1998) assesses ability to produce words belonging to different semantic and phonemic categories. The children must say as many names of animals as possible in one minute, then as many names as possible of things to eat or drink in one minute. They must also produce words beginning with the letter S and then the letter M, each during one minute. This subtest is scored for accuracy. Raw scores were converted to age-corrected standard scores. The scale is from 1 to 20 (M= 10, SD = 3). This subtest has good psychometric properties for its validity and reliability (see Korkman, Kirk and Kemp, 2003).

The *Tower* subtest of the French-Canadian form of the *NEPSY* (Korkman, Kirk and Kemp, 1998) assesses planning, control, self-regulation and problem-solving. The child must move three different colored balls on three pegs by following a prescribed number of moves in order to build a model. This subtest is scored for speed and accuracy. Raw scores were converted to age-corrected standard scores. The scale is from 1 to 20 (M= 10, SD = 3). This subtest has good psychometric properties for its validity and reliability (see Korkman, Kirk and Kemp, 2003).

The *Statue* subtest of the French-Canadian form of the *NEPSY* (Korkman, Kirk and Kemp, 1998) assesses motor persistence and inhibition. The child must remain in a certain position for over 75 seconds and ignore auditory distractors. This subtest is scored for accuracy. Raw scores were converted to age-corrected percentile ranks (M = 26-75). This subtest has good psychometric properties for its validity and reliability (see Korkman, Kirk and Kemp, 2003).

The *Knock and Tap* subtest of the French-Canadian form of the *NEPSY* (Korkman, Kirk and Kemp, 1998) assesses control and ability to inhibit motor reactions in response to a visual stimulus that is in contradiction with a verbal instruction. The children must learn a pattern of motor responses and then maintain that pattern of responses and inhibit their tendency to imitate the action of the examiner. This subtest is scored for accuracy. Raw scores were converted to age-corrected percentile ranks (M = 26-75). This subtest has good psychometric properties for its validity and reliability (see Korkman, Kirk and Kemp, 2003).

Procedure

Administration of the neuropsychological tests took between 90 and 120 minutes, depending on the competence and age of the child. All children were administered each test in the same sequence and at their school. They received a gift worth $10 (Cdn) once they had completed all the tests and were told this prior to beginning the assessment. The tests were administered by psychology undergraduates who had received a 10-hour training session on testing procedures. Testers were also given an instruction booklet, and a supervisor was available at all times to answer their questions. The subjects were randomly distributed to the testers by the research professional in charge of testing. The testers were blind to the group membership of the subjects. The tests were scored by a master's student in neuropsychology, and the scores were counterchecked by a second student before the data was keyed into the SPSS software.

RESULTS

Group Comparisons

The three groups were compared (Neglect, Low SES Control and Mid/high SES Control) by conducting a MANOVA with group membership as the independent variable and the neuropsychological test results as the dependent variables. The scores are shown in detail in Table 1. Univariate analyses were then performed to determine which tests best differentiated the three groups. Least Significant Difference (LSD) post hoc analyses yielded specific comparisons between groups where a main effect was found. These data also appear in Table 1.

The multivariate analysis (MANOVA) showed a significant difference between all three groups when all the tests are considered together (see Table 1).

The F univariate and LSD post hoc analyses (see Table 1) showed significant differences between all three groups.

The neglected children obtained significantly lower scores than both control groups on the tests measuring attention and ability to modify their pattern of response (*Auditory Attention and Response Set*), and visual-motor integration (*VMI*).

The Neglect group and the Low SES Control group obtained significantly lower scores than the Mid/high SES Control group on the tests measuring attention (*Digit Span Forward* and *Visual Attention*) and language (*Comprehension of Instructions*)

The neglected children and the Mid/high SES Control children obtained significantly higher scores than the Low SES Control children on tests measuring verbal memory and learning (*CVLT-C*) and planning (*Tower*).

No differences were observed between the three groups on tests for verbal fluency (*Verbal Fluency*) and motor inhibition (*Statue* and *Knock and Tap*).

Discriminant Analysis

Variables used for the discriminant analysis were the same as those indicated in the section above on group comparisons. The analysis yielded a significant first-order discriminant function ($X^2 = 52.09$ $df = 20$; $p = .000$) and a significant second-order discriminant function ($X^2 = 20.90$; $df = 9$; $p = .013$). Neuropsychological tests therefore did discriminate between the three groups. Table 2 shows the absolute correlation of each variable with the discriminant functions.

Table 1. Mean scores for all tests administered and statistical analysis results

	GROUP							F	F	LSD
	Group 1 Neglect (n = 27)		Group 2 Low SES Control (n = 27)		Group 3 Mid/High SES Control (n = 27)			Multivariate	Univariate	
	M	SD	M	SD	M	SD				
								2.93***		
Digit Span Forward	4.33	1.04	4.59	1.01	5.37	0.88			8.20***	1,2 < 3
Visual Attention	8.96	2.61	8.89	2.63	11.30	3.18			6.35**	1,2 < 3
Auditory Attention and Response Set	8.15	1.70	9.37	1.47	9.56	1.70			5.97**	1 < 2,3
VMI	22.52	18.86	35.30	28.48	38.30	27.04			3.00*	1 < 2,3
CVLT-C	44.33	9.67	39.85	10.38	42.26	10.22			4.69**	2 < 1,3
Comprehension of Instructions	8.70	2.57	9.22	3.12	11.63	1.47			10.68***	1,2 < 3
Verbal Fluency	8.78	2.53	7.93	2.73	9.22	2.36			1.81	-
Tower	12.22	2.23	10.63	3.20	12.15	2.64			2.95*	2 < 1,3
Statue	79.07	22.18	78.11	22.58	85.04	8.12			1.07	-
Knock & Tap	74.67	23.33	68.07	25.56	74.44	20.49			0.70	-

* p < .05.
** p < .001.
*** p < .00.

Table 2. Structure Matrix

	FUNCTION 1	FUNCTION 2
Comprehension of Instructions	.71	.17
Digit Span Forward	.63	.09
Visual Attention	.52	.26
Auditory Attention & Response Set	.45	-.37
VMI	.32	-.24
Statue	.20	.13
CVLT-C	.29	.48
Tower	.05	.48
Verbal Fluency	.14	.32
Knock and Tap	.03	.23

A correlation of .33 (10% of the variance) is considered acceptable (Tabachnick and Fidell, 1996). Function 1: "language capacity and attentional shift". This function is composed of the following tests: *Comprehension of Instructions, Digit Span Forward, Visual Attention,* and *Auditory Attention and Response Set*. It represents the children's language capacity and ability to carry out attention tasks that require ability to shift. Function 2: verbal learning and planning. This function is composed of the *CVLT-C* and *Tower (NEPSY)* tests. It represents the children's capacity for verbal learning and cognitive planning.

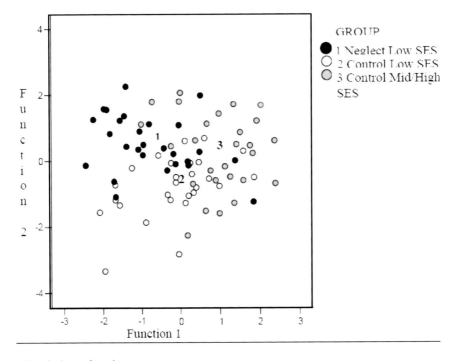

Figure 1. Discriminant functions.

Discriminant analysis confirmed that the neuropsychological tests would differentiate the children according to their group membership. The means for Group 1 for Functions 1 and 2 were -.78 and .51, respectively; the means for Group 2 were -.17 and -.79, respectively; and the means for Group 3 were .95 and .23, respectively. Figure 1 shows the distribution of subjects according to the two discriminant functions and their group membership. It shows that the children in the three groups are distributed around a central point according to their group membership. It also shows that each of the three groups occupies a specific place in relation to the other groups along the two axes representing the two functions resulting from the discriminant analysis.

Classification Statistics

Table 3 shows the group classification results. The discriminant variables predicted group membership in 64.2% of the cases. The neglected children can be differentiated from both control groups on Function 1 by a poorer performance on language, attention and ability to shift. The Low SES Control group also showed a poorer performance for Function 1 in comparison with the Mid/high SES Control group.

Table 3. Classification Results

		PREDICTED GROUP MEMBERSHIP			
		Group 1	Group 2	Group 3	Total
ORIGINAL	Group 1	18 (67%)	4 (15%)	5 (18%)	27 (100%)
	Group 2	3 (11%)	17 (63%)	7 (26%)	27 (100%)
	Group 3	5 (18%)	5 (18%)	17 (63%)	27 (100%)

Function 2, which represents verbal learning and planning, differentiates the Low SES Control children since their performance is poorer than that of the Mid/high SES Control children, in addition to being poorer than that of the neglected children. In fact, the neglected children are comparable to the Mid/high SES Control children for Function 2.

DISCUSSION

The current study had three objectives. The first was to determine whether a neuropsychological assessment would detect specific cognitive deficits in neglected children. The second was to see whether neglected children from low SES families would perform differently on neuropsychological tests in comparison with control children from low and mid/high SES families. The third objective was to determine whether neglected children would manage to develop same-level cognitive performance as control children from advantaged families, which would support the idea that cognitive performance contributes to resilience.

The results of means comparison analyses show that neglect is associated with deficits in attention (ability to modify a pattern of response) and visual-motor integration. The neglected children performed more poorly for those functions than children in the two control groups. Discriminant analysis also shows that the Neglect group can be differentiated from both control groups on Function 1, because of their poorer performance on language, attention and ability to shift (*Comprehension of Instructions, Digit Span Forward, Visual Attention,* and *Auditory Attention and Response Set*). These findings would suggest that neglected children have, at least partially, a specific cognitive profile. Neglect affects certain cognitive functions and not all the functions covered by the neuropsychological assessment; the neglected children showed problems only for the first cluster of cognitive functions (Function 1). However, further studies will be necessary since the profile of the children in the Neglect group is similar in some respects to the Low SES Control children. Furthermore, these results cannot be compared with the findings of previous studies because very few of the latter examined neglect using a neuropsychological approach. These findings do add to previous research that showed poorer performance by neglected children for intelligence (Erikson, Egeland and Pianta, 1989; Palacio-Quintin and Jourdan-Ionescu, 1994) and language (Coster and Cicchetti, 1993). These results also concur with studies that demonstrated the negative effects of poverty on the development of neglected children (Aber and Cicchetti, 1984; Cicchetti and Toth, 1995) since the children in the cohort were socioeconomically disadvantaged. To sum up, the initial objective of the study was to show that neglected children may display a more extensively deficient cognitive profile and not only in terms of intellectual performance; the intensity and extent of damage to cognitive functions may depend, however, on a number of familial, social, individual or other factors. Further exploration of these aspects would be a valuable addition to maltreatment research.

Means comparison analyses showed that both the children in the Neglect group and the Low SES Control group obtained significantly lower scores than children in the Mid/high SES Control group on tests measuring attention, language and mental flexibility (ability to shift). Discriminant analysis also showed that the control children from low SES families performed more poorly on verbal learning and planning in comparison with the neglected children and the children from mid/high SES families.

Associations between socioeconomic environment and the development of cognitive functions have been well documented (Duncan, Brooks-Gunn and Klebanov, 1994; Palacio-Quintin, 1997; Smith, Brooks-Gunn and Klebanov, 1997; Zill, Moore, Smith, Stief and Coiro, 1995). The findings of this study reflect those of previous authors who demonstrated the negative effect of low SES on intelligence, language and other cognitive functions (Duncan, Brooks-Gunn and Klebanov, 1994; Forman, 1979; Gauthier and Richer, 1977; Korenman, Miller and Sjaastad, 1995; Liaw and Brooks-Gunn, 1994; Palacio-Quintin, 1992; 1997; Smith, Brooks-Gunn and Klebanov, 1997; Willis and Pishkin, 1974; Zill, Moore, Smith, Stief and Coiro, 1995;). Furthermore, it is interesting to note the importance of having SES-matched control subjects when studying other at-risk children. The results of this study have demonstrated that different profiles can be observed when neglected children are compared to low or mid/high SES control subjects.

Neglect, Adaptive Capacities and Resilience

Results of the means comparison analyses show that the children in the Neglect group and the Mid/high SES Control group obtained significantly higher scores than the Low SES Control group on tests measuring verbal memory, learning and planning. Discriminant analysis shows similar results: the neglected children and Mid/high SES Control children showed comparable performances, and were both superior to the Low SES Control children. In addition, classification results from the discriminant analysis show that 18% of the neglected children present cognitive profiles similar to those of control children from mid/high SES families. In other words, these results answer the third question as to whether some neglected children are able to develop good cognitive skills. Furthermore, it is important to see how these research results relate to the concept of resilience. Indeed, despite its complexity, the concept of resilience encourages to expand our thinking with regard to neglected children.

Being resilient means pulling oneself together, bouncing back, forging ahead after an illness, trauma or stress. It means surmounting life's trials and tribulations, that is, resisting and then overcoming them and continuing to live as best as one can (Manciaux, 2004).

Resilience is therefore viewed as an individual's ability to face adverse situations and, in doing so, develop and increase his/her skills (Manciaux, 2004). It is the ability to adapt to variable circumstances and environmental contingencies, which translates into the person being able to analyze the level of correspondence between situational demands and behavioral possibilities, and to make flexible use of a repertoire of problem-solving strategies (Block and Block, 1980). For Cyrulnik (1999), there is not such a thing as the socio-cultural profile of a resilient child but rather a profile of traumatized children who have an aptitude for resilience. This ties in with the idea put forward by Banville and Majaron (2005) that protective factors can be categorized into three spheres: affective, environmental and cognitive.

Figure 2 is a diagrammatic representation of protective factors as adaptive mechanisms from the person's point of view. It is also a theoretical representation of the interaction effects that exist between the individual and his/her environment (described in the box on the far right). The section below describes the influence that protective factors relating to the person have on adaptive mechanisms. The model represents an outline that can be used to explain why some young victims of neglect are able to cope better than others.

The *cognitive* protective factors reported in Figure 2 refer to all aspects of cognition (such as memory, judgement, attribution of meaning, interpretation and other executive components) that enable an individual to analyze, interpret and come to a conclusion with regard to a problem encountered. The problem must be sufficiently disturbing that is generates stress which, if not properly managed, can make it difficult for the person to function.

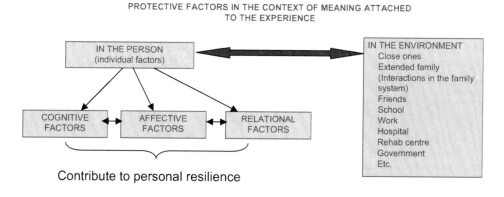

Figure 2. Intervention model based on protective factors (Banville et al., 2002).

Cognitive protective factors therefore play an important role in the attribution of meaning, given that they enable the individual to modulate relevant aspects of perception that can influence thought and memory. Psychologists who use the cognitive approach do the same thing (i.e. modification of perceptions and meaning) in the majority of their treatments. Such modulation of meaning and perceptions has been demonstrated empirically, particularly in victims of mild traumatic brain injury. Studies of mild TBI victims (Mittenber, Tremon, Zielinski, Fichera and Rayls, 1996; Paniak, Toller-Lobe, Durand and Nagy, 1998; Paniak, Toller-Lobe, Reynolds, Melnyk and Nagy, 2000) have shown that knowledge and information provided by people around the victim (which includes case workers) contribute to modifying the meaning attached to the experience. Similarly, these perceptual modifications bring about an improved cognitive management of stress and anxiety. In addition, it would appear that adaptive flexibility also constitutes a protective factor that increases the effectiveness of problem-solving processes. The findings of these TBI studies, which can also be extended to other clienteles, including child victims of neglect, bring to light two main conclusions: Firstly, information and cognitive management of stress enables individuals to distance themselves from and maintain control over events, which influences attribution of meaning and adaptation; secondly, cognitive factors act at varying intensities in most individuals, whatever the ordeals they must overcome. These protective factors can therefore play a particularly important role in the individual's development.

On the affective level, protective factors may enable child victims of affective trauma to modulate their affects and moderate the expression of their emotions. This would promote the use of personality strengths and consequently self-esteem. Lastly, *on the relational and environmental level,* situations that encourage individuals to use their intact social skills and to open up to others, enabling them to get through the ordeal of the moment, with the help of someone who serves as their "resilience tutor".

Certain affective factors and relational and environmental factors have been identified by previous authors. Herrenkohl Herrenkohl, and Egolf (1994) noted the absence of physical abuse, presence of at least one stable adult in the child's life, and positive expectations on the part of the parents with regard to the child's academic performance. Joubert (2004) referred to primitive trust, self-esteem, social skills, optimism, humor, creativity, the ability to give meaning to events, spirituality, willingness to face events, the ability to build a social support network and the ability to ask for and get help.

Cognitive factors are, however, less well targeted. Robin *et al.,* 1996 (cited in Hart, Hofmann, Edelstein and Keller, 1997) pointed to concentration capacities, while Herrenkohl, Herrenkohl, and Egolf (1994) identified level of intellectual performance. If these findings are transposed to the neuropsychological test results of the neglected children in this study, it would suggest that other cognitive functions, such as memory and planning, are also cognitive factors that could influence resilience in neglected children.

Resilience can therefore be considered an ability characterized by a set of personality traits and cognitive functions.

But resilience can also be seen as a *process* – a positive learning process in the face of adversity (Rutter, 1998). Furthermore, for Cyrulnik (1999), resilience is more than resisting, it is learning to live. It is a dynamic process where individuals can develop properly in spite of difficult living conditions or traumatic events. The process is based on the interaction of an individual's internal potential and the support available in his/her environment (Vanistendael and Lecompte, 2004).

Resilience can also be considered the *result* of a process. However, according to Manciaux (2004), it is never absolute, total or acquired once and for all, but varies depending on circumstances, the nature of transformations, contexts and stages in life and according to different cultures.

Above and beyond these definitions, resilience remains a complex and multidimensional concept. Cyrulnik (1999, 2003) explains it as a constant interaction of each of the dimensions mentioned above. Its complexity, however, enables us to formulate questions which need to be answered in the future:

- Do neglected children who develop good cognitive abilities have a psychological profile and personality traits that would enable us to formulate hypotheses as to this positive aspect of their development?
- Do neglected children who have a cognitive profile similar to that of control children from mid/high SES families have personal traits that enable them to seek the help or support they need for their development more easily than other children?
- Are neglected children who develop good cognitive abilities exposed to particular elements in their environment that would explain their development? Even if parents neglect their child, is there someone around them to whom the child can turn and who becomes their "resilience tutor"?
- Have neglected children who developed good cognitive abilities had to overcome ordeals more than the other children? Did the successes they experienced, showing them that it is possible to succeed, in spite of everything, reinforce their confidence in their own abilities?

CONCLUSION

The current study initiates a worthwhile discussion on the cognitive performance of neglected children. These results suggest that most neglected children have cognitive difficulties in language, attention and cognitive flexibility. However, the fact that these children show no significant difference when compared with their non-neglected low SES peers leads us to believe that low SES and the entire context which that entails (improper meals, lack of intellectual stimulation, etc.) significantly influences a child's level of cognitive performance. It is equally surprising to see that the neglected children's cognitive performance (for memory, learning and planning) is equivalent to their non-neglected peers from mid/high SES families. Indeed, these results force us to take a cautious look at our preconceptions since it would appear that neglect and poverty are not necessarily associated with poor cognitive functions, at least for some children.

A valuable contribution to this study would have been to present the "intact" cognitive functions of the neglected children as protective factors promoting resilience, i.e. adaptation in the face of adversity. Clearly, this is a field where research is just beginning and where it has become necessary to further investigate the neuropsychology of neglect, treating cognitive functions as predictors of a child's ability to adapt.

ACKNOWLEDGEMENT

Funding for this study was provided by the Conseil Québécois de la Recherche Sociale, No. RS-3334, Fonds Québécois de Recherche sur la Société et la Culture, No. SR-4709, and Social Sciences and Humanities Research Council of Canada, No 410-2006-2437.

Notes: The authors would like to thank the Mauricie-Centre-du-Quebec Child Protection Services, who facilitated the recruitment of subjects. They would also like to thank Yves Mercure, Daniel Gagnon, Isabelle Frigon, Marie-Eve Nadeau, Louise Bourassa, Cyndie Martin and all the research assistants who made an invaluable contribution to the study.

REFERENCES

Aber, J.L., and Cicchetti, D. (1984). Socioemotional development in maltreated children : An empirical and teoretical analysis. In: H. Fitzgerald, B. Lester, and M. Yogman (Eds.), *Theory and Research in Behavioral Pediatrics* Vol. 2 (pp. 147-205). New York: Plenum.

Banville, F., and Majaron, L. (2005). Intervention psychologique de réadaptation après un TCCL : une approche utilisant la résilience en tant que cadre conceptuel. In : *Recherche interdisciplinaire en réadaptation et traumatisme craniocérébral* Vol. 2, (pp. 169-185). Montréal : Publication du CRIR.

Banville, F., Majaron, L., and Bergeron, C. (2002). *Réflexion sur l'influence de la personnalité dans l'adaptation et dans la réaction aux changements post-traumatiques consécutivement à un traumatisme craniocérébral léger.* Communication par affiche. Congrès international de traumatologie. Québec.

Barahal, R.M., Watermen, J., and Martin, H.P. (1981). The social cognitive development of abused children. *Journal of Consulting and Clinical Psychology, 49,* 508-516.

Baron, I.S. (2004). *Neuropsychological Evaluation of the Child.* New York: Oxford University Press.

Beery, K.E. (1997). *The Beery-Buktenica Developmental Test of Visual-Motor Integration* (4th ed.). Parsippany, NJ: Modern Curriculum Press.

Block, J.H., and Block, J. (1980). The role of ego-control and ego resiliency in the organization of behavior. In: W. A. Collins (Ed.), *Minnesota Symposium on Child Psychology,* Vol. 13 (pp. 39-101). Hillsdale, NJ: Lawrence Erlbaum Associates.

Callahan, C.D. (2000). Stress, coping and personality hardiness in patients with temporomendibular disorders. *Rehabilitation Psychology, 45*(1), 38-48.

Cicchetti, D., and Toth, S.L. (1995). A developmental psychopathology perspective on child abuse and neglect. *Journal of the American Academy of Child and Adolescent Psychiatry, 34,* 541–565.

Chorpita, B.F., and Barlow, D.H. (July 1998). The Development of Anxiety: The Role of Control in the Early Environment. *Psychological Bulletin*, 124 (1), 3-21.

Coster, W., and Cicchetti, D. (1993). Research on the communicative development of maltreated children: Clinical implications. *Topics-in-Language-Disorders, 13*(4), 25-38.

Culp, R.E., Watkins, R.V., Lawrence, H., Letts, D., Kelly, D.J., and Rice, M.L. (1991). Maltreated children's language and speech development: Abused, neglected, and abused and neglected. *First-Language, 11*(33, Pt 3), 377-389.

Cyrulnik, B. (1999). *Merveilleux malheur*. Paris : Presse Odile Jacob.

Cyrulnik, B. (2003). *Le murmure des fantômes*. Paris : Presse Odile Jacob.

De Bellis, M.D. (2005). The psychobiology of neglect. *Child Maltreatment, 10*(2), 150-172.

Delis, D., Kramer, J., Kaplan, E., and Ober, A. (1994). *CVLT-C California Verbal Learning Test for Children*. Toronto: The Psychological Corporation: Harcourt Brace Jovanovich Inc.

Duncan, G., Brooks-Gunn, J., and Klebanov, P. (1994). Economic deprivation and early childhood development. *Child Development*, 65, 296-318.

Dyer, J.G., and Mc Guiness, T.M. (1996). Resilience: Analysis of the Concept. *Archives of Psychiatric Nursing*, X (5), 276-282.

Egeland, B., Carlson, E., and Sroufe, L.A. (1993). Resilience as process. *Development and Psychopathology, 5*, 517–528.

Erickson, M.F., Egeland, B., and Pianta, R. (1989). The effects of maltreatment on the development of young children. In: D. Cicchetti, and V. Carlson (Eds.), *Child Maltreatment* (pp.647-684). Cambridge: Cambridge University Press.

Ethier, L., Lacharité, C., and Gagnier, J-P. (1994). Prévenir la négligence parentale. *Revue Québécoise de Psychologie, 15*(3), 67-86.

Ethier, L.S., Lacharité, C., Desaulniers, R., and Couture, G. (2002). *Informations démographiques (The Family Life Information Questionnaire)*. Unpublished document. Trois-Rivières, QC, Canada: GREDEF, University of Québec in Trois-Rivières.

Forman, S. (1979). Effects of socio-economic status on creativity in elementary school children. *Creative Child and Adult Quarterly, 4*(2), 87-92.

Gauthier, Y., and Richer, S. (1977). *L'activité symbolique et l'apprentissage scolaire en milieu favorisé et défavorisé*. Montreal : PUM.

Hart, D., Hofmann, V., Edelstein, W., and Keller, M., (1997). The Relation of Childhood Personality Types to Adolescent Behavior and Development. A Longitudinal Study of Icelandic Children. *Developmental psychology*, 33 (2), 195-205.

Herrenkohl, E.C., Herrenkohl, R.C., and Egolf, B. (1994). Resilient early school-age children from maltreating homes: Outcomes in late adolescence. *American Journal of Orthopsychiatry*, 64 (2), 301-309.

Hoffman-Plotkin, D., and Twentyman, C.T. (1984). A multimodal assessment of behavioral and cognitive deficits in abused and neglected preschoolers. *Child Development*, 55, 794-802.

Kobasa, S.C. (1979). Stressful Life Events, Personality and Health: An Inquiry into Hardiness. *Journal of Personality and Social Psychology*, 37, 1-11.

Korenman, S., Miller, J., and Sjaastad, J. (1995). Long-term poverty and child development in the United States: Results from the NLSY. *Children and Youth Services Review*, 17, 127-155.

Korkman, M., Kirk, U., and Kemp, S. (2003). *NEPSY Bilan neuropsychologique de l'enfant. Manuel*. Toronto: Psychological Corporation.

Korkman, M., Kirk, U., and Kemp, S. (1998). *The NEPSY Manual*. Toronto: Psychological Corporation.

Larose, F. (2003). Résilience scolaire: État, processus ou produit ? Regards théoriques et considérations méthodologiques sur une « construit valise ». Conférence donnée dans le cadre de la journée d'étude du CRIE : *De la résilience à l'intervention éducative :*

questions d'analyse, accès multidisciplinaires et perspectives d'avenir. Université de Sherbrooke

Lecompte, J. (2004). *Guérir de son enfance*. Paris : Presse Odile Jacob.

Lezak, M.D. (2004). *Neuropsychological Assessment* (4th edition). New York: Oxford University Press.

Liaw, F., and Brooks-Gunn, J. (1994). Cumulative familial risks and low-birthweight children's cognitive and behavioral development. *Journal of Clinical Child Psychology, 23*, 360-372.

Lussier, F. (1996). Normes québécoises du CVLT pour enfants (Quebec norms for the CVLT-C). Unpublished document. St. Justine Hospital, Montreal.

Manciaux, M. (2004). La résilience: Mythe ou réalité ? In : B. Cyrulnik (Ed.) *Ces enfants qui tiennent le coup* (2e Ed.) (pp. 109-120). Revigny-sur-Ornain : Éditions Hommes and Perspectives.

Masten, A.S. (2001). Ordinary magic: resilience processes in development. *American Psychologist, 56*(3), 227-238.

McLoyd, V.C. (1998). Socioeconomic disadvantage and child development. *American Psychologist, 53*(2), 185-204.

Mittenberg, W., Tremon, G., Zielinski, R.E., Fichera, S., and Rayls, K.R. (1996) Cognitive - Behavioral Prevention of postconcussion syndrome. *Archives of Clinical Neuropsychology, 11* (2), 139-14.

Moran, P.B., and Eckenrode, J. (1992). Protective personality characteristics among adolescent victims of maltreatment. *Child-Abuse-and-Neglect, 16*(5) Sept.-Oct. 743-754.

Oates, R.K., and Peacock, A. (1984). Intellectual development of battered children. *Australian and New Zealand Journal of Developmental Disabilities, 10*, 27-29.

Palacio-Quintin, E. (1992). *Test MAME, maturité pour l'apprentissage des mathématiques élémentaires*. Manuel et materiel. Montreal: Institut de recherches psychologiques.

Palacio-Quintin, E. (1997). Facteurs sociaux de risque et facteurs de protection dans le développement cognitif de l'enfant. In: G.M. Garabulsy, and R. Tessier (Eds.), *Enfance et famille: contexte et développement* (pp. 123-135). Ste-Foy, Quebec: Presses de l'Université du Québec.

Palacio-Quintin, E., and Jourdan-Ionescu, C. (1994). Effets de la négligence et de la violence sur le développement des jeunes enfants. *PRISME, 4*(1), 145-156.

Paniak, C., Toller-Lobe, G., Durand, A., and Nagy, J. (1998). A randomized trial of two treatments for mild traumatic brain injury. *Brain Injury, 12*(12), 1011-1023.

Paniak, C., Toller-Lobe, G., Reynolds, S., Melnyk, A., and Nagy, J. (2000). A randomized trial of two treatments for mild traumatic brain injury: 1 year follow-up. *Brain Injury, 14* (3), 219-226.

Perry, M.A., Doran, L.D., and Wells, E.A. (1983). Developmental and behavioral characteristics of the physically abused child. *Journal of Clinical Child Psychology, 12*, 320-324.

Rutter, M. (1998). Resilience Concepts and Findings: Implications for Family Therapy. *Journal of Family Therapy, 21*, 119-144.

Sedlak, A.J., and Broadhurst, D.D. (1996). *Third National Incidence Study of Child Abuse and Neglect*. Washington, DC: U.S. Department of Health and Human Services.

Schore, A.N. (2001). The effects of early relational trauma on right brain development, affect regulation, and infant mental health. *Infant Mental Health Journal, 22*(1-2), 201-269.

Smith, J., Brooks-Gunn, J., and Klebanov, P. (1997). Consequences of living in poverty for young children's cognitive and verbal ability and early school achievement. In: G. Duncan, and J. Brooks-Gunn (Eds.), *Consequences of growing up poor* (pp. 132-189). New York: Russell Sage Foundation.

St-Laurent, D., Nolin, P., and Desaulniers, R. (2003). The *Information on the Primary Environment of the Target Child (0 to 12 years of age) Questionnaire.* Unpublished document. Trois-Rivières, QC, Canada: GREDEF, University of Québec at Trois-Rivières.

Tabachnick, G., and Fidell, L.S. (1996). *Using Multivariate Statistics.* New York: Harper and Collins.

Trocme, N.M., MacLaurin, B.J., Fallon, B.A., Daciuk, J.F., Billingsley, D.A., Tourigny, M., Mayer, M., Wright, J., Barter, K., Burford, G., Hornick, J., Sullivan, R., and McKenzie. (2001). *Canadian Incidence Study of Reported Child Abuse and Neglect.* Ottawa: Minister of Public Works and Government Services Canada.

Vanistendael, S., and Lacompte, J. (2000*). Le bonheur est toujours possible.* Paris : Bayard.

Wechsler, D. (1991). *Manual for the Wechsler Intelligence Scale for Children-Third Edition (WISC-III).* San Antonio, TX: The Psychological Corporation.

Willis, D., and Pishkin, V. (1974). Perceptual motor performance on the Vane and Bender tests as related to two socio-economic classes and ages. *Perceptual and Motor Skills, 38*(3), 883-890.

Zill, N., Moore, K., Smith, E., Stief, T., and Coiro, M. (1995). The life circumstances and development of children in welfare families: A profile based on national survey data. In: P.L. Chase-Lansdale and J. Brooks-Gunn (Eds.), *Escape from Poverty: What makes a Difference for Children?* (pp. 38-59). New York: Cambridge University Press.

Chapter 2

VOLITION: THE MOTIVATIONAL DIMENSION OF HEALTH, ILLNESS AND IMPAIRMENT

Gary Kielhofner[*] and Renee R. Taylor
University of Illinois at Chicago
Chicago, IL 60612 USA

ABSTRACT

Motivation is fundamental to health and to the management of a wide range of illnesses and impairments. Volition, a term based upon existing theories of motivation, connotes the willful or conscious-choice aspect of motivation. The objectives of this chapter are (1) to define volition in relation to health, illness, and impairment, (2) to learn how to characterize stages of volition and to evaluate difficulties with volition using clinical assessment tools, and (3) to demonstrate how re-directing and capitalizing upon volition may enhance quality of life and functioning for individuals with disabilities. Examples within clinical practice situations are provided to illustrate the importance of volition-related concepts, measures, and interventions.

Historically, the topic of motivation has played a prominent role in the understanding of health and illness. Two centuries ago, moral treatment viewed mental illness as a form of demoralization or motivational alienation from life (Kielhofner, 2004). Examples of the importance of motivation in more recent medical and health discourses include discussions of compliance with medical treatment, readiness for change, decision-making related to health and wellness behavior, and discourse in the field of psychoneuroimmunology. These and other discussions underscore that motivation can play an important role in becoming, recovering from, and adjusting to an illness or impairment.

---

[*] Corresponding author: Gary Kielhofner, UIC Department of Occupational Therapy, 1919 W Taylor St. (MC 811) Chicago, IL 60611, phone 01-312-996-3412. fax 01-413-0256. email: kielhfnr@uic.edu

VOLITION: A UNIQUE PERSPECTIVE ON MOTIVATION

In much of the 20th century, views on motivation were rather uni-dimensional; some considered it tissue-related, others libidinal, and others as strictly the result of learning or behavioral conditioning (Freud, 1960). Although with different emphases, a number of theorists in mid-century added to the compendium of human motives a fundamental drive or desire for activity and accomplishment (Berlyne, 1960; DeCharms, 1968; McClelland, 1961; Shibutani, 1968; Smith, 1969; White, 1959).

Based on these revised theories of motivation and other related concepts, a conceptualization of motivation, referred to as volition, was introduced in 1980 and has been subsequently studied and refined (Kielhofner and Burke, 1980; Kielhofner, 2002). The term *volition* connotes will or conscious choice. It was selected to emphasize the deliberate process of willing behavior in contrast to other traditional concepts of motivation which deemphasize conscious choice. For example, psychoanalytic and behaviorist approaches to motivation view behavior as a function of underlying drives which are not under conscious control (DeCharms, 1968; Freud, 1937/1960; White, 1959).

Volition Defined

Volition is as a phenomenon arising from a foundational motive to act that occurs independently of other aspects of motivation, including biological and libidinal drives, and the goal-seeking behaviors they generate (Kielhofner, 2002). Moreover, volition is being grounded both in the nervous system's need for arousal and in an existential opening provided by having a body and mind with the potential for engagement and doing. While this underlying drive for action is considered universal, the concept of volition recognizes that it manifests differently across persons. An individual's unique volition is reflected in ongoing thoughts and feelings an individual has as an actor in the world and in choices and experiences of doing (Kielhofner, 2002). Volitional thoughts and feelings involve concern for one's personal capacity to do things, one's enjoyment and satisfaction in doing them, and the importance or meaning of doing. Three concepts are used to explain the thoughts and feelings that comprise volition:

- personal causation,
- values, and
- interests.

Personal causation, a concept introduced by DeCharms (1992), involves an individual's ever-evolving thoughts and feelings about his or her capacities and efficacy in performance. Values comprise thoughts and feelings about what is important and meaningful to do. Thoughts and feelings pertaining to interest concern enjoyment and satisfaction in doing. In summary, the thoughts and feelings that comprise volition are involved in a cycle of anticipating, choosing, and evaluating the process of acting in the world (Kielhofner, 2002). In this cycle, thoughts and feelings do not only shape choices for action but also are shaped by the doing the selected action. Thus the experience of doing plays a major role in shaping feelings and thoughts.

The concept of volition is used as a guide to understanding people's motivation, including their motivational problems. It offers a way of thinking about both choices concerning what one does in everyday life as well as one's commitment to ongoing and future courses of action (Kielhofner, 2002). A toddler's persistent attempts to take those first successful steps, a child's decision to go for a bike ride with a friend after school, an adolescent's imagining what it would be like to do a particular kind of work, a mother's worry about whether she can balance the demands of her job and a new baby, an adult's reflection on his waning ability to engage in a passionate sport activity, and a grandfather's joy in playing a game of dominos with his grandchildren all illustrate the range of thoughts, feelings, decisions and actions that are a function of volition. In each of these examples, someone is involved in an ongoing process in which motives are being experienced, generated, or expressed (Kielhofner, 2004).

The Role of Volition in Health, Illness and Impairment

An important corollary to volition is the idea that health and well-being are equated not with the absence of illness or impairment, but with the ongoing experience of doing things that provide a sense of capacity and efficacy, that give enjoyment and that allow one to feel a sense of meaning and value (Kielhofner, 2004). Thus illness and impairment are concerns that interfere with the process of doing that gives one a sense of accomplishment. Our very sense of well being is tied to the ease with which we can move into the world. It is important to recognize that not being able to do is its own form of disease.

States of illness and impairment often carry with them pain, suffering, and loss that are direct symptoms or consequences of physiological processes. However, illness and impairment can also bring another type of suffering and loss. This is the suffering that occurs when one is no longer able to do what matters deeply, when one is no longer able to feel the joy or satisfaction attendant to accomplishing things. It is the loss associated with knowing that no longer has valued capacities or opportunities for fulfillment through doing.

Volition is a requirement for authentic engagement in life and also a vital element of therapy change process (Kielhofner, 2002). Volition is essential to change since change requires decision making and commitment to enact and sustain courses of action (Kielhofner, 2002). Whenever a person experiences chronic illness or impairment, volition is always affected and whenever we seek to help people cope with these conditions, volition is always a necessary component.

GATHERING INFORMATION ON VOLITION

Working with volition involves ongoing assessment and discovery. When facing a new or escalating condition, many people may have difficulty resuming activities or identifying new activities that matter to them, and help to restore a sense of personal competence and fulfillment. For clients struggling with issues of motivation, such as values, meaning, capacity, and efficacy, a clear understanding of these complex volitional issues is needed.

Four assessments derived from the model of human occupation can provide critical information about a client's volition and readiness for change (Kielhofner, 2002). They may serve as useful supplements to other measures of cognition and behavior:

- The Occupational Self Assessment (Baron, Kielhofner, Iyenger, Goldhammer, and Wolenski, 2002),
- The Modified Interest Checklist (Kielhofner and Neville, 1983),
- The Occupational Questionnaire (Smith, Kielhofner and Watts, 1986) or the NIH Activity Record (Gerber and Furst, 1992) and
- The Occupational Performance History Interview – Second Version (Kielhofner, Henry, Walens and Rogers, 1991).

Occupational Self Assessment

The Occupational Self Assessment (OSA) (Baron, et al., 2002) is a measure of perceived capacity and importance of a variety of activities. In paper-and-pencil format (See Figure 1 for sample items), clients respond to a series of statements about their performance and about characteristics of the environment that affect performance by indicating how well they accomplish each and how important it is. Then, clients select the activities that are priorities for change in order to voice their own perspectives and shape the goals and strategies of therapy. Though it is relatively brief, this assessment can be broken down into shorter steps and it can be administered verbally for clients requiring accommodation. This tool can be effective in such circumstances because it provides a structured means of reflecting on how well one is performing. It also provides a means of identifying how much different aspects of performance matter.

Often when clients experience many areas of difficulty, it becomes hard to sort out what should be an area of focus. The Occupational Self Assessment provides a concrete means of doing this. It should also be noted that a children's version of the Occupational Self Assessment exists (Keller, Kafkes, Basu, Federico and Kielhofner, 2005). More information about both the adult and child versions of this measure can be obtained in Kielhofner (2007) and at www.moho.uic.edu.

Modified Interest Checklist

The *Modified Interest Checklist* (Kielhofner and Neville, 1983) gives clients an opportunity to indicate what their current interests are, how interests have changed, and whether they participate or wish to participate in an interest in the future. Figure 2 illustrates the format of the assessment. This assessment is helpful in identifying how a chronic illness or impairment has changed interest patterns and participation in activities of interest. It can be completed in sections or administered orally. More information about this measure can be obtained in Kielhofner (2007) and at www.moho.uic.edu.

Step 1: Below are statements about things you do in everyday life. For each statement, circle how well you do it. If an item does not apply to you, cross it out and move on to the next item.					Step 2: Next, for each statement, circle how important this is to you.				Step 3: Choose up to 4 things about yourself that you would like to change. (You can also write comments in this space)
	I have a lot of problems doing this	I have some difficulty doing this	I do this well	I do this extremely well	This is not so important to me	This is important to me.	This is more important to me.	This is most important to me.	I would like to change.
Concentrating on my tasks	a lot of problems	some difficulty	well	extremely well	not so important	important	more important	most important	
Physically doing what I need to do	a lot of problems	some difficulty	well	extremely well	not so important	important	more important	most important	

Figure 1. Sample Portion from the Occupational Self Assessment.

| Activity | What has been your level of interest? ||||||| Do you currently participate in this activity? || Would you like to pursue this in the future? ||
| | In the past ten years ||| In the past year |||| | | | |
	Strong	Some	No	Strong	Some	No	Yes	No	Yes	No
Gardening/Yardwork										
Sewing/Needle work										
Playing cards										
Foreign languages										
Church activities										
Radio										
Walking										
Car repair										
Writing										
Dancing										
Golf										
Football										
Listening to popular music										

Figure 2. Format of the Modified Interest Checklist.

NIH Activity Record and Occupational Questionnaire

The NIH Activity Record (ACTRE) (Furst, Gerber, Smith, Fisher and Shulman, 1987; Gerber and Furst, 1992) and the Occupational Questionnaire (OQ) (Smith, Kielhofner and Watts, 1986) are self-report forms that ask the client to indicate what activity he or she engages in over the course of a weekday and weekend day. Figure 3 shows the format of the OQ; the ACTRE is similar in format.

		Question 1	Question 2	Question 3	Question 4
Time	Typical activities	I consider this activity to be: Work W Daily living task D Recreation R Rest RT	I think that I do this: Very well VW Well W About average AA Poorly P Very poorly VP	For me this activity is: Extremely important EI Important I Take it or leave it TL Rather not do it RN Total waste of time TW	How much do you enjoy this activity? Like it very much LVM Like it L Neither like nor dislike NLK Dislike it D Strongly dislike SD
06:30–07:00		W D R RT	VW W AA P VP	EI I TL RN TW	LVM L NLD D SD
07:00–07:30		W D R RT	VW W AA P VP	EI I TL RN TW	LVM L NLD D SD
07:30–08:00		W D R RT	VW W AA P VP	EI I TL RN TW	LVM L NLD D SD
08:00–08:30		W D R RT	VW W AA P VP	EI I TL RN TW	LVM L NLD D SD
08:30–09:00		W D R RT	VW W AA P VP	EI I TL RN TW	LVM L NLD D SD

Figure 3. Format of the Occupational Questionnaire.

The OQ, on which the ACTRE is based, is the simpler form. It asks persons to report what they are doing during each half-hour waking period of their day. Then they indicate:

- Whether they consider it to be work, leisure, a daily living task, or rest
- How much they enjoy it,
- How important it is,
- How well they do it.

The latter three questions give insight into the volitional characteristics of the activity pattern. That is, they reveal the personal causation, interest, and value experienced in the activity. The questionnaire also provides information about the person's habit patterns (i.e., the typical use of time) and about occupational participation (i.e., the kind of work, leisure, and self-care that make up a person's current life).

The ACTRE, developed for use with persons who have physical disabilities, asks additional questions pertaining to pain, fatigue, difficulty of performance, and whether one rests during the activity. Consequently, in addition to the information provided by the OQ, the ACTRE provides detailed information about how a disability influences performance of everyday activities (i.e., it asks about the level of energy required, the amount of pain and fatigue experienced, and whether rest was taken during the activity). The ACTRE is designed to be used primarily as a 24-hour time log completed at three points during each day. This method helps improve the accuracy of the instrument, since recall is of a very recent past. The forms are ordinarily used to report on an actual period of time, being filled out as diaries during the reporting period. However, it is sometimes more practical to ask clients to report on what is a typical day. In addition to providing details about a client's use and experience of time, these instruments potentially give the occupational therapist important information about the following kinds of problems:

- Particularly troublesome times or activities in the daily schedule,
- Disorganization in the person's use of time,
- Lack of balance in time use,
- Problems such as decreased feelings of competency, a lack of interest, or a lack of value in daily activities.

Occupational Performance History Interview-Second Version

In some cases, it is useful to examine the client's life history, or narrative as a way of exploring volition over time and locating volitional strengths. Often, but not always, clients can draw from past interests and motivators in the process of creating new work roles and finding new activities that they can engage in. A narrative history approach allows for the identification of motivators and strengths that the client may have drawn upon in the past, rather than strictly focusing on negativistic or dysfunctional thinking by continuing to pursue the identification of intermediate and core beliefs. Ultimately, the choice as to whether to pursue a client's narrative, motivators, and strengths versus whether to pursue exploration of intermediate and core beliefs will depend on the time available to treat the client, the client's capacity for narrative exploration, and other unique features of the client-therapist relationship.

If a client and therapist choose to pursue this approach to working with volition, a semi-structured life history interview, the Occupational Performance History Interview-Second Version (OPHI-II) (Kielhofner, 2007) is an effective measure that can guide this process. This measure allows the therapist to collect information about a client's past and present occupational roles, interests and occupational choices, preferred activities, daily routines values, and the life events and settings that can interact with a client's choices and behaviors. It can be broken down as needed to accommodate a person with energy or concentration difficulties. The OPHI-II can be useful for understanding how a chronic condition has changed a client's life, and it reveals how a client perceives her or his life to be unfolding. More information about this measure can be obtained in Kielhofner (2007) and at www.moho.uic.edu.

These assessments can be utilized on a one-time basis as a starting point for identifying strengths and areas of difficulty. Additionally, they may be used for the later establishment of therapeutic goals based on item priorities and importance level. Importantly, they also provide information about the client's *perception* of his or her ability to do things as it contrasts with his or her *actual* ability to do things. Thus, the assessment of volition is critical to the process of evaluating distortions or inaccuracies in thinking as they pertain to a client's performance capacity. Distortions or inaccuracies may be particularly salient for clients with new or escalating chronic illnesses or impairments. These assessments may also be used periodically as follow-up measures throughout the course of therapy to inform turning points or to plan termination. Importantly, these assessments allow the first steps necessary in reclaiming volition that has been affected by illness or impairment. Once clients have identified priorities, capacities, and goals, and have a realistic and accurate perspective of their impairments, activities can be identified, modified, selected, and pursued so that they are more enjoyable and satisfying to perform. This can be characterized as a process of empowering volition.

EMPOWERING VOLITION

The concept of volition recognizes liabilities but emphasizes strengths and motivators Kielhofner (2002). A focus on positive life participation rather than on pathology is used to facilitate authentic involvement in therapy. The following are common empowerment-oriented strategies associated with the concept of volition:

- Building understanding and rapport through careful, narratively-oriented interviewing aimed at revealing how clients interpret their lives and present circumstances coupled with active "checking in" to assure valid understanding[1].
- Actively involving clients in treatment including sharing the concept of volition as a means for self understanding.
- Supporting clients to makes choices to engage in volitionally relevant activities and to reflect on the experience of doing them.

Taken together, these strategies can facilitate clients who are often confused or uncertain about their life circumstance and what the chronic illness or impairment means for their present and future lives. They all focus toward engaging the client in activity planning and problem solving, thereby increasing the client's feelings of control over his or her life.

This approach also emphasizes providing opportunities for persons to experiment, reflect, review and receive feedback on their own capacities and limitations, sense of enjoyment and meaning. This can be accomplished, for instance, through logging their activity patterns and by reviewing their experience of doing. An important process in the management of chronic illness and impairment is for clients to develop a realistic appraisal of their performance capacity and of the effects on engaging in patterns of activity.

Volitional change can also involve values clarification or re-prioritization. With a more restricted capacity for activity, clients are often forced to choose among prior activities of most importance. Therapy may involve assisting clients' re-prioritization of values by identifying what matters to them most.

It can also involve value change. For instance, persons with chronic illness often internalize societal messages that connote illness and disability as essentially "bad". Becoming aware of this internalized oppression can lead persons to re-direct the oppression back to the environment and to focus the parts of self that are essentially valuable. Some persons may need to enlarge the scope of their values to incorporate things that they are still capable of doing. Clients may need to reformulate how they judge their performance making reference to their capacities rather than comparing performance to their past performance and/or to that of others without chronic illness and/or disabilities.

For example, a scenario for many clients with a newly acquired chronic illness or impairment involves which was introduced earlier. Chronic illness is accompanied by the following volitional components:

- Loss of ability to do activities which were previously enjoyable and satisfying,
- Inability to select an activity that is within present capacity because of high standards or expectations of the self.

---

[1] Use of self assessments that allow the client to generate insights to their own volition and identify priorities.

An intervention focusing on volition would suggest the following steps in addressing situations:

- Underscoring the importance of continuing activities that provide enjoyment and satisfaction,
- Acknowledging the reality that some activities and ways of approaching activity are no longer possible,
- Discussing how values (i.e., unrealistically high standards of performance) are making it difficult to chose an activity that might otherwise bring pleasure,
- Identifying why activities were pleasurable activity in the past and what might be enjoyed by them in the present,
- Recommending undertaking old activities in new ways and/or undertaking new activities that are consistent with one's remaining capacities,
- Reviewing how these activities are experienced and proceeding accordingly.

Choosing the right strategy for empowering volition depends, as we have already emphasized, on a careful assessment and understanding of the unique elements of the client's volition. A wide range of examples and strategies for addressing volition can be found in Kielhofner (2007) and in the reference list found at www.moho.uic.edu.

HELPING THE CLIENT WITH LOW OR LOST MOTIVATION: THE REMOTIVATION PROCESS

Sometimes illness or impairment can severely impact volition to the point that the client does not have the resources to engage in the kind of motivational interventions described above. Such clients have for all practical purposes lost motivation. In this case clients must literally be "remotivated". The remotivation process (de las Heras, Llerena and Kielhofner, 2002) is an intervention for people with more severely impaired volition. It was developed over a number of years by clinicians who worked with people with severe and chronic impairments. The remotivation process is predicated on the idea that volition is, in part, socially constructed. That is, the inner thoughts and feelings that come to make up volition are comprised in part of what people see reflected about them by the outside world in social messages. Thus, the social sphere can have a profound impact upon volition and can serve as an important resource for regenerating volition.

The remotivation process is also build on the concept of a volitional continuum comprised of 3 levels or stages of motivation:

- Exploration,
- Competency,
- Achievement.

Exploration is the first level of motivation. At this level persons try out new things and, consequently, learn about their own capacities, preferences, and values. Persons explore when they are learning to do something new, making life changes, or searching for new sources of meaning. Exploration provides the opportunity for learning, discovering new modes of doing, and discovering new ways of expressing ability and apprehending life. It yields a sense of how well one performs, how enjoyable the task is, and what meaning it can have for one's life. Exploration requires a relatively safe and undemanding environment.

Competency is the level of motivation when persons begin to solidify new ways of doing that were discovered through exploration. During this stage of change, persons strive to be adequate to the demands of a situation by improving themselves or adjusting to environmental demands and expectations. Individuals at a competence level of change focus on consistent, adequate performance. Thus they are prone to focus on improving, correcting mistakes, and solving problems. Competency affords an individual a growing sense of personal control and thus affords a sense of pleasure in achieving mastery. *Achievement* is the level of motivation characterized by an even higher level of investment. At this level, people will invest new alteration or energy into an activity. They will take on new responsibilities and challenges associated with the activity.

Underlying the concept of remotivation is the recognition that clients must be met at their current level of motivation. A client who is pre-exploratory (i.e., who shows no curiosity in his environment and cannot take pleasure in action) cannot be expected to spontaneously engage in activity. For such clients, the pleasure of activity engagement may have to be vicarious (by watching someone else do the activity or by having another person perform parts of the activity for the client). Similarly a client at an exploratory level cannot be expected to face mistakes and problems with an attitude of overcoming them. Such clients will be overwhelmed with such challenges and they must be avoided until volition is strengthened. A final point about the volitional continuum is that the highest level of motivation is not necessarily the most desirable for a given client or a given activity. In some instances helping a client move to an exploratory level is simply enough. In other cases a client who has developed new self confidence and discovered news pleasure in doing will want to go on to another level. Supporting volition means supporting the client's choice to go where he or she wants to go motivationally.

Like other volitional interventions the remotivation process is guided by careful evaluation. The information gathered always includes the clients' personal history with an emphasis on his or her volitional experiences (i.e., any past interests, accomplishments, hobbies, cherished activities and so on) and the kind of environments in which this person was most able to do things and happy doing them. When clients are unable to provide this information themselves, it is ordinarily gathered from family members, friends or others who know the client intimately.

In addition, information is always gathered using the Volitional Questionnaire (VQ) (de las Heras, Geist, Kielhofner and Li, 2002). The VQ is based on the recognition that clients, who have difficulty formulating goals or expressing their interests and values verbally, routinely communicate them through actions. For example, persons indicate interest by how much energy they direct to doing something or the affect they display while doing it. Thus, the VQ scale is composed of 14 items that describe behaviors reflecting values, interests, and personal causation. The items that make up the VQ also reflect the volitional continuum that begins with basic behaviors such as being able to indicate preferences and initiate action. Higher levels of volition are indicated by the client's willingness to try to solve problems or correct mistakes and in the display of pride. The highest level of volition is indicated by such behaviors as seeking challenges and new responsibilities.

The items are scored using a four-point rating (passive, hesitant, involved, and spontaneous). The rating indicates the extent to which the client readily exhibits volitional behaviors versus the amount of support, encouragement, and structure that is necessary to elicit them. The scale reflects the fact that persons with higher volition choose action and demonstrate positive affect more readily, whereas persons with more limited volition need additional environmental resources and supports.

The VQ recognizes that a client's motivation may vary in different environments according to how much the features of each environment match the client's interests, values, and personal causation. Consequently, clients are often observed in more than a single context. An environmental form can be used to record information about relevant features of the environment that influences volition. The strategies for selecting the context(s) of observation vary with each client, but the underlying goals are to identify:

- Those factors in the social and physical environment that most affect volition both positively and negatively
- How stable or variable volition is across environments
- The level of motivation a client typically displays,
- The kinds of environmental supports that enhance the individual's volition,
- The client's interests and values

This kind of information allows the therapist to determine the environmental contexts and strategies that will facilitate positive development of the individual's volition.

In addition to learning about the clients' level of motivation and necessary environmental supports the VQ observation also can provide information about:

- The client's interests and values,
- The amount and kind of support required for the client to accomplish a behavior,
- The influence of values, interests, and personal causation on the client's motivation to engage in activities,
- The influence of different environments on the client's volition.

The VQ is used for monitoring the client's level of volition and thus identifying which remotivation strategies should be used with a client.

The remotivation process is divided into three modules as shown in Table 1.

Table 1. The remotivation process

Modules	Goals for the Module
Exploration	Develop a sense of personal capacity, a feeling of security and a realization of personal significance.
Competency	Develop a sense of efficacy and control over decision-making
Achievement	Integrate new areas of performance and new contexts into lifestyle

Each of these modules is further broken down into more specific stages. For example, the exploration module is made up of four stages:

- Validation,
- Environmental exploration,
- Choice-making,
- Pleasure and efficacy in action.

Each of these stages is made up of a set of strategies that is used to remotivate the individual. For instance the stage of validation includes the following two strategies:

- The significant greeting (always encountering the person as a full human being regardless of the persons level of responsiveness) which includes such things as referring to the client by name, announcing oneself and asking for permission when coming into the person's presence, and acknowledging one's awareness of the client's identity or personality, especially by mentioning things that have been of interest to the client or meaningful in some way.
- Introducing meaningful elements (objects or events that have been of interest) into the individual's personal space according to the client's level of tolerance.

The rationale for the use of these strategies is based on the client's level of volition. Thus, for instance if a client is pre-exploratory and shows little or no curiosity in the environment or responsiveness to one's presence, then the strategies of the significant greeting are most appropriate. As the client begins to show a basic level of curiosity, then the strategy of introducing elements of interest and meaning will have the highest efficacy.

The remotivation process is detailed in a manual which also includes case illustrations (de las Heras, Llerena and Kielhofner, 2002). More information on the manual can be found at www.moho.uic.edu.

CONCLUSION

Clients can face challenges to their values, sense of efficacy, and interests at various time points during the course of their illness or impairment. The concept of volition orients us to the importance of understanding clients' volition and of enabling clients to engage in activities that are gratifying, pleasurable, absorbing, and meaningful.

REFERENCES

Baron, K., Kielhofner, G., Iyenger, A., Goldhammer, V., and Wolenski, J. (2006). *The Occupational Self Assessment (OSA)(Version 2.2)*. Chicago: Model of Human Occupation Clearinghouse, Department of Occupational Therapy, College of Applied Health Sciences, University of Illinois at Chicago.

Berlyne, D.E. (1960). *Conflict, arousal, and curiosity*. New York: McGraw-Hill.

DeCharms, R.E. (1968). *Personal causation: The internal affective determinants of behaviors*. New York: Academic Press.

de las Heras, C.G., Geist, R., Kielhofner, G., and Li, Y. (2002). *The Volitional Questionnaire (VQ) (Version 4.0).* Chicago: Model of Human Occupation Clearinghouse, Department of Occupational Therapy, College of Applied Health Sciences, University of Illinois at Chicago

de las Heras, C.G., Llerena, V., and Kielhofner, G. (2002). *Remotivation process: Progressive intervention for individuals with severe volitional challenges. (Version 1.0)* Chicago: Department of Occupational Therapy, University of Illinois at Chicago.

Freud, S. (1960). *The ego and the id* (J. Riviere, Trans.). New York: WW Norton. (Original work published 1937).

Furst, G., Gerber, L., Smith, C., Fisher, S., and Shulman, B. (1987). A program for improving energy conservation behaviors in adults with rheumatoid arthritis. *American Journal of Occupational Therapy, 41,* 102–111.

Gerber, L., and Furst, G. (1992). Validation of the NIH Activity Record: A quantitative measure of life activities. *Arthritis Care and Research,* 5, 81-86.

Keller, J., Kafkes, A., Basu, S., Federico, J., and Kielhofner, G. (2005). *The Child Occupational Self Assessment (version 2.1).* Chicago: Model of Human Occupation Clearinghouse, Department of Occupational Therapy, College of Applied Health Sciences, University of Illinois at Chicago.

Kielhofner, G., and Burke, J. (1980). A model of human occupation. Part one. Conceptual framework and content. *American Journal of Occupational Therapy, 34,* 572-581.

Kielhofner, G., and Neville, A. (1983). *The modified interest checklist.* Unpublished manuscript, Model of Human Occupation Clearinghouse, Department of Occupational Therapy, University of Illinois at Chicago, Chicago, Illinois.

Kielhofner, G., Henry, A., Walens, D., and Rogers, E.S. (1991). A generalisability study of the Occupational Performance History Interview. *Occupational Therapy Journal of Research, 11,* 292-306.

Kielhofner, G. (2002). *Model of human occupation. Theory and application.* 3rd Edition. Baltimore: Lippincott Williams and Wilkins.

Kielhofner, G. (2004). *Conceptual foundations of occupational therapy.* 3rd Edition. Philadelphia: F.A. Davis Company.

Kielhofner, G. (2007). *Model of human occupation. Theory and application.* 4th Edition. Baltimore: Lippincott Williams and Wilkins.

McClelland, D. (1961). *The achieving society.* New York: Free Press.

Shibutani, T. (1968). A cybernetic approach to motivation. In: W. Buckley (Ed.), *Modern systems research for the behavioral scientist.* Chicago: Aldine.

Smith, M.B. (1969). *Social psychology and human values.* Chicago: Aldine.

Smith, N.R., Kielhofner, G., and Watts, J. (1986). The relationship between volition, activity pattern, and life satisfaction in the elderly. *American Journal of Occupational Therapy, 40,* 278–283.

White, R.W. (1959). Excerpts from motivation reconsidered: The concept of competence. *Psychological Review, 66,* 126–134.

In: Positive Approaches to Health
Editors: C. Dumont, G. Kielhofner, pp. 37-46
ISBN: 978-1-60021-800-2
© 2007 Nova Science Publishers, Inc.

Chapter 3

POSSIBILITY SPACES IN EVERYDAY LIFE: ON CREATIVE POTENTIALS IN INTERVENTIONS FOR PERSONS WITH LIFE-THREATENING INCURABLE ILLNESS

Staffan Josephsson[*,1], *Karen LaCour*[1,2] *and Hans Jonsson*[1]

[1]Division of Occupational Therapy, Department of Neurobiology, Care Sciences and Society, Karolinska Institutet, Stockholm Sweden
[2]CVU syd, University College South, Department of Occupational Therapy, Naestved, Denmark

ABSTRACT

The aim of this chapter is to elaborate on how narrative approaches and understanding can be used to create meaning, connections to life, and possible future. The chapter will take its starting point in empirical studies of the meaning of creative activities for the elderly with life-threatening illnesses. Life-threatening illness is often experienced as a disruption of life and the process of meaning-making in human understanding. By being involved in creative activities, this type of engagement provides a platform for experiences of enjoyment and competence in the actual doing, and it further provides opportunities to connect to life both in a more abstract existential way and in concrete ways with the use of the created products. From the analyses of the empirical studies and case descriptions, some important features in narrative understanding will be discussed and exemplified with literature regarding narrative and therapy. These will be: narrative understanding as a human process of meaning-making, the process of emplotment, activities as ongoing stories that are created in communicational acts, co-construction of disrupted narratives between client and therapist.

---

[*] E-mail: staffan.josephsson@ki.se

"So you are working in rehabilitation? And what has brought you into that dysfunction-producing business?" This remark (said by an artist when being introduced to an occupational therapist at a multi professional meeting) might sound a bit provocative for people working in health care or rehabilitation that might have self-images linked to their efforts of enabling possibilities and participation in everyday life for people with disease or disability. Health and rehabilitation professionals prefer not to be identified with views predominately focused on the lacks, needs, and shortcomings among their clients (Mattingly, 1998). However, writers in social science as well as the disability movement have argued that the reasoning and perspectives of health care and rehabilitation, although having good intentions, can contribute to the creation of negative images of disability (Barnes, Mercer, and Shakespeare, 2000; Foucault, 1979; Pfeiffer, 1999). Professionals in health care and rehabilitation can be seen as developing structures, images, and behavioural patterns that might define persons seeking their services by their dysfunctions and shortcomings rather then by their resources and potentials. In addition, the biomedical perspective locates problems in individuals whereas a social focus may locate problems of everyday life in the social domain (Jonsson, and Josephsson, 2005; Mattingly, 1998).

The success of biomedical science has, in understanding dysfunctions and their possible cures, reinforced the approach of creating knowledge about dysfunction and its management. This focus on dysfunction, useful in medicine, has carried over to interventions and rehabilitation efforts that have an impact on how people with chronic disease and impairment live their everyday lives. As a consequence, insufficient attention is often paid to the production of new ways and forms of living under these circumstances. Further, the biomedical perspective tends to classify groups of persons as dysfunctional and different compared to the norms which are supposed to describe healthy or "optimally" functioning people. Consequently, it can be argued that a biomedical perspective has a bias toward theorizing and thinking in terms of problems, suffering, and lack rather than in terms of possibilities, resources, and potentialities among people.

Parallel to the dominant biomedical tradition in health care and rehabilitation, alternative focuses and priorities have co-existed. For example, the notion that patients and clients might benefit from the use of their own creativity brought art and craft into use in rehabilitation clinics more than a century ago. Although this trend, nurtured by the art and craft movement in the western world of that time, had ambiguous rationales (Boris, 1987); it encompassed the belief that individuals and groups have the potential to influence their health through their actions.

The aim of the present chapter is to complement the traditional focus of interventions in rehabilitation and care for persons with chronic illness and impairments. It is not our intention to question traditional biomedical intervention strategies within palliative or rehabilitation care. Rather, the aim is to add to this approach by searching for potential resources to nurture creativity and agency under the challenging circumstances of illness and impairment. This will be done using the tradition of art and craft workshops in health care as avenue of exploration. Specifically, the material from a craft workshop at a palliative care setting for persons with incurable illness such as cancer will be used as an arena of investigation (La Cour, Josephsson, and Lurborsky, 2005). This will allow exploring a contemporary follower of the art and craft tradition within healthcare. The chapter will start with an introduction to the theoretical material used, with a focus on narrative and a possible implication from narrative theory on creativity. Empirical examples from research on spaces for creativity in everyday life for person with life-threatening illness will follow. The chapter will end with some reflections on possible implications of the argumentation presented on contemporary clinical practices.

NARRATIVE AND POSSIBILITY SPACES

In the following, the theoretical resources around the narrative that will be used in our argumentation are presented. Narrative was chosen as theoretical point of departure because it is a philosophical tradition that enables one to reflect and reason in terms of possibilities and creativity rather than lack and dysfunction. In addition, narrative is a concept used widely in contemporary clinical as well as in scientific reasoning (Hyden, 1997; Mattingly 1998). Basically, when narrative is used in reasoning, it refers to a hermeneutic interpretative approach that has to do with how people make sense of material and circumstances. More specifically, in this text, the reasoning is positioned within a narrative tradition developed by Mattingly (1998; 2002), and Mattingly and Lawlor (2001) among others, with Ricoeur (1985) and Bruner (1986; 2004) as central sources. Most definitions of narrative also include a temporal ordering of events. In clinical as well as scientific reasoning, the term has often been identified as a verbal construction with a beginning, middle, and end. However the term is also used in a wider sense as a term for meaning construction (Ricoeur, 1985).

One prominent and classical discussion of narrative, concerns what narrative is about. When Aristotle wrote Poetics (Mimesis) 2400 years ago, he was taking part in a discussion on the very popular performance of tragedies and their relation to everyday life (Aristoteles, 1970). Aristotle's text has been the subject of multiple interpretations; however it could be argued that he used the concept of mimesis to problematize the role of drama and to conclude that dramatic narratives were not an imitation of everyday life. Rather, he identified them as involving the creative construction of possible meanings from the complex and unfolding world of experiences.

The philosopher Ricoeur (1985) has tapped into Aristotle's reasoning on mimesis when theorizing on the human creation of meaning. In his threefold work on time and narrative, he proposes "mimesis" or narrativity as the form in which people sense and create meaning from the myriads of facts, material, and circumstances they encounter in their everyday life. Perhaps, as Ricoeur proposes, humans do not experience life directly. Rather, they apprehend life as stories in the form of the narratives they create. The term used by Ricoeur for this meaning-making is emplotment. Through the act of emplotment, multiple materials such as facts, conditions, events, and wishes are linked to something that makes sense of them. A consequence of Ricoeur's reasoning is the rejection of meaning as an exact mirror of reality. Rather, the creation of meaning is multiple, fluid, and ongoing. That is, one event or happening can be interpreted "emplotted" in multiple ways. This function of narrative has been identified as a function of distanciation (Josephsson, Asaba, Jonsson, and Alsaker 2006; Ricoeur 1973). Ricoeur identifies distanciation as the element of narrative that creates space and freedom in the interpretation of the material in which the narrative is about. Given that Ricoeur identifies emplotment as a possible logic moving out from myriads of contradictory material encountering human beings, each emplotment is an emplotment under negotiation. An interpretative space is created, communicating between the complexity that characterizes life as lived and the meaning created by the plot. Emplotment establishes what might be characterized as possibility spaces in life as lived (Josephsson, 2005). Such spaces for "trying out" might provide arenas to actually negotiate everyday life and find alternative ways to understand life.

If meaning is understood as something that humans constantly construct in communication with their life circumstances, then persons encountering the new circumstance of illness or impairment must create new meanings. It might, therefore, be of value to have arenas or spaces that provide room for this kind of meaning creation. Later we will discuss how a creative workshop at a palliative care facility serves as such space. But first, some further theoretical material will be exposed.

SPACES FOR VULNERABILITY

The literature as well as everyday experience tells us that narrative is not always neat and tidy. Mattingly (1998; 2000) argues that narrative is organised around breaches in life, often about situations and matters where something important is at stake. The narrative landscape is a place were human vulnerability is present. However, it is also a place were salient life matters can be negotiated. In everyday life, when people are involved in enacted stories and dramas, these negotiations becomes embodied (Park, 2005). Rather than separating the body from feelings and reflection about the body, the involvement in enacted stories can be seen as an "ongoing mimesis" that involves communicating and living pertinent life issues (Josephsson, Asaba, Jonsson, and Alsaker, 2006).

Creating Possibility Spaces in Palliative Care

In this section, theoretical ideas concerning narrative will be used to examine stories from a creative workshop for persons with a life-threatening disease at a palliative care facility. We will examine the role of narrative in exploring alternative ways to handle life in the face of an incurable health condition.

Encountering a life-threatening incurable illness can often be experienced as a disruption of life itself or seen, from a narrative perspective, as a breach in life narrative (La Cour, Josephsson, and Lurborsky, 2005). Facing the end of the life narrative in a not too far future, disrupts also the ongoing life narrative. It replaces "life goes on as normal" with a new agenda.

Palliative care in the western societies aims to address the needs of persons living under these conditions. Pain reduction and necessary technical aids are provided as well as physiological and existential support. However, in contemporary literature, there has been a discussion addressing if the focus on reducing symptoms and pain put other relevant issues needed for living everyday life out of focus (Randall, and Downie, 2006). Given that person with a life-threatening illness can live increasingly longer periods of time due to improved medical treatment, it becomes important not only to reduce symptoms of the disease, but also to establish conditions for agency and generative features of everyday life. These issues however have not been the main agenda in palliative care. Nevertheless, they are central issues in the creative workshop for persons with a life-threatening disease at a palliative care facility.

The Creative Workshop

The creative workshop is situated at a hospital/nursing home specializing in rehabilitation, palliative, and geriatric care. Creative activities provided in the setting includes woodworking, pottery, silk painting, soap-casting, knitting, and gardening. It should be noted that the workshop connects to the Scandinavian tradition within geriatric care of using such activities in workshops for therapeutic purposes. The activities are offered both in-group and on individual basis. Within this setting, explorative qualitative studies have been conducted (La Cour, Josephsson, and Lurborsky, 2005). In the next section, some key findings from these studies will be presented and related to the theoretical material presented in the beginning.

Creating Connection to Life

Analyses of interviews from both staff (occupational therapists) and clients at the workshop identified "creating connection to life" as a key functions of activities in this setting. Through creating, participants re-established the role of actor in life rather than simply being a recipient of care. Moreover, processes such as choosing material to visualize an idea, involved making connections between ordinary life and life as a patient within the health care system, drawing together experiences in a multiple context. Life became once again multifaceted and diverse. Clients used phrases such as "finding ways of being yourselves" to describe their experience. For example, choosing colours and making decisions for shape and form gave clients opportunities to bring material from their own life and history into the world of the health care and actively connect to being an actor in life. In light of the earlier theoretical discusion, it could be argued that the workshop established a space for negotiating and testing new emplotments and storylines in life. It was a space for trying out how live could be lived and handled under the new circumstances brought in by the incurable disease.

Challenge and Excitement

Another, and perhaps more complex, aspect of the engagement in the workshop is that many of the participants experienced a degree of challenge in attempting to be creative. To engage in creative activities was more than simply a "positive" aspect of life only. Being creative involves going beyond the given habits and structures, and thus often involves challenges and risks (May, 1994). Several related issues were highlighted by the clients and the staff at the workshop. Clients realized that they had to overcome inner barriers before engaging in the activities at the workshop, since most of them did not identify themselves as creative and skilled in artwork. Notably, for people with terminal health conditions, this "daring" stance needs to be seen in light of the challenges and fears they face from having an incurable disease. That clients brought up the risk of failure if a creation would not turn out as they hoped might sound a bit trivial compared to the other things they face. However, if one considers that activities at the workshop may constitute an emplotting engagement (i.e. that creating links and possible forms is something that is both about the physical creation and about breaches in life), then the workshop can be seen as a try out space for negotiating and processing meaning relating to salient life issues. Following something as it grew and not knowing how the creation would turn out connected to challenges in life outside the disease and health care.

An additional feature of clients' experience was that the concrete work with creations often involved very direct confrontations with limitations caused by the illness. For example, by moulding clay or cutting wood, participants experienced their decreasing physical ability in form such as fatigue and pain. Clients highlighted that in the context of creative activity with a playful approach, such confrontations facilitated participants in experimenting and trying new ways of using their body.

Enacted Social Community

On a social level, engaging in creative activity alongside with others formed a natural meeting place. The social relations were framed in a process of actual doings. There was a reason to be present apart from just sitting and talking. As the process of unfolding provided experiences that in themselves gave material for conversation with others, particularly not only related to health problems. A therapist explained "*[...] it becomes a very good conversation [...] when you do something together you also talk about other things more than you might do when you train specific functions*". This indicates that being together while creating something can ease conversation and the sharing of more in-depth personal issues. While engaged in the creative process and ongoing conversations, the participants unfolded and shared their individual life stories with each other. Through activities, clients could express themselves in a more concrete way, making connection to life before. Participants not only talked, but also used memories of earlier experiences as ideas that were then directly materialized in the creations. For example, one participant explained: "*you consider colours [...], I chose to use the rust-brown and red [...] my best time was when we lived in Africa, much of it comes back*". Choosing these colours of Africa reminded the participant of the best years in her life and memories from that experience became embedded in the creation. Further, the creation provided an occasion for her to share and reflect some of that experience.

Reaching Possible Futures

Engaging in creative activity had implications reaching beyond the tangible acts of making creations. It included reaching for possible futures and alternative meaning horizons. For an idea or a vision of something to be accomplished, a plan had to be made. Thus, creations had the potential to reach beyond the activity in a very immediate way. Plans concerned ideas for what to make in a creation, and to whom it should be given (e.g. creating toys for grand children or making decorative creations for family and friends) constituted possibilities of how things could turn out in the future. Reaching beyond for possible meaning horizons also indicates the symbolic representations embodied in the enactment of the creations. Creations could be seen to carry symbolic meaning, if perceived as actions or representations of dreams, possible endings or as new beginnings. For example, participants created objects representing how life could have been or might become. This can be illustrated by a therapist's story of one client at the workshop:

> "She painted a lot, sat and did sketches. She had one of these dolls where you see the proportions [...] arms and legs and then she dressed it up. Sometimes the doll was a girl dancing ballet; I guess she did that herself in her youth. Then she was careful to give it eyebrows because she herself had no eyebrows now, so much of what she did not have or could do anymore, she created in her paintings".

This example may illustrate both dreams of what once was, but also the person's dreams for the present and a possible future. Reaching to an understanding that the creative activities could provide material representations for possible future and alternative-meaning horizons beyond the concrete creations was a central finding in these studies of experiences from the workshop. Furthermore, reaching beyond the boundaries of this life was expressed for example as participant's choice to create things that they hoped could "live on" as memories for family and friends. In some aspect creations could be seen as a legacy, as a therapist said: *"Maybe it is not just to express oneself but also to still exist in a symbolic way"*. In light of the distanciative functioning of narrative, making objects can be seen as the embodied enactment of narrative plots. This creation might, in line with Ricoeur's reasoning (1985), be something else than what it seems. A space for creative communication is established between the enactment of these objects and the life situations they relate to or will be linked to as gifts, decorations, or objects to use. The engagement in embodied enacted narratives might transcend matters and circumstances serving as possibility spaces.

Pete and the Birdhouse: An Example

At the time when we talked to Pete, he was one of the few men participating in the workshop. The women tended to stick together in a knitting group and Pete found it good to have that group at the workshop as he liked to be around people. Pete stressed that he always had been quite active in his life. *"I never sat still, and to me, it was very strenuous when I first got ill as my whole life changed."* He continued by telling that now it was very difficult for him to activate himself and that he needed someone to push and motivate him under the conditions of being seriously ill. So, for Pete, it was very positive to be at a place where other people gathered; it was so important that he described it as his "life vest". Pete explained that the most important to him was the social contact so he felt less lonely. As he said:

> "Yes it is very positive to come here, meet a few people and have the opportunity to make a few things, after all it would be difficult to just sit and look at each other for several hours, you must have something to do even if it is not much."

Pete was 64 years of age with incurable cancer. He had attended the workshop for about a year. His recent life had been intense. Within a period of three years, he had been divorced, developped serious cancer, and stopped working. Peter told us that he had been in the workforce for almost 40 years and that he always used to be the one to come up with ideas for social events and things to do with colleagues. Now, a lot of these arenas were closed for Pete. He decided to build a birdhouse. Why a birdhouse? Pete did not have an answer. He had no prior experience of the activity, and it was not something that others were building at the workshop. Pete tried to follow instructions from a book, but the right material was not available, so it did not turn out as he had imagined from the beginning. It took him quite a while to build the house. When finished, he brought it home and gave it to his sister for Christmas. He noted that he found it meaningless to create things just to keep occupied. It was important that it was useful and could be enjoyed afterwards.

Pete's story might seem rather common and maybe even dull. Nothing happened really. Especially in the context of life-threatening disease and the other things that have happened to Pete in recent years, the making of a birdhouse seems of little significance. But juxtaposing the story of Pete's birdhouse with the notions of possibility spaces presented earlier brings another perspective. A lot of arenas were no longer available for Pete, because of recent life events and because of his disease. As a consequence he had no other way to find engagement in everyday life and had become passive. The workshop offered him a space for reconnecting to earlier roles (being the social organiser) and involvement in actions that presented challenges for him. Pete could, in a very physical sense, with his work with the birdhouse, approach breaches when life turns out different than expected. Also, the making of the birdhouse confirmed that he was still capable to participate in the ongoing social exchange prominent in everyday life. The making of the birdhouse became a connection to life.

Creating Possibility Spaces/Places

As illustrated above, engagement in the creative activities at the workshop could enable participants to make new connections of past experiences with their present situation and possible futures. Relating to the reasoning on emplotment and possibility spaces addressed in this chapter, the workshop can be understood as a place to create narrative meaning in a non-verbal idiom of creative acts. Engagement in crafts could be understood in terms of how understanding of each individual creation represents multiple stories embedded with meanings that the individual invests in constructing. Creating things can be viewed as materialized narratives. There is a beginning involving daring engagement and formation of ideas. There is a middle of challenges in working with the material, giving shape and holding the suspense of not knowing how the final creation will turn out. Finally, the "ending", with the creation in a materialized form, carries embedded ideas from memories and inspiration from current and future life. Notably, the final creation is no more final than it is about to be given away as a gift or placed at home with the potential of symbolizing another story. Moreover, it is also possible to link the creative workshop to other readings of narrative than the linear with its beginning, middle, and end. Entering into the space of the workshop also involved possibilities to connect to distanciative functioning of emplotment. Bruner (1986, p. 26) identified this functioning of emplotment as stepping into a "subjunctivizing" world of "wandering in human possibilities rather then in settled certainties". Finding alternative ways of living and finding meaning is crucial when having a life-threatening condition.

Conclusion

This chapter highlighted a possible role for narrative and creativity in contemporary palliative care. Drawing observations from a creative workshop at a palliative care facility, we proposed that the workshop succeeds in creating a space for alternative processes than the traditional focus on addressing disease and its consequences. This space is called a possibility space (Josephsson, 2005), and its role is notably to provide those faced with the end of life, an opportunity to experience a connection to life.

REFERENCES

Aristoteles. (1970). *Poetics*. Ann Arbour: University of Michigan Press.

Barnes, C., Mercer, G., and Shakespeare, T. (2000). *Exploring disability: A sociological introduction*. Cambridge, England: Polity Press.

Boris, E. (1987). Dreams of brotherhood and beauty. In: W. Kaplan (Ed). *The art that is life: The arts and crafts movement in America, 1875-1920* (pp 208-222). Boston: Museum of fine arts.

Bruner, J. (1986). *Actual minds, open worlds*. Cambridge, MA: Harward University Press.

Bruner, J. (2004). Life as narrative. *Social Research: An International Quarterly of Social Sciences, 71* (3), 691-710.

Foucault, M. (1979). *Discipline and punish*. New York: Pantheon.

Hyden, L.-C. (1997). Illness and narrative. *Sociological Health Ill, 19*(1), 48-69.

Jonsson, H., and Josephsson, S. (2005) Occupation and meaning. In: C. Christansen and C.M. Baum (Eds). *Occupational therapy: Performance, participation, and well-being.* (pp. 116-132). Thorofare, NJ: Slack.

Josephsson, S. (2005). *The versatile rooms, interpretive possibilities in human occupation*. Society for the Study of Occupation. USA Fourth Annual Research Conference.

Josephsson, S., Asaba, E., Jonsson, H., and Alsaker, S. (2006) Creativity and order in communication: Implications from philosophy to narrative research concerning human occupation. *Scandinavian Journal of Occupational Therapy, 13* (2), 86-93.

La Cour, K., Josephsson, S., and Lurborsky, M (2005). Creating connections to life during life-threatening illness: Creative activity experienced by elderly people and occupational therapists. *Scandinavian Journal of Occupational Therapy, 12* (3), 98-109.

Mattingly, C. (1998). *Healing dramas and clinical plots: The narrative structure of experience*. Cambridge: Cambridge University Press.

Mattingly, C. (2000). Emergent Narratives. In: C. Mattingly and L.C. Garro (Eds): *Narrative and the Cultural Construction of Illness and Healing*. Berkeley: University of California Press.

Mattingly, C., and Lawlor, M. (2001). The Fragility of Healing. *Ethos* 29(1), 30-57.

May, R. (1994). *Modet att Skapa (The courage to Create)*. Stockholm: Natur och kultur (in Swedish).

Park, M. (2005). *The vulnerabilities of re-presenting practice: From clinical gaze to narrative frames of acceptance*. Paper presented at the Society for the Study of Occupation: USA. (Oct) Bethesda, MD.

Pfeiffer, D. (1999). The categorization and control of people with disabilities. *Disability and Rehabilitation, 21* (3), 106-107.

Randall, F., and Downie, R.S. (2006). The philosophy of palliative care: Critique and reconstruction. Oxford: Oxfo d University Press.

Ricoeur, P. (1973). The hermeneutical function of distanciation. *Philosophy Today, 17* (2), 129-141.

Ricoeur, P. (1985). *Time and Narrative*. (Vol. 1). Chicago: University of Chicago Press.

In: Positive Approaches to Health
Editors: C. Dumont, G. Kielhofner, pp. 47-63
ISBN: 978-1-60021-800-2
© 2007 Nova Science Publishers, Inc.

Chapter 4

THEORIZATION OF SPIRITUALITY IN HEALTH CARE: AN ILLUSTRATION THROUGH OCCUPATIONAL THERAPY

Étienne Pouliot[*]
Faculté de théologie et de sciences religieuses,
Université Laval, Cité Universitaire, Quebec City,
Quebec, Canada, G1V 0A6
Director of the *Cahiers de spiritualité ignatienne*
(Centre Manrèse, Québec)

ABSTRACT

Spirituality has become a major interest in health care. Research and publications on this topic indicate that, most often, spirituality is resolved into a theory which makes of it a domain of knowledge. This chapter discusses the apparent need of professions to situate spirituality in an horizon of practice and, consequently, to define it. The chapter further illustrates the change of paradigm necessary to better situate spirituality in health care, by using the field of occupational therapy as a case example.

The place and the role of spirituality in health care are widely discussed in many disciplines or professional practices (Phillips, 2003; Pouliot, 2001). Within the rehabilitation discipline of occupational therapy, publications increasingly point to the importance of spirituality for people with health problems who use these health services (Belcham, 2004; Chan and Spencer, 2004; Christiansen, 1997; Collins, Paul and West-Frasier, 2001; Schulz, 2004; Urbanowski, 2003; Wilding, 2002). Interestingly, spirituality has been included as a concept within an established conceptual practice model used by occupational therapists (Canadian Association of Occupational Therapists, 1997; Chapparo and Ranka, 1997; Do Rozario, 1997; McColl, 2000; Urbanowski and Vargo, 1994).

---

[*] Etienne.Pouliot@ftsr.ulaval.ca

While it has been difficult for occupational therapists to determine what spirituality is, it has been even more difficult to integrate it into the conceptualization and practice of occupational therapy itself (Hoyland and Mayers, 2005; McColl, 2003; Unruh, Versnel and Kerr, 2002; Whalley Hammell, 2001). A certain discomfort results from this situation and many occupational therapists have made this point vehemently. The reasons behind their hesitation and questioning about the place of spirituality in the field of occupational therapy may be summed up as follows. For some, spirituality refers to the sacred and to the religious, thus it concerns chaplains because it is their "speciality". Spirituality is also about private life and personal beliefs. Thus most occupational therapists are afraid of imposing their own beliefs on their clients and choose to act in a way that keeps their intervention free from such personal projections. Additionally, some occupational therapists may feel profound discomfort regarding their own spirituality. And finally, because spirituality has not been part of their professional training, occupational therapists view themselves as not being able to apply any knowledge of spirituality in their practice. They do not feel authorized to manage it in the daily exercise of their profession. Simply stated, they are waiting for certified knowledge on this topic.

In looking at the literature within occupational therapy, I recognized a series of problems similar to my field of spiritual theology and, more widely, practical theology. Thus I plan to illustrate a broader problem by examining how spirituality is problematic in theology and occupational therapy. To limit my comments, I will focus on problems that concern the definition of spirituality and the means of investigating it. This discussion will demonstrate that a theorization of spirituality has occurred in occupational therapy similar to that in theology. But this thesis takes us to a deeper one: fundamentally, spirituality belongs to an horizon of practice. Consequently, it must be defined in terms of competence into a "practice of meaning", which I will qualify differently, as "signifying practice", for reasons I will explain in the last part of this chapter when I will conclude by exposing some major features of the latter hypothesis.

This chapter constitutes neither a complete nor even a systematic review of the literature concerning spirituality and occupational therapy. I examined a limited body of literature identified by a database search and confined to the last fifteen years. The question to which I submitted this literature is: how the problem of spirituality bas been constructed in occupational therapy? This question demands a critical and epistemological analysis that leads precisely to a clarification of the way spirituality is understood, exposed, expressed in theology and in occupational therapy; in others words, the point of view I adopt to examine spirituality is that of its functioning in a (theological or occupational therapy) discourse.

It is important to better understand the meaning of our practices as well as our practices of meaning. By doing so, we can go beyond the simple restoration of health (conceptualized as "normal" states of the body or the soul) and beyond the perpetuation of positivism in health approaches.

1. SPIRITUALITY: A SYMPTOMATIC PROBLEM IN THEOLOGY

How has the problem of spirituality been constructed in theology? The history of theology and spirituality demonstrates how much both were generally understood with reference to a theoretical "order", often an ontological one, in such a way that a practical "order" can be logically deduced or consequently assumed (Pouliot, 2003). This position remains since theology defines itself as a science - that is, as an undertaking of knowledge (*epistemè*). It was done so for a long time but the divorce between theology and spirituality in the second millennium has strongly accentuated this trend.

No one, in theology (to consider only this), can deny the success and the utility of a description of spirituality which establishes the fact of the "internal life", which leads to acquire knowledge of the processes and levels of spiritual life, which help to manage spiritual accompanying, which can become teachings about specific spiritual matters such as unexpected faces of the divinity. But such results refer to some "order": may it be a deterministic one or not. And these elements, based on such "order", are made available for thinking about spirituality, for communicating a spiritual experience, for making spirituality investigable.

Spiritual experience as well as spiritual language turns out to be a major and constant challenge in theology. Why? Because the difficulty is to understand a dynamic in which no "order", theoretical or practical, ever comes to explain once and for all. No positivistic order can ground or serve as foundation to this dynamic; by the same way, no (neutral) knowledge, established in terms of elementary contents associated to an objective "order", can correspond to this dynamic. Indeed, the spiritual or mystic experience involves the simultaneous *procès*[1] of the subject and the object of spiritual life in such a way that no position (role, function, state) can be definitively attributed to them. Through language, mystics tell how they have an unspeakable experience of God (object) while God (subject) acts "inside them" so they are "touched" and transformed (object). Spiritual life functions in a ceaselessly (re-)structuring way, according to practical requirements which the mystic's speech tries to take into account. This challenge may be formulated in this way: "At the beginning is the relationship." It is a challenge to take into account what is at the core of the phenomenon of spiritual life without reducing it to any feeling, knowledge (normative contents), or art which do not fundamentally belong to an horizon of practice. This is what is never left in this *procès*. This is why the status of spiritual/mystic experience or speech is much more difficult to determine than it appears to be – considering only theology here.

My point is that spirituality and theology are constantly and radically questioned when this mystic *procès* is considered and assumed for what it is phenomenologicaly: a practice proceeding from the absence of knowledge – this is to say: not fundamentally like knowledge – while operating through some knowledge. In contrast, there is a trend in theology and even in the specific field of spirituality which has all the characteristics of a theorization of spirituality. More often than otherwise, the problem of spirituality in theology has been constructed from an horizon of theory instead of that of practice. This can be said more abruptly: we (in theology) widely gave in to the temptation to exchange spirituality for knowledge. Or we easily truncate spirituality into knowledge and, paradoxically, presume that this is not only the root of all but what is essential: like a whole valuable in itself. The ambivalence on the sense of spirituality proceeds for the way the problematic of spirituality is constructed.

---

[1] By « procès », I mean the advent of a subject through its structural actualization of his/her identity. I do not mean the actualization of the potentialities of an individual. I do not exactly mean a process, which implies steps in a

The alternative point of view I plan to develop in this chapter concerns a structuring requirement for knowledge. This perspective is more than paying attention to *what* is demonstrated as form of spirituality or to *what* is presented in a spiritual experience in terms of quality, state, or style of spirituality. The difficulty in taking a formal but situated account of spirituality lies in our own capacity (in theology) to grasp it from an horizon of practice where the task is not a quest for foundations (with or without a positivistic "order").

I have previously discussed this difficulty to situate and define spirituality from an horizon of practice in the context of moral theology (Pouliot, 2003). Other authors have also addressed this issue following different theological or philosophical interests (Fiorenza, 1984; Fumerton, 2005; Habermas, 1987). Collectively, these works challenge what is now called foundationalism. They expose it as a system of though which produces an idealized order (positivistic or not) and offers an access to knowledge about the world: an internal or external world that is allegedly reflected so on and which represent to the base for knowledge. The critique of foundationalism reorients us to how speeches and practices (identically) produce meaning and radically engage ourselves. This attention to the construction of meaning itself, in regard to ethics, is a characteristic of postmodernism.

2. SITUATING AND DEFINING SPIRITUALITY IN OCCUPATIONAL THERAPY

I started by exposing a problem that concerns me as theologian or as "specialist" in spirituality. I submit that a similar problem may be recognized through out the discussion about spirituality in occupational therapy. In occupational therapy literature, spirituality is currently situated according to a theoretical horizon and is consequently defined in terms of knowledge about the self (consciousness, "internal world"), or about the world (may it be supernatural or metaphysical). In examining how the problem of spirituality is constructed in occupational therapy, I will draw some conclusions about the position of spirituality in health care generally.

Spirituality: The Issue of Knowledge

Occupational therapy literature offers definitions of spirituality that vary substantially (Engquist, Short-DeGraff, Gliner, et al., 1997; Urbanowski and Vargo, 1994; Wilding, May and Muir-Cochrane, 2005). Some definitions reference a divinity: God, Allah, etc. Others imply a sacred element: supreme and transcending being, mysterious source/power/energy, and feeling of plenitude or connection with the universe. Still others target a quality or a more strictly human condition: spirituality refers to transcendence of the self, to resiliency, to well-being, to some needs.

The main interest of these definitions of spirituality has to establish a distinction between religion and spirituality. Occupational therapists return to this distinction ceaselessly. But why? The aim of this distinction in health care is to command a division of the work.

---

proceeding that has besides a fixed orientation or *telos*. I would rather mean a trial, without any legal or moral presumptions about intention (purely formal description) of an individual.

Religious and/or the spiritual needs should be reserved for corresponding specialists (chaplains) or may become a special task for (some?) health care professionals (particularly nurses, who have already integrated spirituality in their practice; see Henderson, 1994; Scott, Grzybowski and Webb, 1994; Sellers and Haag, 1998).

For occupational therapists, the problem has clearly become the one of supplying adequate knowledge on the topic to allow them to integrate the spirituality into their daily practice (Collins, Paul and West-Frasier, 2001; Dombeck, 1998; McColl, 2003; Phillips, 2003; Unruh, Versnel and Kerr, 2002). Thus the distinction between religion and spirituality in occupational therapists' views also serves the necessity to acquire knowledge: and knowledge before any intervention. The same can be said about health care professionals: whatever the position adopted by them with regard to the religious and/or to the spiritual components, they are assimilated into a domain of knowledge.

It should be mentioned that many practicing occupational therapists do not recognize the distinction between religion and spirituality to be relevant in their professional practice; or, at least, they do not consider it to be a major issue in their practice (McColl and O' Brien, 2003). I have already mention how this can be interpreted: some therapists experience discomfort or ethical reserve for generally related to their personal faith while some others are more tolerant to spiritual/religious attitudes of their patients and even feel concerned by these issues (Collins, Paul and West-Frasier, 2001; Dombeck, 1998). I wonder if the whole situation makes us believe that this distinction is a purely theoretical one. Indeed, what turns out to be useless on a practical level could finally have no value other than speculative. I only want to evoke here the risk of a theorization of spirituality or of any distinctions about it. Knowledge can be strictly valuable for itself and this is an issue which concerns spirituality too.

Spirituality and Disability: Systematic Production of Objects for Knowledge

Professional specialization implies a regionalization of knowledge. Every professional domain is established according to its specific object and the search for relevant determinations of this object. It is only natural that spirituality be considered in this way too.

Several authors in the field of occupational therapy define spirituality in reference to a superior being or a special power (Collins, Paul and West-Frasier, 2001; Unruh, Versnel and Kerr, 2002); McColl (2000; 2003) typifies this perspective. For her, the spirituality includes a transpersonal or even a supernatural aspect and without this sacred and mysterious aspect, spirituality is distorted because it is assimilated to a simply personal (psychological) or interpersonal (sociocultural) component. The spiritual dimension transcends the material and social world; it refers to what exceeds some "natural" or "normal" human experience. In so arguing, McColl (re)builds a so-called domain of spirituality which is not only a different one but a separable one. The domain of spirituality can be examined besides the human, social, psychological, and other, domains. Accordingly it references a specific and separate object (spiritual vs. material, spirit vs. spirituality, the "natural" world and beyond it). Spirituality is explored from the horizon of theory. That is, a domain of knowledge presented through its substantial or functional description, implying data or essential elements of what is then called spiritual; and, of course, these contents are ordered and an organized domain of knowledge is constructed. I choose to explore this latter aspect through secular definitions of spirituality however.

Among the definitions of spirituality in the field of occupational therapy, there are the secular ones which principally refer to the essence of human being, to his/her "internal self", to his/her inner source, to the deep humanity in each of us (Canadian Association of Occupational Therapists, 1998; Kroeker, 2003; Wilding, May and Muir-Cochrane, 2005). These lead to concrete representations of spirituality: spiritual well-being (Collins, 1998; Unruh, Versnel and Kerr, 2003; Urbanowski, 2003), spiritual needs (Hoyland and Mayers, 2005; Wilding, 2002), and spiritual resiliency (McColl and O' Brien, 2003).

It is rather obvious that such definitions associate spirituality to notions (needs, well-being, resiliency, self) coming from other scientific fields: medicine, psychology and their related disciplines. So how cannot expect a production of knowledge in the same way(s), I mean a knowledge corresponding to an "order" of the (internal or external) world? Indeed, life of the soul is sometimes understood according to psychological mechanisms which are not without referring to biophysiological life. Consequently, evidence-based occupational therapy can be requested (Unruh, Versnel and Kerr, 2003; Whalley Hammell, 2003) and, in this reign, spirituality and knowledge about it must be based on empirical approaches. Sometimes, it is the entity of the self that crowns the physical body and gives roots and roof to spirituality. Consequently, the reference to psychosyntheses seems more convenient (Kang, 2003), and spirituality is more clearly understood through a metaphysical point of view. But whatever is the empirical or the metaphysical orientation chosen, an ideal "order" is exposed, I mean constructed. And here are the spiritual, psychological, social, and biophysiological dimensions of the human life, or of the person, or even of the world – as we presume! So the construction of knowledge proceeds by analogy or by correlation, using elements from one level of human life – or person or reality – to expose elements in another one. Spirituality has become the allegedly eminent level/dimension of human beings and of our world. Secular definitions of spirituality finally appear to be constructed similarly to the religious or sacred, since theorization constitute the may we produce objects systematically organized as human knowledge.

I want to say more about secular views on spirituality which especially imply correlations between aspects of the human being: spirituality and self, spirituality and need(s), spirituality and disability, etc. The literature is replete with this. Spirituality refers to a level of well-being or satisfaction (Unruh, Versnel and Kerr, 2002). Spirituality refers to a feeling of connectedness with others or to the cosmos – or even a supreme being (Egan and DeLaat, 1997; Schulz, 2004). Spirituality is related to spontaneity or a special expressiveness (Greenberg, 2003; Schulz, 2004). Spirituality activates personal growth, allowing, for example, the recognition of our own value as person (Egan and Swedersky, 2003). One may insist on the importance of quantitative or qualitative measure of the spiritual phenomenon (Unruh, Versnel and Kerr, 2003), spirituality is still and always viewed through correlations and never understood from itself. This is the way theorization can lead to or may proceed from foundationalism – but theorization can function in a different way by giving place to a fundamental and a practical approach of spirituality, and I will do it later in this chapter.

The major and the most frequent correlation established to understand the spirituality in occupational therapy is about meaning. McColl (2000) summarizes this perspective: disability constitutes a more or less dramatic experience for the self, questioning our own values, our potential of action, our whole existence and finitude. And because disability is manifestly related to a search of meaning, it is advisable to understand this search of meaning from a spiritual point of view – that is, in its spiritual and transpersonal sense rather than psychological (personal) or sociocultural (interpersonal) one (McColl, 2003). I have already indicated that such an effort to distinguish spiritual dimension from other ones may only proceed from a regionalization of knowledge, systematically organized according to specific, different, and hierarchical domains (and data).

Still on this issue of meaning, Whalley Hammel (2001; 2003) seeks to redefine spirituality in a strictly secular way, as being an intrinsically source of meaning. In her evidence-base approach, she pays attention to the meaning experienced in lives, by opposition to a hypothetical meaning of life, and so considers patient personal ability to make sense of his/her experience of disability. For Whalley Hammel, everybody can speak about his or her experience in spiritual or non spiritual terms; meaning concerns production of semantic contents which do not necessarily connote spiritual contents (supreme being, religious values, life after death, etc.). Thus Whalley Hammel tightens the understanding of this function of meaning in people's life and keeps planning to include spiritual values in her professional exercise when she has to. In doing so, she does not escape a theorization of spirituality based on specific or predetermined data which correspond to a pure knowledge on spirituality. Incidentally, Whalley Hammel openly considers that speaking about spiritual crisis simply reflects a particular and predetermined perspective by the therapist. One must then wonder if her position is not, after all, a simple inversion into the same horizon of (deterministic) knowledge, from the client point of view to the therapist point of view.

Similar remarks should be applied to the perspectives developed by Unruh, Versnel and Kerr (2002). They also consider that meaning in life can be experienced and discussed without adding to it any spiritual qualifications. They even claim that secular definitions of spirituality are nonsense; for instance, "Spirit" has inevitably a religious connotation. I would agree with their purpose of integrating spirituality itself into a meaning-making process, which is their way of tightening the understanding of spirituality. But how can we be sure that these perspectives do prevent the kind of theorization I doubt here it could be, especially when the option for an evidence-based occupational therapy is attested as well as it is for Whalley Hammel's perspectives? However I recognize an interesting view – but still an ambivalent one for me – when they oppose an obvious and active character of spirituality to an absent or latent spirituality.

In sum, secular definitions of spirituality in occupational therapy support a double interest: an internal order to human subject (personality) and a search of meaning. This interest is remarkably notified in such definitions, comparing to the more religious and sacred definitions of spirituality. But the fact remains that the spiritual dimension of the human being is then conceived and described as any other dimension of the person, through different correlations. The spirituality and all its concrete instances are situated in a theoretical horizon - rather that a practical one. Knowledge determines spirituality by organizing it among other domains of knowledge, in parallel to all theirs objects of knowledge.

Should it be reminded that Emmanuel Kant (1986 [1790], 2001 [1781]) criticized the postulate of a "wholistic" order, without which nothing concerning the reality can be understand? He limited its validity through theoretical rationality before legitimized it through esthetical rationality – but never from or for the practical use of Reason. Here is a misunderstanding that reflects what we can make of spirituality when we describe it through correlations or by analogy based on ontological perspectives. This misunderstanding often goes with another problem I want to consider now: spirituality in regard to transfer and application of knowledge.

Spirituality and Occupation: Attempts to Transfer and Apply a Set of Knowledge

The appropriateness of spirituality for health professionals is often debated. This is increasingly so for occupational therapists since they claim a holistic vision of the person and health care (American Occupational Therapy Association, 1994; Hubbard, 1991; McColl, 1994). Interestingly, McColl (2003) points out that, in the Canadian Model of Occupational Therapy developed in 1983, spirituality was added as the fourth component of the person. McColl notes that this addition widened more than it specified the practice of occupational therapy. Later, spirituality became a central element in the conceptualisation of the person and, furthermore, the epicentre of the occupational therapy Model (Canadian Association of Occupational Therapists, 1997; Canadian Association of Occupational Therapists, 1998). This is exactly what Whalley Hammel (2001, 2003) as well as Unruh, Versnel and Kerr (2003) criticize. They all claim that their professional mandate concerns first of all and especially the occupation and not spirituality. They also warn that the religious and sacred definitions of spirituality are not so compatible with the mandate of occupational therapists and – as I have already mentioned – that secular definitions of spirituality are not more a solution.

Instrumentalisation is one of the ways to examine this situation. If spirituality has something to do with occupational therapy, it has to answer to purposes established related to health. This is particularly evident for Unruh, Versnel, and Kerr (2003) who assert that investigating spirituality is useful only in order to plan an intervention with a patient. Spirituality is a part of their responsibility and competence only as means to intervene as occupational therapists. Spirituality may become an explicit professional objective for them only when a more secular conception of spirituality is to be considered. Thus, everything is in place for conceiving and using spirituality as a means, among others, to support the healing of sick people or to resolve disability into occupation. When health, disability and spirituality become – or tend to become – a matter of means and goals, "knowledge is power". The instrumentalisation of spirituality still proceeds from a theorization... through technical application and technological success. Indeed, modern science definitively links knowledge and technique, as Kant (2001 [1781]) has so well established.

Besides, occupational therapy and its discussion of spirituality are now frequently associated to the perspectives of phenomenology and hermeneutics. This is certainly an opportunity for occupational therapy to explore and assume a non technical understanding of the profession and of spirituality. But the problem of transferring and applying knowledge is quite the same; I want to show it through some cases I found in the literature.

Urbanowski (2003) conceives spirituality as the experience of meaning in life of people and this meaning-making process evolves with the lived persons' experience. These perspectives, he says explicitly, are based on Heidegger's existentialism which approaches the experience of self and of the world in terms of social construction of meaning. On this philosophical basis, Urbanowski presume that the spiritual transformation which occurs in occupation correspond to successful completion and entrenchment of meaningful occupations; in other words, the meaning-making process is normalized, if not idealized, by Urbanowski. But this does not fit at all to the heideggerian hermeneutics which cannot allow such fixed orientation, recalling instead the fundamental ambiguity of the experience of the self and of the world. Heidegger's project is deformed again when Urbanowski makes of spirituality – understands it as – a measurable phenomenon in spite of its fluctuating character; its holistic nature is simply assimilated to what Heidegger calls the inaccessibility of the "Being", besides technical requirements which are considered in the same constitutive manner. Urbanowski misses the fundamental character of the condition of language exposed by Heidegger. This condition constitutes an horizon from which science and technique can be situated and understood as another gesture-in-language: a second or derived one comparing to a primary or native one (Heidegger, 1986 [1927]). Theses hermeneutics axes are changed when one attempts recovering a set of knowledge and applying it into definite fulfilment.

I keep seeing similar risks when spirituality is assimilated to notions such as the self, especially the authentic one or the one that is deeply human because it implies positive willingness or harmonious transcendence (Kang, 2003; Kirsh and Welch, 2003; McColl, 2003; Wilding, May and Muir-Cochrane, 2005). Kang's psychosynthesis approach is particularly relevant here. He presents the process of the self as a balancing process with a (double) possibility of psychospiritual integration and disintegration. But this system is tricky at least in three manners. First, integration remains the norm if we only considerer his criteria of the spiritual dimensions of psychosynthesis: becoming kinder, finding authentic meaning, being universally humane, centring in calmness, connecting to one and all, and transcending limited agendas revolving around ego, ethnicity, culture, religion or geography. Secondly and consequently, Kang too conceives fulfilment of the self in terms of what may be called authenticity or entrenchment. This positive orientation (integration) is apparently justified by the ontological trend – let's say a trend on the Ego – that characterizes Gadamer's philosophical hermeneutics (1996), which is explicitly the base of all here; Kang suggests, or presumes with Gadamer, that this ontological trend has a specific and normative orientation. Finally and far more important here, Kang clearly take for granted that all the spiritual dimensions are equally fundamental. But these views do not exactly correspond to Gadamer's hermeneutics which exposes the fundamental mediation of language; if language is a common and "ordinary" condition for all of us, it is also a mediation which is not the same of any other ones because interpretation and meaning are produced in a fundamental way. Kang tries to transfer a set of knowledge (a philosophical system) into a psychological frame; furthermore, he imposes theoretical or even instrumental bias to the hermeneutics he applies following a predetermined phenomenology of spirituality and occupation.

In sum, the way spirituality and occupation are linked in occupational therapy is highly instructive. It should serve to warn all of us about any transfer and application of knowledge from a discipline to another one (psychology, philosophy, theology…): and this is what leads to instrumental spirituality. We must pay attention in the way any project seeks to integrate spirituality into a complete (set of) knowledge in order to add new understanding or new tools to professional practice. So I would question and question again projects that conceive and use spirituality as simple means to activate or to promote occupation (McColl 2003). But the same must be done in regard to any phenomenological or hermeneutical notions and systems that we try to import for other specific interests. This is why it is not only spirituality that may have to deal with the ransom of theorization.

3. ON THE EDGE OF SPIRITUALITY: SIGNIFYING PRACTICES

There is another way to construct the problem of spirituality, besides its theorization which is often foundational. I present now some reflections in this respect. I do it in a quite directive and concise way here, initiating moves that can be made then when discussing spirituality in occupational therapy or any other health profession. I discuss issues about meaning and spirituality I found particularly relevant. As a matter of fact, within the literature in occupational therapy, spirituality has become more and more strictly defined in terms of meaningfulness and associated to purposefulness (Beagan and Kumas-Tan, 2005; Collins, Paul and West-Frasier, 2001; McColl, 2000; Whalley Hammell, 2003). It also constitutes a life-sustaining phenomenon associated to the search for meaning in people's lives (Wilding, May and Muir-Cochrane, 2005). It refers to an active meaning-making process which can therefore be latent because specific spiritual contents are not what matters (Unruh, Versnel and Kerr, 2002). In the same perspective of meaning, life stories (narrative), which have pervasive character in person's life, should also be examined (Kirsh and Welch, 2003).

Language as Mediation: An Anthropological Condition for Spirituality

As I noticed before regarding Urbanowski (2003), it is not enough to conceive spirituality as an experience of meaning which is common to all, and which belongs to everyone's ordinary life. Making sense is not a means among other means nor it is grounded in a "funds of sense", may it be an unlimited or a holistic one. Meaning is associated to understanding and constitutes a way of being-in-the-world (Heidegger 1986 [1927]). This is so because language is a unique and an incomparable mediation, at the root of many others (science, art, institutions, etc.). This hermeneutic condition structures everybody's relationship to the world, including what we are (anthropologically speaking). There is nothing above and beyond language for us. Language is constitutive of all phenomena ("reality") we examine and is anthropologically decisive. We all "come-to-the-world" (see Heidegger).

In this horizon of language, spirituality and ethics are fundamentally linked. The meaning-making process by which spirituality can be described (Unruh, Versnel and Kerr, 2002) should be understood in terms of a person's competence to make sense in his/her life and with others. And such a competence cannot be assimilated to any technical competence since it proceeds *like* a "savoir-être" and not from knowledge. Thus spirituality can finally be defined as a signifying practice, I mean a "practice of meaning" that can no more be understood in a pure objective way; spirituality do not represent a process of meaning, a technical or even an esthetical "practice of meaning" which still falls into an horizon of knowledge, with the technical power its gives or the motivational feeling it can indirectly offer. At the same time, ethics (*éthos*) do not simply correspond to deontology and morals (*éthos*), which falls again into an horizon of knowledge because it indicates what to do or not; to advent in intersubjectivity and by reflexivity is what ethics makes of us (through such spirituality).

Since a fundamental difference is made between this constitutive competence to make sense in an horizon of language and any professional competences, it becomes difficult to agree totally with the perspectives developed by Unruh, Versnel and Kerr (2002) about active spirituality, as opposed to latent spirituality. According to them, first, sacred and secular definitions of spirituality are not what matters; it is not beliefs as such (contents of spirituality) but the act of believing ("active spirituality") that constitutes this or that way of being, of thinking, of experiencing life and making sense in one's life. But against these authors' perspectives, if spirituality is an issue of competence for each person because he/she is human, such a competence cannot be latent. How could we speak of a possibility more or less virtual, or of an exercise more or less active in an horizon of language?

My philosophical argument is still closed to Heidegger's views (1986 [1927]) when he explicates how language seeks to let itself being forgotten and even makes itself so. This is why science, technique and arts are put forwards as if they were primarily and fundamentally constitutive for us and for all we do. This hermeneutic condition can only be discovered when is exactly established what derives from what in our understanding of the world/self. This is another way to talk about signifying practices, beyond appearances: that of knowledge, especially when it allegedly coincides with pure objectivity or neutrality. Once spirituality is situated in a practical horizon of language, it can be exposed as a signifying practice. But spirituality is not one signifying practice among many others and I tried to prevent this illusion by overexposing it at the root of all these ones, in terms of (radical) human competence.

There is also an ethical reason to present spirituality in such a radical position from the horizon of language. It is not enough to attach a posteriori some "ethical perspectives" to professional health cares. For instance, Kroeker (2003) calls for virtue in front of scientific disciplines that solely define their views and goals and then evaluate their instruments. Of course, we can no longer let science and technique operate without questioning them with wisdom, I mean from ethical perspectives. But these views can easily repeat theoretical parameters into which Aristotle may have lead us from the beginning of ethics. The ransom here is a principle-based approach which has been seriously criticized in bioethics principally (see Davis, 1995; Emmanuel, 1995; Gert, Culver and Clouser, 2000).

Against such principlism in "ethics", I call for, at least, an ethic of responsibility. Thus the problematic of spirituality and ethics ought to be constructed in a complex way where the question of responsibility can serve to differentiate, again, signifying practice from any technical and any aesthetical practice of meaning. Indeed, our responsibility is engaged not only when come the moment to act professionally but long before the intervention begins: before it is planned and already in the way it is conceptualized. From the horizon of language I try to expose here, all we do correspond to a signifying practice that is anthropologically decisive. I have come to think that ethics and spirituality must be set, together, as conditions of realization of theology (Pouliot, 2003); I suggest the same in health care and in science.

Spirituality and Rationality

The individual perspective of spirituality remains determining in experiencing meaning/spirituality (Unruh, Versnel and Kerr, 2002; Whalley Hammell, 2003). In parallel, it appears impossible to describe the "essence" of spirituality; a single universal concept or a unique definition seems no longer relevant (Schulz, 2005; Unruh, Versnel and Kerr, 2002). What does rationality become then if essences of the world as well as essence of the ego, to what rationality has been linked for so long, are not spiritual issues any more? The solution can be seek in a signifying system where there is no such thing like a centre (world, ego, God) to approach and understand problems. Habermas (1987) has qualified such a system as a decentred understanding of the "self" as well as of the "world". The challenge here is to assume the passage from an idealized objectivity and neutrality to intersubjectivity, from (technical) communication to practices of intercommunication, from multidisciplinarity to interdisciplinarity. In occupational therapy, narratives seem to represent a good step to come to this horizon of practice into language. I discuss it.

Egan, DeLaat, and Vallée (2003) call for a symbolic or a narrative rationality and link it to spirituality. They clearly situate this (specific) rationality besides scientific rationality (*logos*) and besides myth (*mythos*). They mix elements of both fields in another way so to exemplify holistic views. But they only identify, they add a new rationality in a system of complementary rationalities without any indications that would prevent foundationalism in their perspectives. Thus spirituality and narratives coincide in what still looks like a regionalization of knowledge; the frame of narrative approaches appears to fit perfectly to the description of spirituality: which is a symptom of theorization, as I exposed before.

In occupational therapy, narratives are also considered to constitute a modality among others for the investigation of spirituality (Kirsh and Welch, 2003; McColl, 2003; Toomey, 2003) who investigate spirituality through people's creativity and Baptist (2003) who does so regarding daily work). Again an instrumentalization of heuristic models has all the characteristics of a theorization into which spirituality is finally conducted. Furthermore, authors' views do not even fit with Paul Ricoeur's hermeneutic phenomenology from which it is supposedly based. For Ricoeur (1983), narratives concern more fundamentally the condition of human being, who lives in time and space. Narratives are constitutively at stake in human action and thus in the advent of human subjectivity. Narratives cannot be reduced to a (technical) means, nor to a (special, specialized) domain of intervention if we have to respect their status in the philosophical system they come from.

It should be noticed then that Ricoeur's narrative approach has been criticised for its foundationalism by reducing the meaning process itself to a technical step of explanation in a more global and idealistic process of "pre-understanding" (Fodor, 1995). Critics also discuss implications of reducing narratives to a particular kind of speech (Fortin, 1996; Panier, 1991; 2006). Consequently, when Kirsh and Welch (2003) use widely Ricoeur's narrative approach, they too assume that stories offer a representation, ceaselessly reshaping, of the external or internal world of the person. Thus, they perpetuate the foundation of an order reflected through language and somewhat objectified in human action (in time). How cannot assimilate spirituality to a form of imitation of a lived world then, due to a mimetic functioning of meaning (*mimesis*)? Ricoeur's narrative approach is explicitly based on *mimesis*; he overtly admits this option. In a Hegelian philosophy like Ricoeur's one, spirituality cannot constitute necessarily a competence regarding a signifying practice: where the act of signifying (*semiosis*) is formally considered and exposed as anthropologically decisive.

Discussing the status of theory is another way to explain the issue of rationality once articulated to spirituality – understood in terms of a signifying practice (*semiosis*) by opposition to any technical or esthetical "practice of meaning" (*mimesis*). The hermeneutic condition of language does not exclude knowledge and theory. Rather, it requires us to revisit knowledge ceaselessly and to take account to the heuristic function of theory. Saying that the horizon of language is a practical one is to say that theory does not correspond any more to (a possession of) knowledge and that epistemology cannot be reduced anymore to a theory of knowledge. Theorization can lead to something else than a description of the "essences" of the world and/or of an ego (including God); but theorization has to proceeds from a theory of signification (*semiosis*). Thus epistemology can intrinsically include reflexivity on what one's does when he/she says, thinks, makes (and all this is fundamentally equivalent in the horizon of language; see Austin, 1975; Wittgenstein, 2001). This explains why, in hermeneutics, knowledge is for understanding and how a hermeneutic process can constitutes a mode of production... of knowledge (including technology) which radically implies our responsibility. When one is engaged in a complete revision of the status of theory and of what appears to be always at the centre of it (world, ego, God), signifying practices are to be elucidated. And occupational therapy still has to be elucidated as a signifying practice through its condition of spirituality (and ethics).

A major consequence of such a de-centred rationality associated to spirituality is the following one: a client-centred approach, which is widely espoused in health care, must be seriously questioned. In occupational therapy, this principle is aimed at thwarting the risk of imposition of values, faiths, or meaning to the patient by the professional (McColl, 2003; Unruh, Versnel and Kerr, 2003; Urbanowski, 2003; Whalley Hammell, 2001). Everything takes place then as if therapist's spirituality was not involved and must not ever being so. And this is – consciously – for the sole patient's benefit and according to the exclusive patient's requirements. But there is a blind spot, theoretically and practically speaking, in an intervention where one must presume to consider the patient's interest, motivations and goals alone. A question is not asked: how is a therapeutic relationship built? Both poles of the relationship must be considered in an intervention and spiritually expressively submit such question through all the intervention, I mean far before the act of doing this of that. The current distinction between neutrality and non directiveness in a process of meaning – and in counselling – leads to anti-hermeneutical presumption. Theoretical illusion is the most difficult problem to elucidate, even in professional practices.

CONCLUSION

Spirituality is not a medicine nor does it simply represent a domain of knowledge. It has become a major interest in health care as well as in occupational therapy but it is not easy to situate it exactly and to define it in a relevant way. Publications on this topic indicate that, more often than otherwise, spirituality is resolved into an attempt at theorizing all we can intelligibly grasp of our reality. My purpose was to move the problem of spirituality into the practical horizon of language. I hope having indicated new paths for a reflexive understanding of who we are and what we do in our own professional intervention. I consider it to be the first and most important step to establish "positive" approaches to health and intervention: without perpetuating the tacit "positivistic" thinking from which proceed curative approaches in health care.

REFERENCES

American Occupational Therapy Association (1994). Uniform terminology for occupational therapy - third edition. *American Journal of Occupational Therapy*, 48, 1047-1054.

Austin, J.L. (1975). *How to do things with words*. Cambridge (Mass.): Harvard University Press.

Baptist, S. (2003). Gaining awareness of spirituality at work. In: M.A. McColl (Ed.). *Spirituality and Occupational Therapy* (pp. 193-206). Ottawa: Canadian Association of Occupational Therapists.

Beagan, B., and Kumas-Tan, Z. (2005). Witnessing spirituality in practice. *British Journal of Occupational Therapy*, 68, 17-24.

Belcham, C. (2004). Spirituality in occupational therapy: Theory in practice? *British Journal of Occupational Therapy*, 67, 39-46.

Canadian Association of Occupational Therapists (1997). *Enabling occupation: An occupational therapy perspective*. Ottawa: CAOT Publications ACE.

Canadian Association of Occupational Therapists (1998). *Occupational therapy guidelines for Client-Centred practice*. Toronto: CAOT Publications.

Chan, J., and Spencer, J. (2004). Adaptation to hand injury: An evolving experience. *The American Journal of Occupational Therapy*, 58, 128-139.

Chapparo, C., and Ranka, J. (1997). The Occupational Performance Model (Australia): A description of constructs and structure. In: C. Chapparo and J. Ranka (Eds.). *Occupation Performance Model (Australia): Monograph 1*. Lidcombe, Australia: University of Sidney.

Christiansen, C. (1997). Acknowledging a spiritual dimension in occupational therapy practice. *American journal of occupational therapy*, 51, 169-172.

Collins, J.S., Paul, S., and West-Frasier, J. (2001). The utilization of spirituality in occupational therapy: Beliefs, practices, and perceived barriers. *Occupational Therapy in Health Care*, 14, 73-92.

Collins, M. (1998). Occupational therapy and spirituality: Reflecting on quality of experience in therapeutic interventions. *British Journal of Occupational Therapy*, 61, 280-284.

Davis, R.B. (1995). The principlism debate: a critical overview. *The Journal of Medicine and Philosophy*, 20(1):85-105.

Do Rozario, L. (1997). Spirituality in the lives of people with disability and chronic illness: A creative paradigm of wholeness and reconstitution. *Disability and Rehabilitation*, 19, 427-434.

Dombeck, M.T. (1998). The spiritual and pastoral dimensions of care in interprofessional context. *Journal on Interprofessional Care*, 12, 361-372.

Egan, M., Delaat, D., and Vallée, C. (2003). Logos and mythos reasoning in occupational therapy. In: M.A. McColl (Ed.). *Spirituality and Occupational Therapy* (pp. 115-124). Ottawa: Canadian Association of Occupational Therapists.

Egan, M., and DeLaat, M.D. (1997). The implicit spirituality of occupational therapy practice. *Canadian Journal of Occupational Therapy*, 64, 115-121.

Egan, M., and Swedersky, J. (2003). Spirituality as experienced by occupational therapists in practice. *American Journal of Occupational Therapy: Official publication of the American Occupational Therapy Association*, 57, 525-533.

Emanuel, E.J. (1995). The beginning of the end of principlism. *The Hastings Center Report*, 25(4):37-8.

Engquist, D.E., Short-DeGraff, M., Gliner, J., et al (1997). Occupational therapists' beliefs and practices with regard to spirituality and therapy. *American Journal of Occupational Therapy*, 51, 173-180.

Fiorenza, F.S. (1984). *Foundational theology: Jesus and the church*. New York: Crossword.

Fodor, J. (1995). *Christian Hermeneutics. Paul Ricoeur and the Refiguring of Theology*. New York: Oxford.

Fortin, A. (1996). Du sens à la signification: pour une théorie de l'acte de lecture en théologie. *Laval théologique et philosophique*, 52, 327-338.

Fumerton, R. (2005). *Epistemology*. Oxford, UK; Malden MA: Blackwell Pub.

Gadamer, H.G. (1996). *Vérité et méthode: les grandes lignes d'une herméneutique philosophique*. Paris: Seuil.

Gert, B., Culver, C.M., and Clouser, K.D. (2000). Common morality versus specified principlism: reply to Richardson. *The Journal of Medicine and Philosophy*, 25(3):308-22.

Greenberg, N.S. (2003). Spiritual spontaneity: Developing our own 9/1/1: One occupational therapist's spiritual journey across the 9/1/1 Divide. *Occupational Therapy in Mental Health*, 19, 153-189.

Habermas, J. (1987). *Théorie de l'agir communicationnel*. Paris: Fayard.

Heidegger, M. (1986 [1927]). *Être et temps*. Paris: Gallimard.

Henderson, V. (1994). *La nature des soins infirmiers*, St-Laurent (Québec), Éd. du renouveau pédagogique.

Hoyland, M., and Mayers, C. (2005). Is meeting spiritual need within the occupational therapy domain? *British Journal of Occupational Therapy*, 68, 177-180.

Hubbard, S. (1991). Towards a truly holistic approach to occupational therapy. *British Journal of Occupational Therapy*, 54, 415-418.

Kang, C. (2003). A psychospiritual integration frame of reference for occupational therapy. Part 1: Conceptual foundations. *Australian Occupational Therapy Journal*, 50, 92-103.

Kant, E. (1986 [1790]). *Critique de la faculté de juger*. Parin: Vrin.

Kant, E. (2001 [1781]). *Critique de la raison pure*. Paris: Quatridge / PUF.

Kirsh, B., and Welch, A. (2003). Opening expression: The power of narrative in occupational therapy. In: M.A. McColl (Ed.). *Spirituality and Occupational Therapy* (pp. 161-180). Ottawa: Canadian Association of Occupational Therapists.

Kroeker, P.T. (2003). Spirituality and therapy in a secular, pluralistic culture: Toward an ethic of care. In: M.A. McColl (Ed.). *Spirituality and Occupational Therapy* (pp. 55-66). Ottawa: Canadian Association of Occupational Therapists.

McColl, M.A. (1994). Holistic occupational therapy: Historical meaning and contemporary implications. *Canadian Journal of Occupational Therapy*, 61, 72-77.

McColl, M.A. (2000). Muriel Driver Lectureship - Spirit, occupation and disability. *Canadian Journal of Occupational Therapy*, 67, 217-228.

McColl, M.A., and O'Brien, P. (2003). Spirituality and occupational therapists. In: M.A. McColl (Ed.). *Spirituality and Occupational Therapy* (pp. 31-51). Ottawa: Canadian Association of Occupational Therapists.

McColl, M.A. (Ed.) (2003). *Spirituality and Occupational Therapy*. Ottawa: Canadian Association of Occupational Therapists.

Panier, L. (1991). Pour une anthropologie du croire. Aspects de la problématique chez Michel de Certeau. In : C. Geffré, (Ed.). *Merchel de Certeau ou la Différence chrétienne* (pp.37-59). Paris: Cerf.

Panier, L. (2006). Ricoeur et la sémiotique: une rencontre "improbable"? , pro-manuscripto, 22 p.

Phillips, I. (2003). Infusing spirituality into geriatric health care: Practical applications from the literature. *Topics in Geriatric Rehabilitation*, 19, 249-256.

Pouliot, E. (2001). Efficacité thérapeutique des interventions médicales, infirmières, psychosociales et pastorales: mais à quelles conditions? Bilan critique des recherches et publications sur le lien entre santé et spiritualité. Québec: manuscrit déposé au Service régional de pastorale de la santé (SRPS), 208 p.

Pouliot, E. (2003). Éthique et mystique: élucidation de l'acte théologique au revers d'une qualification chrétienne de la morale. In : *Thèse doctorale présentée à la Faculté de théologie et de sciences religieuses*, Québec: Université Laval.

Ricoeur, P. (1983). *Temps et récit*. Paris: Seuil.

Schulz, E.K. (2004). Spirituality and disability: An analysis of select themes. *Occupational Therapy in Health Care*, 18, 57-83.

Schulz, E.K. (2005). The meaning of spirituality for individuals with disabilities. *Disability and Rehabilitation*, 27, 1283-1295.

Scott, M.S., Grzybowski, M., and Webb, S. (1994). Perceptions and practices of registered nurses regarding pastoral care and the spiritual need of hospital patients, *Journal of Pastoral Care,* 48 (2): 171-179.

Sellers, S.C., and Haag, B.A. (1998). Spiritual nursing interventions, *Journal of Holistic Nursing*, 16 (3): 338-354.

Toomey, L. (2003). Creativity: Access to the spirit through occupation. In: M.A. McColl (Ed.). *Spirituality and Occupational Therapy* (pp. 181-192). Ottawa: Canadian Association of Occupational Therapists.

Unruh, A.M., Versnel, J., and Kerr, N. (2002). Spirituality unplugged: A review of commonalities and contentions, and a resolution. *Canadian Journal of Occupational Therapy*, 69, 5-19.

Unruh, A.M., Versnel, J., and Kerr, N. (2003). Spirituality in evidence-based therapy. In: M.A. McColl (Ed.). *Spirituality and Occupational Therapy* (pp. 145-160). Ottawa: Canadian Association of Occupational Therapists.

Urbanowski, R. (2003). Spirituality in changed occupational lives. In: M.A. McColl (Ed.). *Spirituality and Occupational Therapy* (pp. 95-114). Ottawa: Canadian Association of Occupational Therapists.

Urbanowski, R., and Vargo, J. (1994). Spirituality, daily practice, and the occupational performance model. *Canadian Journal of Occupational Therapy*, 61, 88-94.

Whalley Hammell, K. (2001). Intrinsicality: Reconsidering spirituality, meaning(s) and mandates. *Canadian Journal of Occupational Therapy*, 68, 186-194.

Whalley Hammell, K. (2003). Intrinsicality: Reflection on meaning and mandates. In: M.A. McColl (Ed.). *Spirituality and Occupational Therapy* (pp. 67-82). Ottawa: Canadian Association of Occupational Therapists.

Wilding, C. (2002). Where angels fear to tread: Is spirituality relevant to occupational therapy practice? *Australian Occupational Therapy Journal*, 49, 44-47.

Wilding, C., May, E., and Muir-Cochrane, E. (2005). Experience of spirituality, mental illness and occupation: A life-sustaining phenomenon. *Australian Occupational Therapy Journal*, 52, 2-9.

Wittgenstein, L. (2001, [1993]). *Tractatus logico-philosophicus*, Paris, Gallimard.

Chapter 5

ECOLOGICAL APPROACHES TO HEALTH: INTERACTIONS BETWEEN HUMANS AND THEIR ENVIRONMENT

Claire Dumont[*]

Institut de réadaptation en déficience physique de Québec
Laval University, 525 Boul. Hamel, Quebec City,
Quebec, Canada, G1M 2S8

ABSTRACT

This chapter discusses and analyses how ecological models and approaches could contribute to improve human health. In the first section of the chapter, the evolution of human thought will be redrawn, from ancient conceptions of the world up to the most recent ecological models. The second section of the chapter presents a review of ecological theories, models, and approaches relevant to the field of health. The text proceeds in an historical perspective and from general to specific: generic theoretical referents followed by referents specific to a field of practice, a discipline, a population, or a situation. Numerous examples are provided. In the third section, common characteristics of ecological theories, models and approaches are described: 1) the consideration of personal, environmental, and occupational components, and the consideration of interactions between them; 2) the positive vision of health; 3) the focus on empowerment, self-determination, and self-regulation of individuals, and finally, 4) the fact that ecological interventions occur mostly in natural environments, where the person interacts with his or her environment and performs his or her occupations, rather than in institutions or hospitals. The fourth section deepens the concepts of environment and interactions, since these concepts were to date less defined in previous publications. New theoretical referents are proposed for these two elements. The fifth section presents the results of numerous studies with the aim of providing scientific evidence in support of ecological models and approaches. These studies are grouped according to the targeted components, which are the person, environment or occupation, as well as the interactions between these components. Finally, the sixth section brings a different perspective. Some

---

[*] E-mail: Claire.Dumont@irdpq.qc.ca

fundamental ecological mechanisms of interaction are analyzed according to human health and to the current context: demographic changes, climate change, depletion of resources, new diseases, pandemic risks and others. These events will, without a doubt, provoke a budgetary crisis which governments and health care systems will have to face; thus supporting the urgency to adopt ecological approaches. Many research questions are proposed to improve knowledge in the field of human ecology in this section. Concrete suggestions are also identified in order to improve population health. The conclusion presents a lucid and global synthesis of the situation. Humanity is at a stage never reached before, notably because of the presence of so many individuals on earth. Furthermore, human beings possess powerful abilities and technological possibilities but also the awareness and the responsibility which these elements confer to us. All health professionals are called to contribute to necessary efforts in favour of population health, now and for future generations, in a sustainable development perspective.

INTRODUCTION

Among new approaches developed over the last 30 years by many disciplines and in many fields of intervention, ecological models and approaches are increasingly mentioned. This chapter reviews these models and approaches, characterizing their contribution to positive approaches to health. First, the evolution of human thought toward ecological thought will be presented. A brief history of landmarks relative to these models and approaches will permit one to retrace their main foundations. Some generic and interdisciplinary models will allow one to understand the main components of the most recent ecological models. The general characteristics of ecological models and approaches will be described, focusing on person-environment-occupation interactions. Scientific evidence supporting their use and application will be demonstrated in various disciplines and domains of intervention. Finally, the conclusion will address the potential contribution of ecological models and approaches in knowledge evolution and improvement of population health in general.

This chapter intends to make a contribution in demonstrating the urgency to adopt professional practices that respect the principles defined in ecological models and approaches, such as sustainable development and "thinking globally and acting locally". Numerous economical sectors are challenged to modify their practices by following these principles, for example: agriculture, forestry, industry, or transportation. The health sector must not be excluded from these discussions. All aspects and all levels of the health sector are targeted: laboratory research, social research, professional education and training, clinical practices in hospitals or clinics, interventions in the social domain, public health, services organization, health systems management, governments, insurance companies involved in the process of decision making concerning health care, food production, and others. All disciplines involved in the field of health, as well as those in related sectors, can participate in reflecting on professional practices with the aim of improving population health.

1. THE ECOLOGICAL THOUGHT: HISTORICAL PERSPECTIVE

Ecological models and approaches are grounded in a way of thinking and of conceiving the world that make it possible to retrace origins. Indeed, the thought evolved over centuries. The state of knowledge contributes largely to our conception of the universe, to our way of thinking, and to our way of acting. From an historical perspective, certain famous philosophers, several representatives of religions, scientists, and artists brought alternately various insights on the conception of the world. Particular events also brought, directly or not, their contribution. The next paragraphs will illustrate the progress made to reach ecological thought as observed at the beginning of the 21st Century.

During the Middle Ages, the world was seen as enchanted. All unexplained phenomena were interpreted by delights, witchcraft, magic or religion mainly because of limited scientific knowledge (Taylor, 2002). Religion proposed various symbols to try to integrate some rationality into this type of conception of the world, and to make it more explicable and controllable. It was then all about amulets, holy water or miracles. The planet earth was at that time described by scientists as the centre of the universe: a stable universe, of which the limits were known and perceptible. Later, the conceptions were revised in accordance with the *post newtonian* science, which excludes that superior meanings can express themselves through the universe encircling us. The scientific rational thought invaded gradually our conception of the world (Taylor, 2002).

The more formal ecological thought was born with Charles Darwin in the 19th Century. His theory of evolution appeared in 1859, and can be considered as the first real ecological theory. According to this theory, life evolved through continuous interactions between living species and their environment. The best combinations have persisted and life has evolved this way until today. This theory was revolutionary because of its completely new perspective of the human being, situating it at the same level as other living species. It was going further than the simple description of phenomena; it provided explanations about fundamental mechanisms. It was so revolutionary that, even in the 21st Century, in spite of multiple evidences, its adoption meets numerous resistances, notably with what is called *Intelligent Design* (Gould, 1999).

Other scientific events enlightened the influence of the environment on human beings, and contributed to the development of ecological thought. Thus, the importance of environment for human health was first demonstrated in the 19th Century, when a physician named John Snow demonstrated the relationship between the contagion of wells of drinking water and the cholera epidemic in London (Rosen, 1993). He associated the number of deaths in each area of London to the degree of pollution of the part of the Thames River from which the company obtained its water. This event took place in 1854, 30 years before the discovery of the bacillus by Koch, and even before the knowledge of the existence of micro-organisms. Public health considers this fact as one of its foundations, which emphasizes the importance of environmental factors for population health (Green, and Kreuter, 1999).

During the same period, in the field of nursing, Florence Nightingale's work was remarkable as she recognised that the healthiness of the environment was a fundamental cause of numerous deaths and diseases. This woman focused on hygiene and established hospital practices which allowed the saving of an incalculable number of lives. These practices are still part of the foundations in the field of nursing (Nightingale, 1869; Salazar, and Primomo, 1994).

In sociology, the first analogy between the development of a human being and the growth of a plant, which grows in a favourable or unfavourable environment, was made in 1921. More recently, the link between the growth of populations and the capacity of environments to support this growth was established. These ideas contributed to birth control, health education, and control of diseases. Medical sociology also developed in the 1960s, notably by studying the social, institutional, and cultural contexts which affect people (Green, and Kreuter, 1999; Rosen, 1979).

During the 20th Century, spectacular technological breakthroughs have been observed (automobile, plane, telephone, radio, television, computer, internet, etc.), and particularly in the field of biology (vaccines, antibiotics, insulin, DNA, genetic, etc.). These spectacular successes in science and technology have made the rational thought triumphant and have influenced our conception of the world. The body has been conceived as a machine, and medicine as the science which has to repair this machine. Science developed extra organs, drugs or medicines to cure health problems, or to compensate for dysfunctions. It has been the golden age of the reductionist thought, and of the linear chain of causality. Everything has come down to recognizable, controllable and reproducible elements. It has been the domination of the biomedical model in the field of health.

Besides, in industrialized nations, the world wars contributed to the development of the production line work and to bureaucratic work organization. All human activities have been affected: feeding, leisure, home routines, etc. Furthermore, the mechanization limits physical efforts necessary to carry out different tasks. We travel in automobiles, robots and machinery perform numerous tasks, we often remain seated in front of the television or the computer, and we live in food overprofusion. The use of fossil fuels, mainly petroleum, allows a way of life without any common measure with all which could have occurred since the beginning of the humanity: efficient transportation, industrial development, resources exploitation, manufacturing and use of oil by-products, etc. (Homer-Dixon, 2001).

During the 1970s, one event resulting from progress in technology contributed to change our conception of the world: it was to see pictures of the earth, the blue planet, photographed by astronauts from space missions. These pictures exposed the "finitude" of the planet, the vulnerability of life on it, and it gave impulsions to ecology in the 1980s. Indeed, as fundamental science, ecology studies distribution and abundance of organisms, not without revealing the effects of human activities and technologies on the environment (Campbell, 1995).

Some perverse effects of science, technology, and their associated conceptions of the world and the human being, appeared at the end of the 20th Century and beginning of the 21st Century. Industrialization provokes global warming and its consequences: hurricanes, smog, pollution in cities, reduced ozone layer, populations' displacements, etc. To improve on an economical level, to ensure survival or sometimes simply for comfort or by greed, humans overexploit their environment, which results in deforestation, desertification, resource depletion, famine, loss of biologic diversity, and loss of lands and seas that were previously productive. We attend to the extinction of numerous plants and animals, including many yet undiscovered living species and ecosystems. Humans then loose resources, sources of knowledge, and probably undiscovered medicines (Last, 1993; McMichael, 1993; Reeves, and Levoir, 2003; Staples, Ponsomby, Lim, and McMichael, 2003).

Toxic products in the environment cause different health problems such as cancers and lung problems (Jerrett, Burnett, Willis, Krewski, Goldberg, DeLuca, and Finkelstein, 2003; Martin, Latorre, Saldiva, and Braga, 2002; Schreinemachers, 2003; Steiner, 2002; Willis, Krewski, Jerrett, Goldberg, and Burnett, 2003). Pesticides, antibiotics, and hormones are used in food production with powerful side-effects including carcinogenesis and neurological damage. They also provoke insect as well as bacterial resistance which requires the use of increasingly more potent cocktails. More and more bacterial resistance to antibiotics by humans is observed that diminishes the possibility to cure infectious diseases (Andremont, Brun-Buisson, and Struelens, 2001; Barrett, Kuzawa, McDade, and Armelagos, 1998). There is a danger of epidemics or pandemics like influenza and there is a real risk of rapid transmission especially in the context of global travel, trade, and over-population.

New diseases also appear following human interventions or human lifestyles, of which one of the most known and spread is AIDS, but many others are also observed. Sedentary lifestyles and food overprofusion (mainly composed of fat and sugar) provoke obesity and premature ageing in a large part of the population (Cope, and Allison, 2006; Hensrud, and Klein, 2006). Our way of life, notably food and smoking, is clearly associated to the majority of cancers (Canadian Cancer Society, 2007). Our sterilized environment causes difficulties in the development of the children's immune system. The incidence of allergies has never been so high, notably because young are not exposed enough to different bacteria or other natural substances existing in the environment and overly exposed to other kinds of toxic products (Aubier, Neukirch, and Annesi-Maesano, 2005; Petronella, and Conboy-Ellis, 2003). The incidence of developmental delays among children is increasing in industrialized countries and became an important concern for the World Health Organisation (WHO). Consequently, neonatal medical practices are questioned as well as parent-child relationships and certain environmental factors (Blanchard, Gurka, and Blackman, 2006; Mead, 2006; Zimmer, and Panko, 2006). Globally, our way of life is not adapted to our genetics stemming from millions of years of evolution: a physically effortless life in overprofusion, using various technologies and with the presence of multiple unusual chemical products (Gross, Li, Ford, and Liu, 2004; Pickett, Kelly, Brunner, Lobstein, and Wilkinson, 2005).

Some authors identify the use of petroleum, an energy concentrated during millions of years, as one of the main sources of these problems. Indeed, petroleum allows a way of life among which the advantages and the comfort exceed our real needs, and it leads to abuse and waste. It is a source of conflict and war, stimulates human greed, contributes to global warming, and allows resources exploitation which exceeds levels of possible renewal. For these authors, the use of petroleum destroys the balance which was previously in place on this planet (Homer-Dixon, 2001; Simmons, 2006).

Facing these events, many authors speak about a third epidemiological transition produced by all these changes, after one of infectious diseases related to hygiene and over-population in cities and one of chronic diseases related to industrialisation during the 20th Century (Barrett, Kuzawa, McDade, and Armelagos, 1998; Cook, Jardine, and Weinstein, 2004). This time, our way of life is the cause of health problems, what could be considered as an anthropological origin (Barrett, Kuzawa, McDade, and Armelagos, 1998).

On the other hand, we have discovered that causes and risk factors of many diseases are multiple and they include personal and environmental factors. It is the case notably of autoimmune diseases like multiple sclerosis or type I diabetes (Baird, 1996; Mead, 2004; 2006) and chronic diseases such as hypertension, obesity, and type 2 diabetes (Barker, 2004a;

2004b; Gluckman, and Hanson, 2005; 2006; Gluckman, Hanson, and Pinal, 2005; Nathanielsz, 1999). We have also learnt that genes interact with environment in complex ways; they are activated and shaped by the environment of the cell, as well as the personal environment of each individual, which includes emotions and behaviours. In addition, research revealed that early life events shape the developing nervous system and influence the risk for diseases (Mead, 2004; 2006).

In this context, the curative traditional biomedical model based on biological causes and risk factors has limits and it cannot explain the origin and the evolution of numerous diseases necessary to discover appropriate treatments. Medications have improved life expectancy for diseases such as type I diabetes and AIDS, but they have failed to cure these diseases. To improve our understanding, to analyse situations and intervene efficiently in order to improve human health, it is necessary to use new theoretical referents. Ecological models and approaches could potentially bring a new perspective that could favour the evolution of knowledge and the discovery of new solutions.

Ecology is a science which occupies a more and more important place in our societies. More and more scientists and people in general have become aware that we need to live in harmony with our environment to ensure health, quality of life, and long-term survival (Brundtland Commission, 1987). In many sciences, reductionist thought and the linear chain of causality tend to be replaced by a more systemic thought, taking into account multiple factors and their reciprocal interactions. An ecological approach notably allows a better understanding of the complexity of the world and avoids the trap of misleading simplifications (McMichael, 1993). However, it is only recently that ecology has tended to influence thought and actions. The next section presents ecological frames of reference relative to the health or social fields, demonstrating the evolution of thought toward a better understanding of its complexity, which notably states an innovative ecological thought.

2. ECOLOGICAL FRAMES OF REFERENCE IN THE HEALTH AND SOCIAL FIELDS

Human beings acquired the refinement of language and communication which we know. Very young children have high abilities to learn languages, but they will not learn to speak if adults do not teach them, for example if raised by primates. Research on primates also demonstrates that primates cannot develop our ability of speaking, even raised in a human being's family. Recently, an association was established between a defective gene and a problem of language, demonstrating the possible genetic origin of our language skills. Language development in human beings requires both personal factors, notably from the point of view of genetics, and environmental factors, that is an environment where adults communicate and use language. The capacity to learn any language results from a complex brain which develops in a particular environment, according to the directives of a human genome.

Ecology is a new science in the early stages of development. Ecology studies interactions between living species and their environment (Krebs, 2001). Ecology can be applied to humans as they are shaped by their environment and they also shape it resulting in a mutual adaptation or construction (Kondrat, 2002; Satariano, and McAuley, 2003).

In the next paragraphs, ecological frames of reference, which consider humans, environment, and interaction between both, are presented: 1) the first ecological models in social sciences; 2) the Ottawa charter for health promotion; 3) the social cognitive theory; 4) frames of reference in the rehabilitation field; 5) practice models of occupational therapists, and 6) a model describing patterns in origins of diseases.

2.1. The First Ecological Models Applied to Humans in Social Sciences

One of the first models that qualified as ecologic and applied to humans in social sciences was Bronfenbrenner's ecological model (1977; 1979). This model put the focus on environment, which was a new perspective compared to previous models, centred uniquely on the person. In an attempt to better describe human development within the framework of the relation between the person and the environment, Bronfenbrenner (1977; 1979) proposes a conceptualization of the environment which he names "ecological environment". It consists of a set of four imbricated structures, one into the others, which is a juxtaposition of systemic levels where interactions are mutual. It includes the microsystem, mesosystem, exosystem, and macrosystem.

The microsystem represents the smallest of the systems. Bronfenbrenner describes it as being the immediate environment of which the person is a part, such as home, school or working environment. The microsystem includes the complex interrelations between the person and the environment. It is in this environment in which the person assumes roles (relative, parent, girl, professor …) and undertakes activities at precise moments. The environment also includes physical and social characteristics which are relevant for the person. The mesosystem consists of a set of microsystems of which the individual is a part. The interest of the mesosystem concerns mainly the relations between these microsystems. The exosystem is different from both precedents because the person is not directly integrated into this component. It is a continuation of previous systems and it makes reference to formal and informal social elements. It does not include the person, but it influences him/her indirectly through its social constituents. The exosystem includes the main institutions of the society such as neighbours, media, governmental organisms, systems of transport, among others. Finally, the macrosystem heads the previous three systems. It represents a kind of "blueprint" of the society. It refers to the culture in which individuals live. According to Bronfenbrenner, the macrosystem is informal and implicit. It includes the political, social, legal, and economic systems and so it influences the previous three systems. The macrosystem refers to attitudes and ideologies.

Bronfenbrenner's model is one of the main foundations for social work. In addition, this conceptualization of the environment was adopted in numerous models and domains of intervention, such as psychology, nursing and occupational therapy (Corcoran, Franklin, and Bennet, 2000; Eckert, and Murrey, 1984; Law, 1991; Salazar, and Primomo, 1994).

Another series of models which also qualified as ecologic were published in social sciences. These models applied to ageing people who were progressively loosing their autonomy. They focus on the interaction between the ageing person and the environment, with the aim of improving autonomy at home and quality of life. Three of these models are briefly presented in the next paragraphs. They are: Lawton's "Ecological Model" (Lawton,

1980; 1982; 1986), Kahana's "Congruence Model of Person / Environment Fit" (Kahana, 1982), and the "Ecological Model of Housing" (Eckert, and Murrey, 1984).

Lawton (1980; 1982; 1986) highlighted that the individual is not in a passive relationship with the environment, but rather can create and change this environment which, in turn, affects his/her behaviour. His "Ecological Model" emphasizes the concepts of competence, environmental press, and adaptation. The person is represented as a set of "competences" (i.e., biologic health, sensory and perceptive abilities, cognitive skills, motor skills, and the strength of the "Me") (Lawton, 1982). The environment places demands on the person (referred to as "environmental press") (Lawton, 1980). Every person presents a given level of competence when he/she is in an environment offering a specific level of demand (Lawton, and Nahemow, 1973). The person reaches his/her level of "adaptation" when the environmental press is neither too much nor too little, given the person's level of competence (Kiernat, 1983; Lawton, 1980).

Another model, the Kahana's "Congruence Model of Person / Environment Fit" (Kahana, 1982), resumes elements of Lawton's "Ecological Model", and adds the concept of "preference". Kahana's model does not focus on physical characteristics of the person, but rather on his/her preferences. Kahana's model also demonstrates the complexity and the congruence of the physical, social, and psychological environments.

Finally, the "Ecological Model of Housing", by Eckert and Murrey (1984), was developed to structure research and discussions about the possible alternatives in terms of housing for ageing people. This model is also based on Lawton's model. The premise of the model testifies that the knowledge of the context in which the person lives leads to a better understanding of his/her psychological state and behaviour. Eckert and Murrey present the person as a set of competences, as proposed by Lawton (1982). To this conceptualization, they added elements such as person's life history and demographic characteristics. They presented the person as being a part of many environments and related systems, getting close to Bronfenbrenner's conceptualization of the environment.

2.2. The Ottawa Charter for Health Promotion

The "Ottawa Charter for Health Promotion", published in 1986, has determinedly adopted an ecological perspective by defining health as: "a state of complete physical, mental and social well-being [...], an individual or a group must be able to identify and to realize aspirations, to satisfy needs, and to change or cope with the environment. Health is therefore seen as a resource for everyday life, not the objective of living. Health is a positive concept emphasizing social and personal resources, as well as physical capacities". Thus, health is not seen as the absence of diseases or impairments, but as the possibility to live harmoniously in an environment which presents adequate resources. This charter was translated in more than 30 languages and was adopted by numerous countries. More recently, the "Charter of Health Promotion of Bangkok" (WHO, 2005) develops concrete strategies and proposes solutions at various levels (local, regional, political, industry ...) to improve human health.

2.3. The Social Cognitive Theory

According to Bandura's (1986) social cognitive theory, internal and external factors harmonize to shape the thoughts, feelings, and social behaviour of an individual (Bandura, 1986). From this theoretical perspective, human functioning is viewed as the product of a dynamic interplay of personal (cognitive, emotional, biological), behavioural, and environmental influences (see Figure 1). People are viewed as self-organizing and proactive, rather than reactive organisms shaped and shepherded by environmental forces or driven by concealed inner impulses.

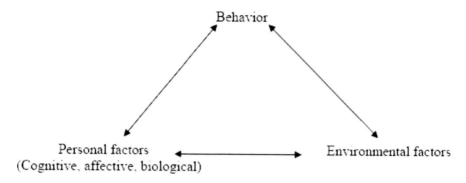

Figure 1. Interactions between the person, environment and behaviour (Bandura, 1986).

Rooted within Bandura's social cognitive perspective is the understanding that individuals are imbued with certain abilities that define what it is to be human. Primarily among these are the abilities to symbolize, plan alternative strategies (forethought), learn through vicarious experience, self-regulate, and self-reflect. These capabilities provide human beings with the cognitive means by which they are influential in determining their own destiny (Pajarez, 2005).

By drawing on their symbolic capabilities, humans can extract meaning from their environment, construct guides for action, solve problems cognitively, support or anticipate courses of action, gain new knowledge by reflective thought, and communicate with others at any distance in time and space. Symbolizing also enables people to store the information required to guide future behaviours. It is through this process that they are able to model observed behaviour. Through the use of symbols, individuals solve cognitive problems, and engage in self-directedness and forethought. People plan courses of action, anticipate the likely consequences of these actions, and set goals and challenges for them to motivate, guide and regulate their activities. It is because of the ability to plan alternative strategies that one can anticipate the consequences of an action without actually engaging in it.

Individuals have self-regulatory mechanisms that provide the potential for self-directed changes in their behaviour. The manner and degree to which people self-regulate their own actions and behaviour involve: 1) the accuracy and consistency of their self-observation and self-monitoring; 2) the judgments they make regarding their actions, choices, and attributions: and 3) the evaluative and tangible reactions they make regarding their own behaviour through the self-regulatory process. This last function includes evaluations of one's self (self-concept, self-esteem, values) and tangible self-motivators that act as personal incentives to behave in self-directed ways. For Bandura (1986), the capability that is most "distinctly human" (p. 21) is that of self-reflection, hence it is a prominent feature of the social cognitive theory. Through self-reflection, people make sense of their experiences, explore their own cognitions and self-beliefs, engage in self-evaluation, and modify their thinking and behaviour accordingly.

Self-efficacy is one of the fundamental elements of Bandura's theory (Bandura, 1986; Pajarez, 2005). Self-efficacy beliefs are defined as: "people's judgments of their capabilities to organize and execute courses of action required to attain designated types of performances" (Bandura, 1986, p. 391). Self-efficacy beliefs provide the foundation for human motivation, well-being, and personal accomplishment. Indeed, unless people believe that their actions can produce the outcomes they desire, they have little incentive to act or to persevere when facing difficulties. Much empirical evidence now supports Bandura's contention that self-efficacy beliefs touch virtually every aspect of people's lives, their vulnerability, and the life choices they make. Self-efficacy is also a critical determinant of self-regulation. Moreover, numerous studies have demonstrated, within different populations presenting various health problems, that self-efficacy beliefs are health determinants (Bandura, 2003; Schwarzer, 1992; 1994).

2.4. Models of Reference in the Field of Rehabilitation

Rehabilitation is a sector of intervention which was developed mainly after the Second World War, notably because of the improvement in survival rates of war wounded soldiers. In this sector, intervention models evolved from a biomedical perspective in the sixties, towards a biopsychosocial one in the 1980s, and now toward an ecological approach (Fougeyrollas, 2001). In the biomedical model, rehabilitation interventions consisted of removing or reducing impairments and helping one become the "most normal possible". In the biopsychosocial model, the environment is taken into account in the interventions, but the main objective is still to cure or to reduce impairments. The environment is seen as a means to contribute to goal attainment or to compensate for persistent sequelaes. The "independent living movement" contributed significantly to the evolution of models in the field of rehabilitation (Craddock, 1996). This movement focuses on the social dimension of handicap, in opposition to the biomedical one, and proposes interventions targeting the environment rather than individuals (Fougeyrollas, and Beauregard, 2001).

Ecological approaches in the field of rehabilitation retain elements from both biopsychosocial and social models. The purpose of interventions is not to cure, but is to put the person in interaction with his/her environment so that he/she continues to develop. The intervention consists of a mutual adaptation of the person and environment to favour social participation. It is thus possible to intervene on the person by improving abilities, or on the environment by setting up enablers, facilitators, or by eliminating obstacles. Finally, it is possible to observe an improvement in abilities or a reduction of impairments and disabilities once the person is in interaction with the environment, because he/she is so going to continue to progress and evolve. The normative perspective often associated with the curative biomedical model would be also removed from interventions in ecological approaches. These approaches rather encourage open-mindedness to differences (Fougeyrollas, and Beauregard, 2001; Trickett, 1994). This situation can be illustrated by interventions that occurred several decades ago in the treatment of deformities resulting from thalidomide. A person could be considered cured after having corrective surgeries on his/her deformities and/or with the use of prostheses which made him/her, from a normative perspective, seemingly similar to other people. On the other hand, the person could be more limited in his/her activities and social participation after these surgeries and/or while using prostheses.

More specifically in the sector of intellectual disabilities, Gagnier and Lachapelle (2002) described the evolution of concepts associated to the foundations of interventions. Until the years 1960-1970, people with intellectual disabilities were placed in institutions. Following important reforms, these people gradually started to leave the institutional milieu to integrate into society. Further to this "uninstitutionnalisation", the focus was on "normalization" in the 1970s, and in the 1990s, it was on promoting the value of social roles, social integration, and social participation. According to this evolution, Gagnier and Lachapelle (2002) recommend an ecological approach for interventions.

In the mental health domain, in the case of chronic diseases like schizophrenia, the notion of restoring replaces the notion of curing (Cnaan, Blankertz, Messinger, and Gardner, 1988). Thus, it is not a question of being cured of the disease, but it is one of learning to live with it, to be able to participate in life socially, and to reach a certain quality of life. This mental health perspective has been developed following claims by people with mental health problems for more humanized care, and treatment approaches that are less centred on biomedical aspects.

To illustrate these new perspectives, two ecological, generic, and interdisciplinary theoretical referents, widely spread and used, are presented here: the Disability Creation Process (DCP) Model (Fougeyrollas, Cloutier, Bergeron, Côté, Côté, and St-Michel, 1996), and the new model of the WHO (WHO, 2001a).

2.4.1. The Disability Creation Process Model

The DCP Model was developed by Fougeyrollas and his colleagues (1996) following two international consultations, including meetings, conferences, and questionnaires. It is widely used throughout the province of Quebec, and is rapidly becoming popular throughout America and Europe. According to the DCP Model, social participation corresponds to the accomplishment of *life habits*. *Life habits,* as defined in this model, are current activities and social roles that are valued by the person or his/her socio-cultural context according to his/her characteristics (age, gender, socio-cultural identity, etc.). They ensure the survival and growth of a person within his/her society, throughout his/her existence. The extent to which life habits are accomplished (social participation), or not accomplished (handicap situation), is a function of the interaction between personal and environmental factors. According to this model, personal factors consist of personal characteristics (demographic characteristics, personality, etc.), the level of integrity or impairment of *organic systems* (nervous, circulatory, etc.), and *capabilities* (cognitive, language, etc.). These personal factors are influenced by *risk factors,* which may influence risk for a disease, such as trauma, or any other disruption to a person's integrity, capabilities, or development. On the other hand, *environmental factors* are comprised of social (family, services, etc.) and physical components (climate, architecture, etc.), that may act as facilitators or obstacles to social participation (see Figure 2) (Fougeyrollas, 1997; Fougeyrollas, Noreau, and Boschen, 2002).

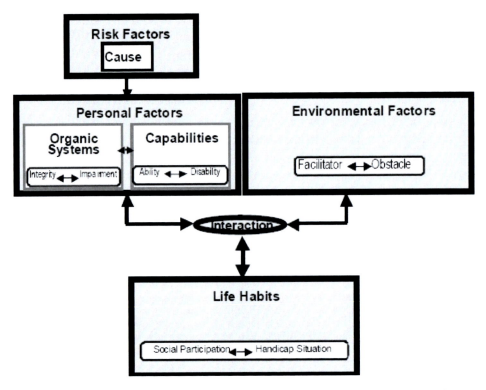

Figure 2. Disability Creation Process: Explanatory model of the causes and consequences of disease, trauma and other disruptions to the integrity and development of a person.

2.4.2. The International Classification of Functioning, Disability and Health

In 1948, the WHO published the International Classification of Diseases (ICD), which is still used today in its tenth version (ICD-10). In the purest biomedical tradition, the aim was to classify all diseases and disorders by systems (bone, muscular, digestive, etc.). Its first interest is the codification of diagnoses with the focus on aspects of morbidity and symptoms (Fougeyrollas, 2001). This model presented several gaps, notably by its normative vision of human beings and by the lack of consideration of the consequences of chronic diseases on the person. Indeed, it was possible to diagnose a "disease" without the person being disturbed by it, simply in reference to a defined norm. On the other hand, many diseases could not be cured or are cured but result in limitations, disabilities or sequelaes for the person. The classification did not take into account these dimensions. A new classification was thus elaborated: the International Classification of Impairments, Disabilities and Handicaps (ICIDH) (WHO, 1980). This classification had the advantage to distinguish the biologic level of the organic systems (impairments) of their consequences on the person (disabilities) and on his/her activities (handicaps). This classification proposes an understanding of the handicap according to a linear relation of causality between different levels: diseases appear in organic impairments or function disabilities, generating limitations from the point of view of behaviour or person's skills, and resulting in handicaps from a social point of view. The ICIDH widened the strictly biologic perspective of the ICD. Nevertheless, this model did not take into account the environment; it remained linear and reductionist, and its terminology was negative. Thus, it cannot be considered as an ecological model.

In the spring of 2001, the WHO officially adopted a new classification of functioning, disability, and health (WHO, 2001a), which is a new version of the ICIDH. The development of this new classification took place over a period of thirty-some years. The work and debates surrounding its development have constituted a place where its conceptual evolution, its different paradigms, and the relationships between socio-political forces which make up the foundations of "scientific" knowledge - the science of "disability" within a modern context - could be brought to the fore (Fougeyrollas, and Beauregard, 2001). The model finally attained its independence from the family of health classifications under the name of International Classification of Functioning (ICF) (WHO, 2001a) (see Figure 3). Compared to the ICIDH, the new model proposes a systemic approach, a positive definition of components, and introduces environmental factors. The concept of occupation is represented by two entities: activities and participation. Activities refer mainly to usual daily tasks, such as feeding and walking, and occupation refers mainly to social roles, such as working, parenting, and so on. Within this model, health is not considered as the absence of disease; it applies to everybody, not only to people with disabilities or impairments (Stewart, 2002).

This model presents a new perspective in the field of health. Compared to the previous classifications of the WHO, it illustrates the evolution until the adoption of an ecological thought. While traditional health indicators are based on population mortality rates, the ICF shifts focus to "life", i.e., how people live with their health conditions and how these can be improved to achieve a productive, fulfilling life. It has implications for medical practices, laws and social policies, to improve treatments, and for the protection of the rights of individuals and groups (WHO, 2001c).

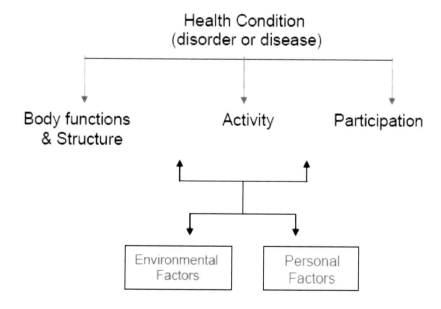

Figure 3. The International Classification of Functioning (WHO, 2001a).

Many other authors have elaborated models which include personal and environmental components in the last decades. One of those is the model of Evans and Stoddard (1996) which, however, emphasizes the curative health system and cannot be considered as ecological. Another one, the Whitehead/Dahlgren Model (Dahlgren, and Whitehead, 1991;

Popay, Williams, Thomas, and Gatrell, 1998) focuses on different levels of the environment, defining the following categories of factors affecting health: 1) individual (age, sex, heredity); 2) individual lifestyle; 3) social and community influence; 4) living and working condition, and 5) general socioeconomic, cultural and environmental conditions. These levels have many similarities with the categories defined in Bronfenbrenner's ecological model. In addition to these generic and interdisciplinary models, numerous disciplines and fields of intervention have adopted this type of theoretical referent. The next sub-section presents three of the most important ones developed by occupational therapists.

2.5. Models of Practice for Occupational Therapists

Occupational therapists have developed many ecological conceptual models which constitute the basis of professional practices and research for their discipline. The ecological approach in occupational therapy was developed partially as an answer to the "independent living movement" (Craddock, 1996). One perspective of this movement which was retained by occupational therapists states that people with chronic diseases have to learn to live with their limits and with the resources available in the environment to improve their social participation. The person is not a patient who must be cured and who must be the most autonomous possible, he/she is a partner who has to express his/her self-determination. In this context, occupational therapists become a consultant, and a facilitator. They act to eliminate obstacles from the environment, according to the choices expressed by the person and to his/her lifestyle (Craddock, 1996; Thibeault, and Hébert, 1997).

Models of practice for occupational therapists have the same three principal components: 1) an intrinsic component, the person; 2) an extrinsic component, the environment, and 3) occupation. They also demonstrate the interrelationships between each component (Polatajko, Mandich, and Martini, 1999). Three of these models will be briefly presented: the Model of Human Occupation (Kielhofner, 2002; 2004), the Canadian Occupational Performance Model (COPM) (Canadian Association of Occupational Therapist, 1997; 2002), and the Person-Environment-Occupation-Performance (PEOP) Model (Christiansen, Baum, and Bass-Haugen, 2005). The specific contribution of occupational therapists in ecological approaches is to focus on occupation and its interactions with the person and environment.

The Model of Human Occupation draws upon concepts from psychology, anthropology, philosophy, sociology, and social psychology regarding human needs and motives (Kielhofner, 2004). Concepts from early occupational therapy literature have been incorporated to understand how occupation is organized into everyday patterns. This model uses systems theory to frame how these factors are organized together in human action and experience. The model conceptualizes humans as being comprised of three elements: volition, habituation, and performance capacity. Volition refers to the process by which individuals are motivated towards and choose what they do. It includes a deep human drive for action, combined with thoughts and feelings about doing things, which are shaped by previous experiences and linked with the future. The sets of thoughts and feelings are referred to as personal causation, values, and interests. Habituation refers to a process whereby "doing" is organized into patterns and routines. These habituated patterns of action are governed by habits and roles. Performance capacity refers to both underlying objective mental and physical abilities, and subjective interpretation of experience that shapes performance. This model conceptualizes the environment as providing opportunities, resources, demands, and constraints. The physical environment consists of natural and human-made spaces, including objects within them. The social environment consists of groups of persons, and of occupations that the individuals belonging to those groups perform. How the environment affects each person depends on that person's values, interests, personal causation, roles, habits, and performance capacities. "Volition, habituation, performance capacity and environmental conditions always resonate together, creating conditions out of which our thoughts, feelings and behavior emerge." (Kielhofner, 2004, p. 151).

The COPM (Canadian Association of Occupational Therapists [CAOT], 2002; Law Cooper, Strong, Stewart, Rigby, and Letts, 1996) includes a statement of values and beliefs, in association with a conceptualization of occupational performance and factors affecting occupational performance. The values and beliefs relate to occupation, person, environment, health, and client-centred practice. Occupational performance is the result of a dynamic relationship between persons, environment, and occupation over a person's lifespan. Occupation is conceptualized as including self-care, productivity, and leisure. It is further described as: 1) a basic human need; 2) a determinant of health; 3) a source of meaning and purpose, choice and control, balance and satisfaction; 4) a means of organizing time, materials, and space, and 5) a descriptor of human behaviours that provides a unique perspective on human life. The person is seen as an integrated whole, which includes emotional, cognitive, physical, and spiritual components. Spirituality is presented as the central core of the person and is defined as "a pervasive life force, manifestation of a higher self, source of will and self-determination, and a sense of meaning, purpose and connectedness that people experience in the context of their environment" (CAOT, 1997, p. 182). Environment refers to contexts and situations which occur outside individuals and elicit responses from them. The environment includes institutional, physical, social, and cultural dimensions.

The PEOP Model (Christiansen, Baum, and Bass-Haugen, 2005) is a client-centred model organized to improve the everyday performance of necessary and valued occupations of individuals, organizations, and populations, and to improve their meaningful participation in the world around them. The model describes an interaction between personal factors (intrinsic factors, including psychological/emotional factors, cognition, neurobehavioural, and physiological factors, as well as spirituality) and environmental factors (extrinsic factors, including social support, societal policies and attitudes, natural and constructed environments, and cultural norms and values) that either support, enable, or restrict the performance on the activities, tasks, and roles of the individual, organization, or community (Baum, and Christiansen, in: Christiansen, Baum, and Bass-Haugen, 2005, Chap. 11, p. 244). One particularity of this model, compared to those previously presented, is that it adds the concept of well-being, which is associated to the personal dimension, and the concept of quality of life, which is associated to the environmental dimension. These two elements constitute additional targets for intervention.

Other ecological models were developed for specific purposes by occupational therapists. This is the case for the Ferland's "Ludic Model" (1994). This model describes the importance of playing for children as an element of social participation and as a tool of global development. Playing would be as essential to the child as work and leisure activities are for adults. It is a key means for the child to learn to interact with the environment.

2.6. Patterns in Human Development and Origins of Diseases

Research from the 1990s, referred to as "the decade of the brain", suggests a means for understanding the role of complex factors such as life experiences and stress in the origins of health problems and disease. Mead (2004; 2006) is a physician who proposes a model for explaining interactions between humans, life experiences, and the evolution of disease. This model integrates scientific results from multiple disciplines such as developmental neurobiology (Kennel, and Klaus, 1998; Klaus, and Kennell, 1976; Schore, 1994; Siegel, 1999), critical period programming, and traumatic stress (Scaer, 2005; van der Kolk, 1996a; 1996b; 1996c). The model demonstrates that the capacity of self-regulation and perception are inherent in all of us, and are individually shaped by interactions between genes and their environments. This process, referred to as "experience-dependent maturation", occurs during critical periods of brain development in the first years of life and appears to be evolutionarily designed to maximize adaptation to one's unique environment. Parent-child relationships have been found to play a crucial role in shaping our developing nervous systems, exerting a particularly strong influence in early life during pregnancy, labour, and delivery. Their vital role continues through infancy, adolescence, and beyond. These relationships affect us across multiple generations, influencing our nervous systems, physiologies, and genes. Because the nervous system regulates and interacts with all other organic systems, factors that influence its regulatory relationships and patterns may also affect risk for disease. These factors include chemical, physical, as well as emotional events, which appear fully capable of interacting with genes to shape our capacities for physiological, behavioural, and emotional self-regulation. These factors also influence how we respond to life in general, and particularly to stress (Mead, 2006).

Mead proposes a four phase model in the origins of chronic disease in which disease is initiated during periods of critical growth in organic system development during prenatal and early life, when patterns of organic system regulation are highly influenced by their external environment. This model can explain the presence of diseases such as type I diabetes, multiple sclerosis, inflammatory bowel disease, asthma, post traumatic stress, and other (Mead, 2006). According to the experiential chronic illness model, all diseases, whether mental, physical, or both, are influenced by interactions between the developing organism and its environment (Mead, 2004; 2006) (Figure 4). Environmental contributions to the origins of disease appear to follow common patterns involving: 1) predisposition to altered states of regulation following exposure to environmental events during critical periods of development in early life; 2) perpetuation of risk following exposure to stressful events, or failure to progress if stressor intensity is insufficient and presence of buffers (understood as a resource) is strong; 3) precipitation of clinically overt symptoms after sufficient exposures to stress, and 4) variation in symptom expression with exposure to idiosyncratic stressors and buffers. Risk is passed on to offspring through transgenerational transmission, for example when psychobiological regulation is altered due to disruptions in bonding, lack of proximity, or parental states of altered regulation.

The parent-child relationship has been grossly underestimated by the biomedical approach. It is now demonstrated that the adult brain initially regulates the immature infant brain and gradually facilitates the learning process of self-regulation for the child. The roles of parental availability, parental support, and social networks have consequently been underestimated as well. When parents are physically unavailable or become emotionally dysregulated following traumatic events, such as a violent attack or the loss of a loved one, their children lose their ability to effectively self-regulate as well.

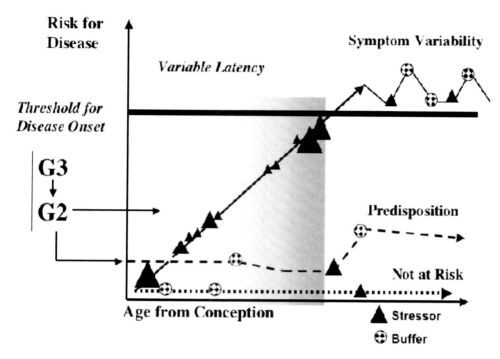

Figure 4. Patterns in origins of diseases (Mead, 2006).

According to the model, such events can train the developing nervous systems to operate in suboptimal patterns of regulation or may place the individual at risk for becoming more easily dysregulated following stressful events later in life. With sufficient exposure to stressful life experiences, patterns of dysregulation may progress to full-blown disease. Patterns of dysregulation represent attempts by a self-organizing system to adapt to an overwhelming environment and may be addressed, even in adulthood, by facilitating a return to the inherent capacity for self-regulation. The model provides perspectives for identifying preventive and curative strategies in chronic illness. It recommends changes in current health care practices, such as reducing obstetrical interventions during pregnancy and birth (such as amniocentesis and caesarean sections). These medical interventions are indeed stressful events that interfere with parent-child bonding and carry the highest risk for negatively influencing developing patterns of regulation in immature organic systems. The model also provides recommendations for the early treatment of traumatic stress in all family members as a form of prevention for later dysregulation problems.

In synthesis of this section, we observe that the effect of environment and of person-environment-occupation interaction on health and human development is more and more recognized and understood. These interactions appear to involve the smallest molecules of our cells, as well as the organs, the entire person, his/her relatives, and all the components of the environment. Numerous disciplines adopt this kind of theoretical referent. It is indeed more in accordance with the reality of the living world than reductionist models. These theories and models can thus lead to discovering or identifying promising solutions to

3. SYNTHESIS OF THE GENERAL CHARACTERISTICS OF ECOLOGICAL THEORIES, MODELS AND APPROACHES

On Borneo Island, an orang-utan called Kousasi is now famous. After becoming an orphan at the age of 2 because he was captured by men, he escaped several months later and he survived by using his exceptional abilities. Usually the orang-utans live with their mother up to the age of 6. We do not know how he survived with the multiple dangers of the forest during his childhood. All his life, he was next to human beings as well as other orang-utan orphans in an establishment dedicated to the reintegration and survival of orang-utans. He so well led his fate that, once grown-up, at about 19, he became the dominant male in his territory and he has numerous descendants. He continues to maintain relationships with the orang-utans he had met during his childhood and his adolescence. In some difficult moments during his life, he required help from human beings. His successes demonstrate his exceptional qualities of tenacity, determination, and resilience all along his life. An environment strewed with obstacles was not sufficient to overcome his strength of character, and maybe it even contributed to make him exceptional. We know more about his species because of him. His exceptional life thus contributes to the survival of his species.

Many important convergences can be observed in ecological theories, models, and approaches presented previously. This section enlightens four of their main common characteristics.

The first general characteristic of these theoretical referents is to include at least three components: the person, environment, and interactions between them (Frohlich, Corin, and Potvin, 2001; Satariano, and McAuley, 2003). In addition, ecological models applied to humans include, most of the time, another component: occupation. Occupation is expressed by behaviours, life habits, activities, social roles, and/or life events (Bandura, 1986; Fougeyrollas, 1997; Law, Cooper, Strong, Stewart, Rigby, and Letts, 1996; Letts, Rigby, Stewart, 2003; Mead, 2006; Stokols, 1992; 1996). The person is presented under many facets: the molecules inside the cells, the organs, the entire body, and also the psychological, social, and spiritual dimensions. The environment, as well as the interactions between components, includes many different sub-components and facets, which will be discussed in Section 4. These components can be targeted by interventions based on ecological approaches, using different strategies in different situations (Richard, Potvin, Kishchuk, Prlic, and Green, 1996).

The second common characteristic is to adopt a positive vision of health, in opposition with a negative vision focusing on diseases. Health is not defined as the absence of diseases in many theoretical referents (Ottawa Charter for Health Promotion, 1986; WHO, 2001a). More precisely, Bandura's theory adopts a positive perspective of human and health, besides the DCP model and Mead's model (Mead, 2006) include both positive and negative visions of health and humans. In the field of rehabilitation, health and recovery are seen as the integration in the community and the possibility of interacting with the environment (social participation) and not just as the absence or reduction of diseases, impairments, or disabilities (Harvey, 1996).

The third characteristic is that the individual is considered capable of taking care of him/herself. Interventions adopt an empowerment perspective and aim at developing people's self-determination, self-regulation, and self-defence mechanisms (Bandura, 1986; Kahana, 1982; Kar, Pascual, and Chickering, 1999; Mead, 2006; Minkler, and Wallerstein, 1997; Ottawa Charter for Health Promotion, 1986; Richard, Potvin, Kishchuk, Prlic, and Green, 1996; Sprague, and Hayes, 2000; Whitney-Thomas, and Moloney, 2001). People's objectives and perceptions guide interventions (CAOT, 2002; De Hope, and Finegan, 1999; Kielhofner, 2004). The person is considered in development, capable of involving him/herself in an adaptation process (Dumont, and Rainville, 2006), able to make the necessary actions to improve his/her functioning in the environment by him/herself, according to his/her evolution.

Finally, in ecological models and approaches, interventions are conducted mostly in natural living environment (home, school, workplace ...) where people interact with their natural environment, and not in hospitals or clinics. It is thus possible to involve the person, environment, occupation, and interactions between these components, with the aim of improving health, social participation, or quality of life. These kinds of interventions are often called community-based practice. Many types of community-based interventions have been developed in the last years. Some of these interventions will be presented in Section 5. Before that, the following section will provide an in-depth look at the concepts of environment and interaction which were less clearly defined in the theoretical referents presented previously.

4. ENVIRONMENT AND INTERACTIONS

Researchers noticed that the colder the water in which eels live, the higher their blood sugar concentration is. In cold water, they become diabetics according to medical definitions. Eugnio Rasio is a researcher who uses this characteristic of eels to study the effects of diabetes. For the eel, which can live in deep and cold waters, assimilating sugar in this way constitutes a protective factor that prevents so their blood from freezing. The eel thus possesses a gene which makes it react to an environmental factor. This factor has a direct effect on its metabolism.

The human genome includes a gene which is associated to type I diabetes. The type 1 diabetes is an autoimmune disease which appears only in presence of a genetic factor associated to an environmental factor. This environmental factor is undifferentiated and constitutes a stressor for the body, as the cold water can be for the eel. For people living in cold countries, like Inuits, this gene can constitute a protective factor more than a disease, as it is for eels. For example, in their traditional way of life, Inuits ate foods that were exempt from sugars, which at times consisted mainly of raw meat and fish. These people also perform intense and regular physical activities, for example hunting, and generally the fight for the survival. It is also necessary for them to protect their body against cold weather. The fact of not secreting enough insulin and of having a high concentration of blood sugar can protect them from chilblains. In addition, they usually do not have high concentration of blood sugar because of their food and activities. This personal characteristic (low assimilation of blood sugar) is, on the other hand, harmful and can even cause death in the context of the way of life which prevails in industrialized nations. This way of life involves food overprofusion, high levels of sugars in food, and low physical activities. Genes associated with insulin production, probably inherited from the evolution of the genome over billions of years, can thus be at the same time a protective or a harmful factor, depending on environmental conditions and individual's occupations. It is an example of interaction between a personal factor, an environmental factor, and an occupation.

Ecological models and approaches take into account the complexity of human situations more than most of the simple traditional models. In spite of the numerous advantages of these models, of the new perspective they bring, and of the large consensus around them, two of their main constituents still need to be explained and deepened: they are the concepts of environment and interaction. This section proposes a frame of reference for a better understanding of these two concepts.

Environments and interactions between person and environment could be analysed in different ways, depending on the disciplines and the defined targets. Human beings, human environments and their mutual interactions are probably more complex than the equivalent components of other living species. The human environment is indeed comprised of numerous facets, compared with that of insects or bacteria for example. We are part of several environments, we can change from an environment to another, and we can transform our environments in a radical way. Our environments have different characteristics: physical, social, cultural, economic, and other. Human beings also have specific characteristics and powerful skills (symbolization, communication, rational thought) which can be multiplied tenfold by our tools and our technical means. The interactions between person and environment are thus more complex than for other living species. In addition, the occupation component must be added as it is a major determinant of the person's development and health.

Many models presented previously provide definitions and a classification of elements included under each concept. Many conceptualisations of the environment are available in the literature, but an absence of consensus is noted. In addition, the concept of interaction is most often mentioned without being precisely defined and consequently remains unclear. A better theoretical understanding of these components could lead to improve knowledge about health problems and help to find solutions, notably by identifying the most influential components.

4.1. A Conceptualisation of the Environment

Bronfenbrenner's (1977, 1979) ecological model presents a conceptualization of the environment which consists of a set of four imbricated structures: the microsystem, mesosystem, exosystem, and macrosystem (see Section 2.1). Law (1991) proposes to add the ontosystem (the individual) to an extremity and the chronosystem (the temporal dimension) at the other extremity of Bronfenbrenner's systems. The ontosystem is the individual seen as a whole, with his/her general characteristics: gender, age, race, height, capacities, personality, interests, values, etc. The chronosysntem refers to patterning of environmental events and transitions over the life course, to effects created by time or critical periods in development, and to sociohistorical conditions.

The conceptualization of the environment from several previously mentioned models is different from Bronfenbrenner's one, and divides it into at least two components: the physical and the social environment. Other models add components like culture or institutions. Law (1991) suggested integrating these two conceptualizations, and she presented the different components of the environment in two axes: contents and dimension. The crossing of both axes gives a mosaic of components of the environment. From the point of view of contents, Law proposed the physical, social, cultural, and institutional components. From the point of view of dimension, she retained Bronfenbrenner'systems, to which she has added the ontosystem and the chronosystem (see Table 1).

This idea of crossing axis is retained in the conceptualisation of environment proposed here. All components previously mentioned are included in one or the other axis, the vertical or the horizontal one. One system is added at the vertical axis: the intrasystem, which include the person's internal parts: organs, cells, and all molecular elements inside the body (proteins, lipids, etc.). Table 1 presents this perspective of the environment, from the smallest to the largest components. Considering actual scientific knowledge, it would be possible to identify smaller or larger components in the vertical axis of the proposed model, considering for example physics of subatomic particles and physics of the universe. Nevertheless, these two extreme dimensions are not retained in this proposal, because their direct relationship with human health has not been documented yet. In the horizontal axis, the components proposed by Law (1991) are retained.

As the individual is considered a part of several environments, the notion of ecological transition can be used when a person changes environment, for different reasons. This period of transition requires important mutual adaptations between the person and his/her environment. It is notably the case of people who undergo an important traumatism or disease which changes drastically their usual occupations (Dumont, and Rainville, 2006). This situation was also studied for refugees experiencing a drastic change of their occupations (Connor Schisler, and Polatajko, 2002). Other examples can be someone who becomes an adult and leaves his/her parents to live his/her own life, a student who changes school, or an adult who becomes retired.

Sciences involved in the intrasystem and ontosystem are numerous and varied. Disciplines in biomedical sciences often scrutinize the individual in a microscopically perspective. Many disciplines in the health or social fields usually adopt a larger perspective when considering mainly the microsystem, like psychology, social services, nursing, occupational therapy, and anthropology. Sciences involved in the mesosystem, exosystem or macrosystem are for example public health, health promotion, sociology, political sciences, economic, management, history, or geography.

Table 1. Components of the environment

	Physical	Socio-cultural	Institutional and Organisational	Politico-economical
Intrasystem				
Ontosystem				
Microsystem				
Mesosystem				
Macrosystem				
Exosystem				
Chronosystem				

To improve understanding of this proposal, the reader is invited to choose a situation of interest and to identify the relevant elements in each of the sections of the Table 1. For example, it is possible to locate family, laws, government, or climate. This conceptualization of the environment can facilitate the adoption of an ecological approach, because it allows targeting more clearly relevant elements of the environment involved in a situation. Consequently, social or health professionals do not have to look only at the person with a health problem, but to consider all relevant components of the environment of which he/she is a part. To find solutions, it is thus possible to target the person as well as one or more other components, such as family, workplace, transportation, etc. This analysis of the environment can also contribute to more efficiently articulate interventions in partnership with different resources in the environment, notably by identifying their potential contribution. In addition, it is also possible to define a global intervention strategy aimed at the environment. This strategy would consist in promoting the creation of favourable environments. Section 5 provides several examples of these types of strategies.

4.2. A Conceptualisation of Interations

> Love constitutes a particular interaction situation. It can totally change one's occupations. Love can be considered as a transformer, and it can also involve mutualism, protection, communication, production and synergy at the same time. It could even involve perturbation or domination in certain circumstances. It asks for adaptation most of the time. Many personal constituents are involved in love, for example, cognition, hormones, senses, values, or identity. Fortunately, love is still mysterious, powerful, and uncontrollable ...

Interactions were not, until now, clearly and specifically defined and discussed in a theoretical referent concerning the health or social domain and they constitute a field of knowledge in development. First, it is possible to say that the interaction situation is often opposed to the linear chain of causality. The linear chain of causality is relevant when it is possible to establish a causal relationship between two elements. In the interaction situation, it is not possible to foresee the effect of an element; it depends on the way that other elements react.

Interactions are briefly conceptualized in different manners according to the authors. For many occupational therapists, they simply correspond to occupations (CAOT, 2002). In the DCP model, interactions are mentioned without being defined (Fougeyrollas, Cloutier, Bergeron, Côté, Côté, and St-Michel, 1996). Satariano and McAuley (2003) noted the importance of considering interactions when assessing a person's disabilities, and not only personal characteristics, without defining these interactions. Frolich, Corin, and Potvin (2001) consider mainly interactions as relationships between people. As a unit of analysis of interactions between people, dyads and triads were proposed, like a couple, family, or the relationship between a worker and his/her superior (Racine, 1999). For Lawton (1980), the interaction corresponds to the subjective experience of the environment, which is the internal representation of the external environment. Interactions are then mainly at a cognitive or emotional level. Keysor and Jette (2001), as for them, suggest considering the mediator effect of beliefs, emotions, and coping strategies, in addition to the physical and social environment, when investigating interactions. For Mead (2006), stressors and buffers interact with genes during critical periods and can provoke diseases. In addition, according to the previously mentioned models, interactions also vary according to the environmental component involved (social, cultural, microsystem, macrosystem, etc.).

In the domain of pharmacology, drugs interactions are well known and documented (Bachman, 2004; Tatro, 2006). Drug interaction is a response that is different from the one that is anticipated by each of the drugs, when taken separately. It is possible to observe an increased effect (synergy), a decreased effect (antagonism), and a modified effect (idiosyncrasy) of a drug in the presence of another. These are new effects, side effects or unexpected effects, and these interactions can be beneficial or not. The level of interaction is also taken into account in pharmacology. Drugs can interact together, but can also interact with individual characteristics. Indeed, many studies demonstrate different drugs effects depending on gender, or by introducing drugs at different times of day, or even during different periods of a treatment. As a result, they can have very different effects with the same or smaller doses (Gandhi, Aweeka, Greenblatt, and Blaschke, 2004; Meilbohm, Beierle, and Derendorf, 2002).

Ecology defines several interaction situations which can serve as foundation for a better understanding of this concept. Interactions defined in ecology are, for example, predation, parasitism, mutualism, commensalism, herbivorism, and allopathy. As mentioned previously, interactions in human ecosystems are more complex, because the main elements which interact (person, environment, and occupation) include numerous components, which in turn are also complex. For example, it is possible to find interactions in various environments in which a person is part of; in all his relational systems, with his family, friends, colleagues, and so on. Resources, services, community, and events can influence a person, as well as formal or informal social rules. In addition, we begin to understand how the intrasystem reacts in front of external situations, like it happens in experience dependent maturation (Mead, 2006). All components and all levels of the person or environment can interact with any other component or level. It is thus possible to imagine a constellation of interaction situations. In spite of this complexity, an attempt of conceptualization of person-environment-occupation interactions will be proposed here. As it was mentioned before, occupation must be taken in a wide sense, and it includes activities, life habits, social roles, behaviours, and life events. The list of interaction situations proposed below must be considered as a first attempt. Future reseach projects should be conducted in order to validate and improve it.

Fundamentally, in the interaction situation, it is not possible to anticipate a result only by the presence of a unique element. For example, the fact of having a given personal characteristic would not be enough to predict any result. It would also be necessary to consider environmental factors, characteristics of occupations, and the way they interact together to predict the result of this personal characteristic.

A series of interactions between personal, environmental, and occupational components can be defined, corresponding to the various possible combinations of a positive, negative or neutral effect on the person, environment or occupations, for a theoretical possibility of 27 different situations of interaction (3^3). A situation of interaction was defined here for 22 of the possible combinations. For example, when components interact and results in a positive effect on the person, environment, and occupation, we speak about "synergy". The least plausible combinations were not retained in this list, for example, negative effects on the person and environment associated with positive effects on occupation. Note that these interactions can be present for all levels of the environment (see Table 1), that is from the intrasystem to the macrosystem or even chronosystem. This deepening of interaction situations allows adding targets of interventions: besides acting on the person, occupation, and on one or several constituents of environment, it is possible to look for a favourable interaction or to use the interactions in place to reach an objective. Changes in the person, environment or occupation can modify the initial interaction. Consequently, the situation of interaction is not necessarily stable, it evolves.

1. Synergy: elements in the three components strengthen themselves mutually; positive effects are observed for the person, environment, and occupation. For example, a person's abilities are used optimally in a favourable and supporting environment, and positive effects result from this for the person, environment, as well as occupation.
2. Antagonism: an element of a component cancels another element; no effect is obtained for any of the three components. Occupations are effortless, just like the person's reactions or the reactions of the environment. For example, a person cannot use his/her capacities in an environment where they are not used advantageously; or an environment is not adapted to a person's characteristics, thus his/her efforts are useless.
3. Adaptation: an element of a component modifies itself to fit with another element, and this adaptation can be mutual. Compensation constitutes a specific variant of adaptation, and happens when a component compensates for a limit in another. Positive effects are observed at least from one component (person, environment or occupation). For example, a workstation is modified to fit a person's characteristics. The person is now able to perform various tasks at work. The environment becomes more secure for all employees because of this adaptation of the environment. The person could also develop new skills to fit the requirements of an environment with the same positive consequences. Furthermore, the working methods of all employees could change, following these adaptations.
4. Transformation: an element of a component is transformed by another, which constitutes a particular and extreme situation of adaptation. Possible effects for all components can be observed. For example, a person is transformed by certain events in his/her life; the social environment is transformed by the significant contribution of some people.
5. Resilience (resilience is the rate at which a system returns to a single steady or cyclic state following a perturbation): an element of a component is modified by the negative effect of another component, but it bounces back, and even is reinforced by this negative effect. For example someone surmounts life's tribulations and is reinforced by traumatic events, is able to overcome them. A resilient environment or ecosystem can withstand shocks and rebuild itself when necessary. Following a perturbation, the attacked element reacts for survival; sometimes it is not possible to foresee the result. For example, the effect of over-utilisation of antibiotics was not known when penicillin was discovered, but some bacteria have become resistant in reaction.
6. Protection: an element of a component protects another element. Positive effects are observed in at least one component. For example, laws protect against discrimination, or prevent people from damaging physical environments, vaccines

prevent diseases, etc. Numerous behaviours and occupations aim at protection: battles for territory, mothers protecting children, etc.

7. Repair: an element of a component is repaired (fixed, cured, relieved) by another. The repair can be necessary when the protection was not effective. For example, a supporting environment helps the healing process of a person following a depression.
8. Disturbance or perturbation: an element of a component is disturbed by another. Changes in other components can be observed, according to the degree of disturbance. These changes are harmful. For example, the arrival of a person in an environment disturbs other people and harms functioning, or a modification in an environment modifies the customs of people and harms their functioning. A disruptive element can lead to its exclusion, when possible, because no positive effects result from the presence of this element. On a larger scale, numerous human occupations disturb the environment, and people, like climate warming.
9. Destruction: an element of a component is so disrupted by another that it is destroyed. A loss is observed, and can be extended to all components in some circumstances. For example, a harmful environment provokes diseases or deaths, or the harmful behaviour of a person destroys a community. On a larger scale, certain human occupations destroy ecosystems.
10. Inclusion: an element of a component accepts the presence of another having particular characteristics, without being disturbed or disrupted. Positive effects are possible for the person, environment, and occupation. The inclusion may be considered as a kind of global adaptation of the environment.
11. Exclusion: an element of a component is avoided or rejected by another. Positive or negative effects are possible. Exclusion can be used for protecting a component from an element which could be harmful.
12. Competition: when two elements are in competition for the same third element, there will be a winner and a loser. Competition for a territory or for females is frequently observed in nature. The domination is a particular situation of competition. For example, the presence of a person in a particular environment deprives another person in the same environment, because there can be only one who benefits from it. The effects on occupation can be positive or negative.
13. Cooperation: two elements of one or another component work together to reach the same objective. Together they have more chances to reach it. For example, enablers or facilitators are set up in the environment to allow performing some occupations. The person uses these facilitators and even proposes new ones which are going to facilitate the realization of the targeted occupations.
14. Mutualism: two elements of one or another component help mutually; positive effects are observed for both. For example, a person improves some characteristics of the environment, and it helps him/her by improving his/her own capacities.
15. Parasitism: an element of a component is dependent on another for maintaining itself. Positive effects are observed on one side but negative effects on the other one. For example, a person lives in an environment where he/she constantly asks for help, that harms the environment and does not bring any benefits regarding occupation.
16. Exploitation: an element of a component uses another, but this other one does not receive something in return. The hunting or predation is an example of exploitation; human beings exploit numerous resources of their environment (other human beings,

forests, minerals, oceans, etc.). An individual can also be exploited by elements of the environment. Positive effects are present for the one who exploits and it can favour occupation.

17. Over-exploitation: an element of a component abuses another, what bothers or is harmful to this element. Over-exploitation is a variant of disturbance. A person who burns him/herself up in a community and abusive resources exploitation of the environment are examples. Even if positive effects can be observed in the short run, in a long-term perspective, all components are in a losing situation.

18. Production: an element of a component obtains positive results with the intervention of another. For example, someone improves his/her capacities by going to school; or interventions on the environment, like forest management, make it more productive. Procreation may be considered as a type of production.

19. Over-production: an element of a component wears itself out at the request of another. Losses are observed for the person, environment, and occupation at short, mid_2 or long-term. Over-production is a variant of disturbance. For example, over-production leading to resource depletion can be considered as a harmful disruptive element for the environment. Another example is when someone is exhausted because of too demanding work occupations.

20. Consumption: an element of a component is used by another one but it receives something (a payment) in exchange; positive effects are observed for both. Consumption may be considered as a kind of mutualism. Consumption improves production.

21. Over-consumption: an element of a component abuses another for elements which are not essential, causing negative effects for all components (person, environment, and occupation). The fact of consuming useless things can be considered as a disruptive element for the person and can alter his/her occupations.

22. Communication and knowledge transfer: two elements of components exchange information that can or cannot bring positive effects. This type of interaction will, most of the time, be favourable. For example, positive effects can be observed by the acquisition of new information or knowledge.

4.2.1. Concrete Examples of Interactions

To understand and deepen interaction situations, three examples from the health domain will be brought. The first interaction situation will be illustrated in regard to traumatic brain injuries. The nature and the severity of traumatic brain injury explain only a relatively small part of social participation of affected individuals, and these variables are not good predictors of social participation (Dumont, Gervais, Fougeyrollas, and Bertrand, 2004). This linear perspective (i.e. trying to explain a variable with others variables), is situated at this moment in a reductionist causality relationship which does not allow a complete understanding of the situation. On the other hand, if the situation is analyzed from the perspective of interactions between different components, it is possible to improve this understanding. For example, it is difficult to predict return to work for someone who has sustained a traumatic brain injury by considering only the characteristics of the trauma. The requirements of the employment and the possibilities of mutual adaptations must also be considered (Crépeau, and Scherzer, 1993; Crisp, 1992; Evans, 1999; Sherer, Madison, and Hannay, 2000; Wagner, 2001; Wehman, West, Kregel, Sherron, and Kreutzer, 1995; Yasuda, Wehman, Targett, Cifu, and West,

2001). In a situation of synergy or adaptation between the person, environment, and occupation, the person would be able to return to work. A transformation (for example of the workplace) could also make it possible. In the case of parasitism, over-exploitation or exclusion, it will not be possible.

The situation of a woman faced with the decision to have children or not is another example illustrating interactions between various factors. A woman may desire to have children (personal factor concerning the volition), but this desire can be modulated by resources in the environment (environmental factors). If environmental resources are limited, the woman is not likely to have the required help and may decide not to have children. The child may be perceived at this moment as a disturbance for the person, environment, and occupation. In the case of a supportive environment, a child can bring adaptations which will be favourable for all components. The fact of desiring children only might not be enough to take action, and it is the same for the presence of facilitators in the environment: both will affect results. In the situation of protection or resilience, she may decide to have children; in the case of disturbance or domination, she may decide the contrary.

Post-traumatic stress disorder is another health problem which illustrates the person-environment-occupation interaction. Anxiety or stress is a fundamental mechanism of survival which allows one to avoid potentially harmful situations and to react quickly. This mechanism is located in autonomic regulation zones of the brain (Levine, 1997; 2005; Scaer, 2001; 2005). The physiological reactions which it engenders (high blood pressure, increased cardiac frequency, sweating, pupils' dilation) aim at mobilizing the organism to fight or flee from a difficult situation. These reactions are not under the control of the will or cerebral cortex. When the environment is overwhelming, like in a traumatic situation, regulatory processes can become extreme, as it is seen in the physiological and emotional responses of fight (anger), flight (dissociation, anxiety, the need to keep doing or moving), and freeze (the immobility response). In front of the same stressful event, an individual might have a normal stress reaction and another one might develop post-traumatic stress disorder. Personal and/or environmental factors will determine if the person will develop a post-traumatic stress disorder when facing a stressing situation (Mead, 2006). It can arise when a person does not have enough resources in face of a situation which is perceived as dangerous, without a means to escape or life-threatening (Levine, 1997; 2005; Scaer, 2001; 2005). Someone who has fewer personal or environmental resources will be more vulnerable to post-traumatic stress disorder following a traumatic event. These resources can be regarding personal capacities, environmental protection or support available, time available, occupational requirements, perception of control which one has over events and others. In the interaction situation of cooperation, mutualism, protection, repair, resilience or inclusion, the person will not develop post-traumatic stress disorder. In the case of over-production or destruction, the person may develop it.

Interactions are complex phenomena from which their effects are usually not possible to predict while considering each element separately. Some interactions are favourable to the person, environment or occupation, like synergy, mutualism, adaptation, inclusion, or cooperation. Some interactions are favourable for at least one component, such as protection, resilience, repair, exploitation, production, or consumption. Some interactions are favourable for a component but unfavourable for another, like parasitism or domination. Some interactions can be harmful for a component, but not necessarily for another, like exclusion. Some interactions can have a positive effect or no effect, according to the situation, for instance communication. Finally, some interactions are always harmful, such as disturbance, destruction, over-exploitation, over-production, and over-consumption. It is obviously necessary to look for favourable interactions in any intervention. After this theoretical analysis, scientific evidence supporting ecological approaches in order to improve population health will be provided.

5. SCIENTIFIC EVIDENCE SUPPORTING ECOLOGICAL MODELS AND APPROACHES

Incas did not seem to use sophisticated writing, but knew how to read sunlight and natural phenomena. For example, they knew that the presence of a particular type of shell on the beaches of the West coast of South America meant the return of El Niño, something that so many contemporary scientists try to predict. The modern science in industrialized countries produces a new form of illiterates: those who do not know how to read the numerous messages of natural phenomena and of lay knowledge. That constitutes a loss of an inestimable source of information.

To adopt a theoretical referent, it must have demonstrated its descriptive, explanatory or predictive value in various situations. Moreover, professionals in all disciplines are asked to adopt practices based on scientific proofs and best evidences (Barnard, and Wiles, 2001; Pain, Magill-Evans, Darrah, Hagler, and Warren, 2004; Welch, 2002). The relevance of theoretical referents presented previously is demonstrated at least partially because they are abundantly used and recognized in health and social domains. This section presents scientific proofs and evidences supporting ecological models and approaches in the context of population health. The listed studies are grouped together in four categories: those who target the individual in an ecological perspective, those who target the environment, those who target occupation, and finally those who target interactions between individual, environment, and occupation.

5.1. Person Targeted Interventions

When we speak about interventions aiming at the individual, health professionals mostly make reference to traditional curative approaches which are abundantly described. However, ecological models and approaches adopt another perspective, which is a positive one. They target empowerment of individuals and the development of different personal skills in order to reach long-term results. Furthermore, many interventions ask for a personal implication, notably to adjust the environment and adapt to it; this emphasizes the importance of the person's strengths, such as will, self-determination, self-control, self-regulation, and self-efficacy (Bandura, 1986; CAOT, 2002; Dumont, Gervais, Fougeyrollas, and Bertrand, 2004; Dumont, and Rainville, 2006; Kar, Pascual, and Chickering, 1999; Kielhofner, 2004; Mead, 2006). Numerous interventions can target these constituents of the individual, rather than focusing on disabilities or impairments reduction, especially in the case of chronic diseases with limited possibilities of an effective cure. The next paragraphs present different situations of interventions of this type.

5.1.1. The Social Cognitive Theory and Self-Efficacy Beliefs

The social cognitive theory was successfully applied and has demonstrated its efficiency in numerous contexts. It is considered as a positive psychology or as the psychology of optimism, competence and of the 21st Century (Bandura, 2003). Its central organizing concept is self-efficacy. According to this theory, the system of beliefs, which forms the feeling of self-efficacy, is the foundation of motivation and action. The hypothesis under this theory is that if people do not believe they can succeed in something, they indeed have few reasons for acting or persevering in face of difficulties. More than 1800 studies and articles which support this general hypothesis were listed (Bandura, 2003), covering a large variety of fields of practice and social domains: psychology, education, orientation, health services, mental health, rehabilitation, ageing, sports, management, social intervention and others. Bandura's (2003) recent volume supplies details about this theory, as well as research which ensued from it. As mentioned previously, this theory has a significant contribution for positive approaches to health and is congruent with the ecological perspective (Satariano, and McAuley, 2003).

Numerous studies have undoubtedly demonstrated the importance of self-efficacy beliefs for health. In an intrasystemic perspective, several research results suggest that psychosocial factors modulate the immune system, which can in turn influence diseases susceptibility (Hebert, and Cohen, 1993; Kiecolt-Glaser, and Glaser, 1988; O' Leary, 1990). This immune regulation influences neuroanatomical, neurochemical, and neuroendocrine links between the central nervous system and the immune system. Perceived self-efficacy can affect the organic system through stress, depressive affects, or self-regulating mechanisms situated in the central nervous system. It has been observed that exposure to stress weakens the immune system (decreased number of lymphocytes, and activity reduction by T lymphocytes and killer cells). Furthermore, in the presence of stress, the autonomous nervous system is activated; catecholamines and endorphines can be secreted (Kelly, Hertzman, and Daniel, 1997). On the other hand, stress has no unfavourable physical effects on the individual, if he/she has a perceived capacity of control over the stressor (Bandura, 1991). The absence of perceived control increases the risk of diseases (Peterson, and Strunkard, 1989; Schneiderman, McCabe, and Baum, 1992). It has also been observed that antibody blood levels are higher during pleasant days compared to stressful days (Stone, Neale, Cox, Napoli, Valdimarsdottir, and Kennedy-Moore, 1994), and that stressed people are more vulnerable to infections like colds (Cohen, Tyrrel, and Smith, 1991). Several studies also demonstrated that competence in stress management can improve the functioning of the immune system (Antoni, Schneiderman, Fletcher, Goldstein, Ieronson, and Laperriere, 1990; Gruber, Hall, Hersh, and Dubois, 1988; Kiecolt-Glaser, et al. 1985; 1986).

Considering pain control, Ross and Ross (1984) demonstrated the efficiency of cognitive opioid mechanisms, such as occupying the mind, counting, or mentally reciting a remembered text. Perceived self-efficacy also has an effect on pain (William, and Kinney, 1991). The development of the person's perceived self-efficacy to control pain can thus contribute in a significant way to decrease it. Furthermore, a placebo can have the effect of increasing self-efficacy beliefs and can act like cognitive strategies of self-regulation for pain control (Bandura, O' Leary, Taylor, Gauthier, and Gossard, 1987). It is thus possible to use one or the other of these two strategies for pain control.

Psychotherapy based on social cognitive theory demonstrated its efficiency in the treatment of anxiety, phobia, depression, eating disorders, alcoholism, and drug addiction. In the case of depression, medicines being less expensive, the therapy often turns in this direction. The long-term beneficial effects of a psychological treatment are lost, on the other hand. The social cognitive theory notably supports the recognized fact that if we undertake an enhancive and distractive activity, we can decrease depression, but if we brood, we increase it. In the treatment of drug addiction, the theory particularly exploits the importance of an ecological perspective. It was indeed demonstrated that it is necessary to act on three elements, which are person, environment and behaviour consumption, in order to obtain a sustained effect (Bandura, 2003).

In the case of chronic diseases, interventions based on the social cognitive theory also demonstrated positive effects (Bandura, 2003). In heart diseases for example, walking on a treadmill allows to resume gradually one's confidence in one's cardiac capacities. This test gives a lot of information about the level of effort which is possible to reach, and also demonstrates the person's capacity to relatives. So, a spouse can be reassured about her husband's capacities in making efforts by observing him while he is performing on the treadmill. Besides, similar to the case of depression, the theory recognizes that the fact of participating in significant activities is favourable for people with chronic diseases.

Many other examples of applications of this theory in the field of health were published. For arthritics, this theory was successfully used in pain control. For people having sustained a traumatic brain injury, some models of intervention are based on it (De Hope, and Finegan, 1996). Seigley (1998) deepened personal and environmental factors which can influence behaviour associated to the health of ageing people using Bandura's social cognitive theory. This theory is also widely used in health promotion to favour the adoption of healthy behaviours. Furthermore, the theory invites in interventions that do not only aim at the person and his/her behaviours, but also on the environment.

5.1.2. Client-Centred Approach

The client-centred approach is an orientation of practice situated in an ecological perspective. This type of approach is more and more recognized in several disciplines. It is notably supported by the CAOT and is associated to the MCRO presented previously (CAOT, 1997; 2002; Sumsion, 1999; Thownsen, 2003). The CAOT made a gathering of postulates for client-centred occupational therapy practice. These postulates are: 1) occupation gives sense to life and is an important health determinant; 2) each person is unique, has an intrinsic value, has the capacity to choose for him/herself, is a social and a spiritual being; 3) the environment transforms the occupation and is transformed by it; 4) health is influenced by the capacity of the person to make choices regarding occupations, and 5) client-centred occupational therapy practice asks for the recognition of an active partnership in intervention (CAOT, 1997; 2002).

Occupational therapists from England also elaborated a definition of client-centred occupational therapy (Sumsion, 1999). It gets closer to characteristics from ecological approaches, notably by considering the notion of empowerment, and it reads as follows:

> "Client-centred occupational therapy is a partnership between the therapist and the client. The client's occupational goals are given priority and are at the centre of assessment and treatment. The therapist listens to and respects the client standards and adapts the intervention to meet the client's needs. The client participates actively in negotiating goals for intervention and is empowered to make decisions through training and education. The therapist and the

client work together to address the issues presented by a variety of environments to enable the client to fulfil his or her role expectations."

The client-centred approach is not specific to occupational therapists. Moreover, Thibault and Hébert (1997) demonstrated the resemblances between the client-centred approach adopted by occupational therapists and the principles generally admitted in health promotion, like empowerment, social justice, autonomy in the environment, importance of adopting active and significant lifestyles, and respect of cultural diversity. The client-centred approach is also recommended in physiotherapy (Potter, Gordon, and Hamer, 2003; Struber, 2003). It supports family centred practice in the case of children and young people having health problems (Jirikowic, Stika-Monson, Knight, Hutchinson, Washington, and Kartin, 2001).

5.1.3. Self-regulation and Empowerment Approaches

According to Bandura (2001), some of the most important peculiarities of the human being are self-control, self-reflection and self-regulation capacities. The frontal lobe of the brain is associated to these typically human capacities (Johanson, Risberg, Tucker, and Gustafson, 2006; Kennedy, and Coelho, 2005; Stuss, and Levine, 2002). This zone of the brain can regulate cognition, behaviour, and feelings (Gutierrez, 2001; Posner, 2005; Rueda, Posner, and Rothbart, 2005). The development of these skills is generally made between 2.5 and 7 years of age (Koschanska, Coy, and Muray, 2001; Posner, 2005). As for the whole human brain, genetic and environmental factors condition the maturation of this zone of the brain. Both relatives and society would thus play an important role in the development of self-control and self-regulation (Baumeister, DeWall, Ciarocco, and Twenge, 2005; McCartney, and Berry, 2005; Posne, and Rothbart, 2000; Ylvisaker, and Feeney, 2002).

The theoretical foundations of interventions based on self-regulation are now established and their applications in several fields of intervention are observed, like in nursing, rehabilitation, psychology, and medicine (Barkley, 2001; Johnson, 1999; Johnson, Fieler, Wlasowicz, Mitchell, and Jones, 1997; Mead, 2006; Molden, and Dweck, 2006; Reuille, 2002; Siegert, McPherson, and Taylor, 2004). The self-regulation theory is used in numerous studies involving specific pathologies (Fortune, Smith, and Garvey, 2005; Green, Payne, and Barnitt, 2004; Harman, and Clare, 2006), and human development (Buckner, Mezzacappa, and Beardslee, 2003; Ryan, and Deci, 2000).

Self-regulation is also associated with empowerment, and approaches based on those elements were described as essential in several diseases, like type I diabetes (Gonder-Frederick, Cox, and Ritterband, 2002; Jacqueminet, Masseboeuf, Rolland, Grimaldi, and Sachon, 2005), traumatic brain injury (Kennedy, and Coelho, 2005; Ownsworth, and Fleming, 2005), asthma (Zimmerman, Bonner, Evans, and Mellins, 1999), stuttering (Finn, 2003), depression (Beauregard, Paquette, and Levesque, 2006), eating disorders (Kitsantas, Gilligan, and Kamata, 2003), addiction to smoking (Bayot, Capafons, and Cardena, 1997) and more globally in several chronic diseases (Frentzel-Beyme, and Grossarth-Maticek, 2001). Interventions improving self-determination may focus for example on the skills of decision-making and problem solving. According to Sprague and Hague (2000), the most empowering interventions are the ones that enable the creation of mutual support groups and advocacy. According to these authors, people's empowerment requires an equalitarian therapeutic relation, respect, and mutual confidence. Empowerment can also mean intervening on the environment by setting up facilitators or providing resources (Kar, Pascual, and Chickering,

1999; Spragues, and Hague, 2000). Furthermore, some authors applied empowerment not only to individuals but also to organizations, groups, and communities (elements of social environment), emphasizing the ecological perspective of empowerment (Sherraden, and Ninacs, 1998; Trickett, 1994).

One of the possible effects of a lack of self-regulation is the dissociation between mind and body. Body-oriented (somatic) psychotherapies look at the role of dissociation which occurs between mind and body or between parts of the self (Caldwell, 1996; Ogden, Minton, and Pain, 2006; Ogden, Pain, and Fisher, 2006; Scaer, 2001). The body contains memory fragments for movements, images and sensations associated with traumatic events (van der Kolk, 1996). It provides an access route for reconnecting parts that have become dissociated, and which are therefore inaccessible to conscious recall (Scaer, 2001; 2005). Some authors suggest that dissociation, which can result from life experiences such as trauma, is a form of dysregulation that influences the expression of symptoms (Caldwell, 1996; Scaer, 2001; 2005) and the development of chronic disease (Mead 2004; 2006; Scaer, 2001; 2005). Our increasing scientific understanding regarding interactions between mind and body supports the use of approaches that address symptoms by repairing and reconnecting links between mind and body (Scaer, 2001; 2005; Schore, 1994).

Finally, David Servan-Schreiber was a psychiatrist who advocates therapy in an ecological way, without using drugs or medicines. His book demonstrates the efficiency of his therapeutic methods (Servan-Schreiber, 2005).

5.2. Environment Targeted Interventions

> Studies trying to identify what affects cows' stress at the time of going to the slaughter house are performed with the aim of obtaining the softest meat possible. An autistic person collaborates in these research studies because his particular cognitive capacities make him able to understand the feelings of cows. He demonstrated that cows were frightened by everything metallic as well as long and rectilinear corridors. Slaughter houses have thus eliminated metallic objects and built curved corridors, so the cows are put under less stress. We can wonder if we treat human beings in a right way, some hospitals seem to have been designed especially to increase stress ...

The ecological approach suggests acting not only on the individual, but also on components of the environment. Numerous interventions involving the physical or social environment can affect health: improvement of life conditions, availability of drinking water, absence of war, healthy food, decrease in toxic products, among others. Notably, it is demonstrated clearly that food and toxic products cause various health problems, like cancers (Grant, 2002; 2004; Gulis, Czompolyova, and Cerhan, 2002; Jerrett, Burnett, Willis, Krewski, Goldberg, DeLuca, and Finkelstein, 2003; Martins, Latorre, Saldiva, and Braga, 2002; Saez, Figuerias, Ballester, Perez-Hoyos, Ocana, and Tobias, 2001; Schreinemachers, 2003; Steiner, 2002; Willis, Krewski, Jerrett, Goldberg, and Burnett, 2003). To create favourable environments, the most important characteristic would obviously be not to be harmful (absence of toxic products, of violence, etc.) (Stokols, 1992), but in a positive perspective, this environment should also possess qualities which will now be explained.

5.2.1. Qualities of the Environment in Ecological Approaches

When we speak about qualities of the environment in ecological approaches, we mean that environment should be more inclusive (this refers to the notion of social inclusion), should be more resilient, adaptable, as well as more cohesive. In the same way, Whiteneck, Fougeyrollas and Gerhart (1997) identified four elements of the social environment which exerts a significant influence on the social participation of people with impairments. These are accommodation, availability of resources, social support, and equity. These characteristics are close to the concepts presented here, and these notions will now be clarified.

Inclusion is the opposite of exclusion and segregation. An inclusive society allows each individual to evolve and progress, no matter what his/her personal characteristics are. It means that each individual, no matter what his/her peculiarities are, has a place in various environments. Even if he/she presents differences, he/she is considered the same as the others at school, at work or while participating in leisure activities (Rousseau, and Bélanger, 2004). An inclusive society allows each individual to make a contribution to social life, according to his/her capacities. So, people having impairments should not be considered only as users of services, but as full-fledged citizens. More specifically for children, the concept of school inclusion replaces, henceforth, that of school integration. It means that all children must attend schools in their neighbourhood, village or city. Rousseau and Bélanger (2004) notably discusses issues, obstacles and enablers or facilitators of school inclusion, from the point of view of teachers, other professionals, directors, families, and the general community. Creating inclusive schools obviously implies interventions on the environment, and not only on children.

Another favourable characteristic of the environment is to be resilient or adaptable. A resilient environment adapts itself to a "different" individual without being disrupted by the adaptations required by the presence of this individual. Certain environments are more resilient than others, like schools and work organisations allowing flexible schedules, with various tasks, which are possible to perform in various ways and are distributed in an efficient manner. Other environments are less resilient like in very structured working organisations, or where people work on an assembly line or under pressure.

However, creating inclusive and resilient environments constitute a challenge (Rousseau, and Bélanger, 2004). Among the characteristics of resilient and inclusive environments, the structures in place would notably have to be conceived according to principles of barrier-free design (Letts, Rigby, and Stewart, 2003). A resilient and inclusive environment must be conceived in a way that allows every person to carry out occupations and social roles, no matter what his/her personal characteristics are. It should allow access to public utilities for all, to public transportation for all, including adapted transportation, as well as offering possibilities of different adaptations at the workplace or at school, like part-time or adapted workstations.

Finally, an environment demonstrating cohesion, conceptualized by certain authors as the "social capital" is another characteristic of the environment which can be favourable to population health. Social cohesion is defined as the social support, wealth distribution, presence of social programs, and access to different education, health, work and other services (Bartley, Blane, and Smith, 1998; Elstad, 1998; Evans, Barer, and Marmor, 1996; Syme, 1998). Bélanger, Sullivan, and Sévigny (2000) define social capital by referring to structures and characteristics of social organizations, like the density of networks or civil associations, standards of reciprocity and interpersonal confidence between citizens which facilitate coordination and cooperation for mutual profits, resilience of people and groups, self-esteem and feeling to exert control over the environment. These concepts (social cohesion and social capital) were used in several studies about inequalities, demonstrating their association with population health (Kawachi, 1997; Kawachi, Kennedy, and Glass, 1999; Kawachi, Kennedy, and Wilkinson, 1999; Lynch, Smith, Kaplan, and House, 2000; Syme, 1998). Public health also emphasizes that the important decrease of child mortality rates and the improvement of life expectancy in the 20th Century are not mainly attibutable to medical progresses, vaccines or antibiotics, but in fact to the improvement of life conditions (food, hygiene, better social and work organization, etc.). Hundred of studies in many domains have demonstrated without a doubt the association between low economic status, risk factors and health. The quality of the environment has always been a major health determinant.

Social support is mentioned to be a type of cohesion which is favourable to health by numerous authors, for all levels of the social environment (Delgado, 1996; Levy, and Wall, 2000; Nash, and Bowen, 1999; Whiteneck, Fougeyrollas, and Gerhart, 1997). It is about individual and family support (Calvert, 1997; Kelton, 2001; Wolkow, and Ferguson, 2001), community support or networks support (Aitken, and Morgan, 1999; Calvert, 1997; Delgado, 1996; Nash, and Bowen, 1999; Wolkow, and Ferguson, 2001) and finally, work environment support which can be cohesion between employees or supervisors' support (Aitken, and Morgan, 1999). The beneficial effects of health professional's support as well as the one of peers with similar health problems are also reported (Kelton, 2001).

In order to carry out interventions aiming at building environments that are as close as possible to the previously mentioned characteristics, several fields of knowledge must be mastered. Many interventions imply partners of various disciplines, besides those of health or social domains, for example industrial hygiene, ergonomics, architecture, management, urban economic planning, civil security, toxicology, community organization, or education. Thus, the ecological approach implies, most of the time, interdisciplinary and intersector-based interventions (Stokols, 1992).

Some health disciplines adopt intervention models focusing on the environment, for example social workers or occupational therapists. In addition, Effken (2001) defines, by means of an ecological model, one of the aspects of the nurses' professional practice which is sometimes considered as intuitive. What is called intuition could correspond to the perception and analysis of personal factors reported by the patient as well as environmental factors. This source of information would be one of the constituent of the science of nursing. Salazar and Primomo (1994), as for them, developed a generic model based on that of Bronfenbrenner for nursing. They considered a hierarchy from the microsystem to the macrosystem, and therefore defined interventions for each level.

5.2.2. Interventions Targeting Specific Components of the Environment

Interventions targeting the environment can be varied, given the complexity and the numerous facets of this concept. Several types of interventions target, however, mainly one or the other of the components of the environment.

Families and proxies are the main elements of the microsystem (Bronfenbrenner 1977; 1979). Members of the family are, most of the time, essential partners in ecological approaches for health professionals. The importance of the environment is noticed by the influence of family and relatives on the development of a child's language (Bornstein,

Haynes, and Painter, 1998; Sylvestre, Cronk, St-Cyr Tribble, and Payette, 2002). Moreover, Sylvestre and colleagues (2002) used Bronfrenbrenner's model as a foundation for their interventions in speech therapy. According to these authors, interventions involving the family and school environment would be more relevant and more effective than direct interventions with the child.

Other applications of Bronfenbrenner's model involving the microsystem are found in various domains, such as adolescent pregnancy (Corcoran, Franklin, and Bennet, 2000) and for young people who are rejected by their peers in schools (Margolin, 2001). Reifsnider (1995) presents a specific application of Bronfrenbrenner's ecological model in the case of children suffering from malnutrition. Cowen (2001) uses an ecological model for interventions with abused children and their family. Social services interventions in the field of health can also be based on an ecological model which includes interdisciplinarity (Germaine, 1994), notably for the intervention with children who have behaviour regulation problems (Bagley, and Mallick, 2000).

Other interventions are situated in the mesosystem, like the creation of a support network for the person (Rauch, and Ferry, 2001; Rowlands, 2002), the integration in a peer support group (Hibbards, et al., 2002) or the creation of supporting environments such as the "Clubhouse" (Jacobs, 1997).

Furthermore, the physical environment can even be designed to improve health. Several studies demonstrated the effects of urban planning on health, simply with the possibility of being able to walk or use a bicycle, what can notably reduce obesity and numerous health problems which ensue from it (Berrigan, and Troiano, 2002; Ewing, Schmid, Killingsworth, Zlot, and Raudenbush, 2003; Satariano, and McAuley, 2003; Zlot, and Schmid, 2005). Indeed, people are more incited to exercise if the environment is facilitating, which is favourable to health. In addition, an environment is probably less stressfull when designed for people rather than for cars.

Considering hospitals, physical management is also favourable to individuals' health. So, children's hospitals are out fitted to facilitate the cohabitation of parents with their sick child; this can reassure the child and facilitate his/her therapy. The maternity facilities are built out of hospitals, in pleasant environments that look like a house, with labour rooms, and the possibility for the cohabitation of children with both parents. Moreover, these elements are recommended by the United Nation Children's Fund (UNICEF), and are recognized to improve children's health (UNICEF, 2006). As for ageing people, the management of the environment can help keep them at home and be more effective than interventions aiming at the individual to attain this objective. The concept of prosthetic environment is used to identify housing which is especially designed to facilitate orientation and autonomy, in order to compensate for cognitive impairments of residents and improve their quality of life. For example, familiar objects are set up, cupboards that allow the residents to manipulate various objects are placed in visible and accessible places, and there are numerous indications which are easy to understand and help one to move around (Day, Carreon, and Stump, 2000; Rule, Milke, and Dobbs, 1992). Furthermore, a group of hospitals are designed according to the Planetree Model, which recognizes the importance of architectural and design factors which are home-like and pleasant to improve patient outcomes. These hospitals seem more like a day spa. There is a piano in the lobby, carpets in the hallway and mood lighting around every corner. There is no restriction to visiting hours: relatives can come and go and visit patients as they please. The Planetree Model of care is also associated to patient-focused care, family-centred care and cooperative care (Byers, 1997; Planetree, 2006).

Other interventions target the macrosystem. It can turn out to be convenient to act on a political plan to favour peace, to facilitate the adoption of laws favouring healthy environments, for example by reducing discrimination and violence, or developing full employment strategies, including a better recognition of part-time jobs and promotion of flexibility at work to accommodate the greatest number of persons possible. Other types of interventions can consist of creating associations, or lobbying for a cause, among others. The fields of knowledge of public health and health promotion can be relevant in these types of interventions that are more political, and they will be described in more depth in the next sub-section.

5.2.3. Ecological Approach in Public Health and Health Promotion

Public health considered environmental factors in a biomedical perspective at its beginning. So, the concern about physical environment associated to chemical agents (toxins, quality of the air) and biologic elements (infectious agents) began after the Second World War. The increase of chronic diseases after the sixties brought some consideration about social environment (behaviour, life conditions, wealth ...). In the 1980s, AIDS firmed up the perception of the importance of the social, economic, political, and organizational environments on health. Since then, the new public health adopts an ecological perspective, and considers all personal and environmental determinants (physical, social, political, economic or organizational), as being able to influence health (Ashton, and Seymour, 1988; Chu, and Simpson, 1994; Evans, Morris, and Marmor, 1996; Macintyre, and Ellaway, 2000; Stokols, 1992). Public health interventions based on ecological approaches therefore target personal and environmental factors (McLeroy, Bibeau, Steckler, and Glanz, 1988).

Health promotion is an important sector of public health. Several authors demonstrated the ecological roots of health promotion (Best, Stokols, Green, Leischow, Holmes, and Buchholz, 2003; Green, and Kreuter, 1999; Green, Richard, and Potvin, 1996; McLeroy, Bibeau, Steckler, and Glanz, 1988; Newes-Adeyi, Helitzer, Caulfield, and Bronner, 2000; Stokols, 1992; 1996; Stokols, Allen, and Bellingham, 1996; Stokols, Grzywacz, McMahan, and Phillips, 2003; Struber, 2003). One of the foundations of health promotion is to favour the adoption of healthy behaviours (food, exercises, etc.). By basing itself on different theories, like Bandura's social cognitive theory, it is now admitted that the adoption of behaviours is conditioned not only by the individual, but also mainly by the environment. Indeed, sectors of intervention in health promotion which emphasized the individual are blaming the victims and neglecting social aspects which can influence behaviour and health. For example, Ruffing-Rahal (1994) uses an ecological well-being model in a health promotion program for old women by putting the emphases on environmental factors. However, health promotion interventions targeting the environment are complex and are still in development. They are also inevitably interdisciplinary and intersector-based according to some authors (Stokols, Allen, and Bellingham, 1996). According to others, they necessarily involve several components of the environment (Richard, Potvin, Kishchuk, Prlic, and Green, 1996). Health promotion strategies aim at managing environments which are, notably, going to facilitate the adoption of healthy behaviours by acting on social organisation and infrastructures (bicycle paths, barrier-free design, security, public transportation, creation of associations, education, smoking banned in public places, etc.) (Best, Stokols, Green,

Leischow, Holmes, and Buchholz, 2003; Stokols, 1992; Stokols, Grzywacz, McMahan, and Phillips, 2003). A concrete example of intervention in the socio-political domain is the Healthy Cities Movement which originates from the health promotion sector. This movement adopts an ecological perspective by focusing on community participation and intersector-based cooperation (Green, Richard, and Potvin, 1996).

5.3. Occupation Targeted Interventions

The positive effects of occupation, its therapeutic or preventive value, as well as its impact on health and well-being have been studied mainly by occupational therapists. In the next paragraphs, studies reporting the impact of various occupations are presented. Work, volunteering, going to school, leisure activities, sports, physical activities, arts and crafts, ritualized activities, as well as the use of objects will be discussed.

5.3.1. Work

Work constitutes one of the main occupations, and it is valued (Strong, 1997). In a study by Thorén-Jönsson and Möeller (1999), participants expressed their values and purposes in life through their choices of occupation. One of the most important purposes for them was to have a paid employment.

The results of a study by Strong (1997) highlight the numerous positive effects of success in integrating into the workforce people with mental health problems. Work allows these people to be identified as "normal", to move away from labels in mental health, to become a capable person, and to find a place in the world. Success at work gradually transformed participants' self-image. Participants redefined their person because of their perseverant efforts at work, by demonstrating to themselves that they were capable and that they were a person, not just an illness, and by transcending social labels. Work is described as a bolster in their daily battle against illness, and reinforcement to counteract negative societal attitudes. Work inspires hope in future possibilities. It becomes a modality for practicing and developing new interests, skills and customs that are necessary for the development of new roles, such as those of friend and worker. At the workplace, people contribute to a common objective, thus giving rise to feelings of membership and acceptance (Strong, 1997).

In her studies, Charmaz (1994; 1995; 2002) explored the importance of work for people with a disease or disability. She proposed that they can maintain their self-esteem and their identity through employment. Nevertheless, to ensure success for these persons, the employment had to allow for a certain amount of flexibility. Bambrick and Bonder (2005) had similar comments in their study about elderly adults' perception of work and volunteering.

According to Westwood (2003), going to school can increase self-esteem, socialization, self-confidence, and motivation for adults with mental health problems. This occupation is generally recognized for its beneficial effects on health because it promotes the development of various skills and the development of identity. It also supports the person's evolution, and promotes personal fulfillment.

Craft work contributes in establishing and maintaining personal and social identity (Dickie, 2003). A study by Reynolds (2003) demonstrated that arts and crafts contribute to constructing one's self, notably for people with chronic illness. These occupations appear to play a significant role in supporting coping and achieving a satisfactory identity for them. It provides a socially recognized identity - an "able" identity. An artistic identity seems to become a major positive source of self-image. Artwork has facilitated development of and renewed interests, satisfaction, and hope about the future.

5.3.2. Sports and Leisure Activities

Physical activity is clearly associated to health, and its benefits are abundantly described for cardio-vascular, muscular, digestive and other systems, as well as for autonomy and cognitive function (Heyn, Abreu, and Ottenbacher, 2004). In addition, sports and leisure activities present occasions to develop self-esteem, self-confidence and self-efficacy, by showing one's skills to oneself and to others, which is particularly the case for athletes taking part in competitions (Specht, King, Brown, and Foris, 2002).

Along the same lines, Wickham, Hanson, Shechtman, and Ashton (2000) demonstrated that sports and leisure activities can constitute a source of motivation for people with a spinal cord injury. According to Passmore (2003), leisure enables commitment to a pleasant activity and fulfillment. Participation in these activities is a determinant of social inclusion and health. It develops one's potential. Leisure can also help develop feelings of self-efficacy, competence and self-worth, as well as decrease mental health problems.

Ratcliff, Farnworth, and Lentin (2002) studied the situation of women survivors of childhood physical abuse. These women suffered a traumatic body-mind experience that can have long term effects. A common response to physical and emotional trauma is dissociation from the experiencing of one's body. Dissociation is a coping mechanism that affects one's sense of self. It is not valuable to keep this coping mechanism into adult life because it may result in a fundamental alteration of a persons' experience of him/herself within his/her environment. Engaging in physical activities such as martial arts and circus performances appears to have supported participants in achieving a body-mind connection. For these participants, physical activity was an integral experience to their development, an experience of embodiment that was safe, empowering and life affirming (Ratcliff, Farnworth, and Lentin, 2002). Another example is a study by Graham (2002), which demonstrated how dance can transform life and provide meaning. The benefit of this activity for elderly people has also been demonstrated (Connor, 2000; Lloyd, and Chandler, 1999).

5.3.3. Objects

Objects constitute mirrors of self and identity: cellular phones, clothes, cars, etc. They have meanings and thus the power of the symbolic use of objects. They may be symbols of awards, gratifications, and statements. Objects can transform us. They widen one's perception of self and develop one's sense of ownership. Objects in the home provide meaning and opportunities for action, and encourage insight (Alsaker, and Josephsson, 2003; Hocking, 2000). In some cases, objects can be more important than occupation. According to Stone (2003), sources of identity and sense of self is derived less from work than from resulting consumption and leisure. For Dickie (2003), objects must be recognized by family, close relationships or society in order to contribute to one's identity.

5.3.4. Ritualized Occupations

Ritualized occupations offer possibilities for identification, related to values and meaning that rite confers to these occupations. Howie (2003) studied the rites relative to a book club.

These activities have particular conventions, rules, routines, and communal practices that are respected by group members. This type of occupation can be reassuring in difficult times (Howie, 2003). "The efficacy of rituals in drawing attention to ordinary existence lies in their ability to enact and promote reflection on life and its inevitable complexities and contradictions" (Howie, 2003, p. 137).

Rites of passage are another type of ritualized activity and are used by Gutman (1997) in her interventions with young male adults with traumatic brain injury. These interventions are carried out with the aim of restoring their identity and improving roles accomplishment. They are based on social learning theories, role acquisition theories, and role gender theories. They use activities associated to role accomplishment and rites of passage (sport, parenting, volunteering, membership in associations, work, etc.). For example, it could consist of getting a drivers' licence, moving to an apartment, getting married or obtaining a diploma (Gutman, 1997).

Purves and Suto (2004) studied how activities such as rites of passage contribute to renegotiating identity from the person-environment-occupation perspective for elderly people in transition from a previous living situation to another one that is more appropriate to their level of functioning. Participants in this study were able to find a new identity within this transition because they put into place occupations linked with past habits and rituals. Rituals and rites of passage can add "symbolic efficacy" to occupation, a concept from medical anthropology (Bourdieu, 1990).

5.4. Interactions Targeted Interventions

Another possible intervention target to favour health is to act on interactions between the person, environment, and occupation. This section presents only interventions which seem the most promising because of the numerous facets of the concept of interaction previously presented.

The person-environment-occupation interaction suggests a perspective of empowerment. Indeed, the person has to be, as much as possible, able to act on his/her own environment in order to obtain the desired results. In addition, as mentioned previously, the creation of resilient, cohesive and inclusive environments also facilitate positive interactions.

However, when considering interactions, a favourable environment will not be inevitably the easiest one or the one which allows avoiding problems and efforts. The concept of resilience explains this phenomenon. Resilience is the capacity to resist when facing difficulties and even to be strengthened by obstacles. The favourable environment is the one which allows the person to develop his/her skills, to meet challenges, and to grow. There are numerous examples of situations where persons improve various abilities and skills after having surmounted important difficulties. In certain circumstances, some people will be broken or reduced to nothing, whereas others will leave having gained from it. It is once again a situation of interaction; it is necessary to find the best combinations between the person, environment and occupation, combinations which are going to allow the person to develop (Resnick, 2000; Scaer 2005; Wolkow, and Ferguson, 2001).

5.4.1. Interactions in the Intrasystem

Considering biomedical sciences, the person-environment interaction is more and more used to explain the origin of diseases. Indeed, several diseases arise only in the presence of a genetic predisposition associated to an environmental factor. It is the case, notably, for autoimmune diseases like type I diabetes, multiple sclerosis or arthritis (Staples, Ponsonby, Lim, and McMichael, 2003; Mead, 2004, 2006). Baird (1996) even affirms that most of the current diseases are due to interactions between the genotype and environmental factors.

For the unborn child, interactions with environment inevitably passed on by the mother, mainly by the placenta. These interactions would principally be at the origin of health problems, rather than genetic aspects (Begley, 1999). For example, children born with mothers who had preeclampsia have been found to have abnormalities in blood pressure and cortisol (Tenhola, Rahiala, Martikairen, Halonen, and Voutilainen, 2003). Several studies also demonstrated the links between socioeconomic levels and child's health, nevertheless without clarifying any underlying mechanisms (Macintyre, 1997; Rahkonen, Lahelma, and Huuhka, 1997).

Furthermore, personal factors that are not genetic, interacting with environmental factors, could explain the occurrence of diseases, like cardiac problems, cancers or psychiatric problems. The biologic bases of numerous psychiatric problems are then searched (Mohr, and Mohr, 2001). For example, some authors spoke about neuroplasticity or about the effect of events on brain and behaviour; that lead to the use of new intervention models, which integrate all dimensions affecting mental health, including contextual factors (Mohr, and Mohr, 2001).

It has also been discovered that numerous environmental factors interact with the human genome and modify it (this phenomenon is called epigenetics), and there is a transgenerational transmission of these alterations. Numerous current health problems may then come from the way of life, nutrition and exposure to various substances or stressors by the parents and grandparents (Crews, and McLachlan, 2006; Junien, Gallou-Kabani, Vige, and Gross, 2005; Titus-Ernstoff, 2006; Whitelaw, and Whitelaw, 2006). This also means that our current way of life will affect future generations. In addition, the study of the effects of life events and parenting behaviours across generations suggests that transgenerational transmission of disease may be influenced by interactions between life experiences and patterns of nervous system self-regulation, which appear to influence genetic expression (Meaney, Weaver, Wu, Hellstrom, Dioro, and McGown, 2006).

Scientific research increasingly demonstrates that life events influence patterns of regulation of the nervous system and other organ systems (Klaus, and Kennell, 1976; Kennel, and Klaus, 1998; Schore, 1994). From this perspective, disease is seen as a form of dysregulation at the emotional, behavioural, and/or physiological level and can be influenced by life events, which shape and alter patterns of self-regulation. Examples of significant events include prenatal maternal stress (Huizink, Mulder, and Buitelaar, 2004) which influences birth weight and can alter hypothalamic-pituitary axis regulation in the baby in ways that can last for his/her lifetime (Barker, 2004a; 2004b; Gluckman, and Hanson, 2005; 2006; Gluckman, Hanson, and Pinal, 2005; Nathanielsz, 1999). Studies demonstrate that low birth weight, which is increased by prenatal stress, is also linked to a growing number of chronic adult diseases including hypertension, hypercholesterolemia, type 2 diabetes, obesity, asthma, and chronic lung disease, among others (Gluckman, and Hanson, 2005; 2006; Gluckman, Hanson, and Pinal, 2005; Nathanielsz, 1999). Individuals who develop chronic diseases such as asthma, diabetes, and inflammatory bowel disease, for example, are more likely to have experienced complications at birth, like being born by caesarean section, even when the caesarean was performed for convenience and not for medical indications (Mead, 2004; 2006). It is also observed that experiences of traumatic stress are more common in adults suffering from chronic pain, fibromyalgia, and chronic fatigue (Scaer, 2005), as well as individuals with skeletal fractures, diabetes, liver disease, depression, chronic lung disease, and other symptoms (Felitti et al., 1998). These experiences refer to events that are perceived as life-threatening and inescapable, and also include highly stressful early family environments.

According to Steinhauer (1997), nothing influences a child's development more, after his/her genetic, than the quality of the parental care given during the first three years of life. The proliferation of synapses as well as the "operationnalisation" of neuronal circuits is remarkable at this age, and it is known that synapses are shaped by the stimuli of the environment (Direction des communications du ministère de la Santé et des Services sociaux, 2005). In this context, the birth and child care domain rediscovers the importance of parent - child bonding (Bolwby, 1969; Goldberg, Blokland, and Myhal, 2000). The interactions between the child and his parents from the birth - some will also say during the intrautero life - are naturally the foundations of this bond (Cassidy, 1999; Mead, 2006). The professional practices are thus revisited in order to favour this interaction as well as parent-child bonding (Direction des communications du ministère de la Santé et des Services sociaux, 2005) for example by providing greater support for women and families during pregnancy and when their children are young, and reducing obstetrical interventions during pregnancy and birth (such as amniocentesis and caesarean sections). This constitutes a long-term strategy which aims at maximizing the health of the next generation, including the increase of IQ (Klaus, and Kennel, 1976). In addition, these interventions probably reduce risk for chronic illness (Mead, 2006). The parent-child bond is also recognized for its role in the healthy development of self-regulation (Klaus, and Kennell, 1976; Schore, 1994).

Our still too limited knowledge about the complexity of interactions involved in the development of human beings encourages the adoption of ecological approaches which respect fundamental life mechanisms, even if it is not yet possible to understand and explain all of them.

5.4.2. Interactions in the Ontosystem and Microsystem

Interactions in the ontosystem and microsystem take place mainly in the person's immediate environment and include close relatives. They can affect many components as will be illustrated below for a variety of fields of practice.

Psychologists generally target the individual in their interventions. On the other hand, some authors from this discipline, like Bandura, underlined the importance of the environment (Cloutier, 1996). Behavioural approaches, which have been used since the beginning of the 20th Century, focus on the effect of environment on the individual. Later in the century, psychologists have increasingly considered the human development following an ecological approach, often using Bronfenbrenner's conception of the environment (Bronfenbrenner, 1977; 1979). Ecological psychology, which considers person-environment relation as a unit of analysis, is now well documented (Barker, 1968; Gibson, 1977; 1988; Schoggen, 1989). According to this ecological perspective, personal and environmental aspects mix together to influence the individual's behaviour. Notably, the effect of media on individual's behaviour was recognized. For this discipline, the ecological perspective distinguishes itself from biologic perspectives (centred on the person) or sociological perspectives (centred on the environment) because it does not favour one pole to the detriment of the other, rather it integrates both. This approach distinguishes itself from other theories by its focus on the global context. Each of us would be different if we had developed in another physical or social environment, or in another century. According to Cloutier (1996), there are ecological laws governing relationships between individuals and environment, and this domain of knowledge is still in development. In addition, community psychology also bases itself on ecological principles by developing interdisciplinary and inter-sector social strategies of transformation based on the empowerment of communities (Maton, 2000).

More specifically in counselling and orientation for career choice, the person-environment interaction is one of the foundations of professional practice, and is recognized as a determinant of career choice (Bujold, 1989). This fact has been demonstrated in numerous studies (Bujold, 1989). In this perspective, Holland's theory defines six types of personality and six types of different environments. The interaction of a type of personality with a type of given environment will lead to the career choice. A given environment can have a different effect on an individual according to his/her personality. Holland's theory also states that it is important to consider the perception of the environment by an individual as well as the formal and informal environment (Bujold, 1989).

In ergonomics, the fundamental object of this science is the man-machine interaction in the accomplishment of a task. The machine can be conceived according to the tasks to be carried out, but also according to the needs, morphology, and physiology of human beings (Grandjean, 1988). Numerous mutual adjustments are possible.

More specifically in auditory impairments, an ecological model of communication was developed. It integrates the dimensions of the signal, the message and the behaviour of both persons in a situation of communication, as well as the physical and social environment into which is situated the communication (Borg, 2000).

Many paediatric models of intervention target interactions in the microsystem, given that the parents and the family are strongly involved in almost all types of intervention which concern children. For example, a model of interdisciplinary intervention, which integrates a developmental approach as well as an ecological approach, was developed in the field of rehabilitation. It is called the "Life Needs Model". In this model, child's needs are seen in a holistic perspective. The concepts of resilience and protective factors in the family and the environment are considered, as well as social participation and quality of life (King, Tucker, Baldwin, Lowry, LaPorta, and Matens, 2002).

Again considering child-family interactions, a psychologist in California suspected that asthma was influenced by bonding disruptions occurring at birth (Madrid, 1991; 2005). When mothers were treated for bonding disruptions using hypnosis or eye movement desensitization and reprocessing (EMDR), the child's asthma resolved on the same day, even if the child had been severely ill for years. Although not all children with asthma recovered when their mothers were treated, the majority had complete recoveries and stopped needing medication. So, when treating an individual with psychotherapy to promote a return to self-regulation, the effects may also benefit the broader "system", such as children and family members in the family system, whose capacity for self-regulation may increase when another family member improves (Madrid, 2005). Based on many studies, Mead (2006) recommends the use of trauma therapy, to provide early treatment after a trauma to the whole family system or the parents, not only the individual who is symptomatic.

Another concrete example is kangaroo care. Kangaroo care is a new kind of postnatal transportation that bears some analogy to in utero transport and may be safer than incubator transport. It consists of transporting the infant on the mother's or other caregiver's chest. It is a natural intervention that humans appear to have been designed to do, and it may be the kind of things that could be used to maximize health and even prevent or decrease risk for disease. Apparently it is helpful with babies of all ages and not only premature babies. Kangaroo care notably helps to regulate the child's nervous system (Charpak, et al., 2005; Johnston, et al., 2003; Ludington-Hoe, and Swinth, 1996). It has also been demonstrated that greater contact between parents and babies in the first 24 hours after delivery in general, and in the first hour in particular, generates benefits for child development, even many years later (De Chateau, 1984; Klaus, and Kennel, 1976).

Besides, when someone becomes ill in a family, its balance is broken. To reinstall homeostasis in a family where one of the members presents an impairment or illness, it is necessary to foresee the support required for all family members and to avoid excess burden on one or some of its members. This search of homeostasis can involve various resources around the family. Supporting families aims at making sure that homeostasis is satisfactory for all of its members (avoid burden). It can mean involving families in decisions about the ill person such as choices of interventions, teaching them and giving them explanations so that they can make enlightened choices, in an empowering perspective (Law, 1998; Pelchat, and Lefebvre, 2002).

5.4.3. Interactions in the Mesosystem and Exosystem

The curative biomedical model, centred on reduction of diseases and impairments, structured on a one to one intervention (professional and patient), based on providing prescriptions followed by periodic meetings in the professional's office, turns out as not being really adapted to reach some health objectives, particularly in the case of chronic diseases. In this case, it is more about empowerment, self-regulation, autonomy at home or social participation than about specific curative interventions. In this context, health professionals have to meet the needs of persons by means of community-based services, in interdisciplinary and intersector-based teams, by emphasizing coordination of care and access to services, rather than on mastering modalities of curative treatments or therapy. However, service organization and professionals are not well prepared for this type of practice (Craddock, 1996; Dreiling, and Bundy, 2003; Hébert, Maheux, and Potvin, 2002). New effective models of intervention are thus looked for, among which those who ensue from an ecological perspective of intervention (King, Tucker, Baldwin, Lowry, LaPorta, and Matens, 2002; Struber, 2003).

Acting on the person-environment-occupation interaction requires intervening in the natural environment, the mesosystem itself, where interactions between the person, environment, and occupation can come true. Community-based programs, in opposition to those in institutions, can allow this interaction. Such programs aim, for example, on integration into the community, social participation, school integration or integration of labour force. There are several examples of this type of service organization in the literature and some of them will now be presented (Freeman, 1997; Gadoury, 1999; Naylor, and Buhler-Wilkerson, 1999; Remondet Wall, Rosenthal, and Niemczura, 1998).

Community-based interventions are used more frequently because of their seemingly lower costs and superior results. So, it has been demonstrated, without a doubt, that child development is superior in a family environment compared to institutional environment. Besides, several studies have demonstrated that it was more effective to intervene directly in the environment where the person lives in order to reduce behaviour problems, rather than intervening in an institutional environment where real interactions are absent (Bagley, and Mallick, 2000; Freeman, 1997; Peters, Gluck, and McCormick, 1992; Yody, et al., 2000). However, in some cases, it has not been scientifically demonstrated that it is more effective than the traditional approach in institutional environment, for example for people having sustained a traumatic brain injury (Freeman, 1997; Remondet, Rosenthal, and Niemczura, 1998).

Willer and Corrigan (1994) expressed ten ecological intervention principles which support community-based interventions for people with impairments in their model called "Whatever it takes model" (Willer, and Corrigan, 1994). These principles were used in other models of intervention such as the de Hope and Finegan's (1999) "self-determination model". These principles are:

1. No two individuals with injury are alike, it is thus necessary to adapt intervention to each person and to his/her specific context;
2. Skills are more likely to generalize when taught in the environment where they are to be used;
3. Environments are easier to change than people;
4. Community integration should be holistic;
5. Life is a place-and-train venture (traditional interventions consist most of the time of doing "train and place");
6. Natural supports last longer than professionals support;
7. Interventions must not do more harm than good;
8. The service system presents many of the barriers to community integration; for example the reimbursement of services or equipments by insurance companies sometimes does not respond to person's needs;
9. Respect for the individual is paramount;
10. Needs of individuals last a lifetime; so should their resources; nevertheless, interventions in health institutions last a short period of time.

Condeluci (1995) proposes the model of interdependence in order to favour community integration of people with impairments. The principles which he expresses have several common elements with those of the "Whatever it takes model" presented previously. He defines interdependence as the process by which the persons share their talents with others for the profit of the community. His model emphasizes the capacities of the person and not his/her disabilities. The process is individualized; every intervention must be specific to the person. It is centred on the person, in a perspective of unconditional acceptance and empowerment. Interpersonal relationships are considered, and this model meets the challenge of social inclusion by acting on the environment.

Integration in the work force for people with impairments is an objective of social participation which requires, most of the time, an ecological approach (Jacob, 1997; Kowalske, Plenger, Lusby, and Hayden, 2000; La Marche, Reed, Rich, Cash, Lucas, and

Boll, 1995; LeBlanc, Hayden, and Paulman, 2000). Supported employment is a strategy which consists in facilitating work integration by offering to a person the required long-term support so that he/she can keep this employment, by providing, for example, surveillance, assistance or help. The environment thus adapts itself to the individual to allow him/her to work. This approach, abundantly described and studied in the literature, turned out to be beneficial for the person and effective in terms of costs (Goodall, and Ghiloni, 2001; Remondet Wall, Rosenthal, and Niemczura, 1998; Wehman, West, Kregel, Sherron, and Kreutzer, 1995; Yasuda, Wehman, Targett, Cifu, and West, 2001). Implications of the person in decisions as well as motivation were identified, among others, as factors of success in this approach (Wehman, West, Kregel, Sherron, and Kreutzer, 1995; Yasuda, Wehman, Targett, Cifu, and West, 2001). In the same way, Goodall and Ghiloni (2001) made a review of the American governmental programs which were set up to favour work integration of people with impairments. They notably considered laws, financial incentives, and flexibility in programs such as possibilities for part-time jobs or the possibilities for prolonging the training and support period. These creative measures turned out to be beneficial. Moreover, a study reported the advantages of this ecological model of intervention compared to a traditional model in institution: a better integration in the community, an improved independence, and the improvement of the vocational status (Torrey, Becker, and Drake, 1995).

In addition, Stokols (1996) proposes the following steps in ecological interventions aiming at work integration of people with impairments: 1) to analyze the links between socio-physical conditions and person's abilities; 2) to see the influence of personal and environmental conditions on people's and community's well-being; 3) to develop the adaptation between the person and environment (i.e. architectural barriers, adaptation of workstation); 4) to make actions on the individual and on the environment according to what is the most effective (fit out a workstation or modify the entire place to get more security for everyone in the workplace); this can imply conducting consultations and working in association with various disciplines (i.e. consultations and exchanges with supervisors concerned by job organization, school integration, or integration into a group); 5) to be aware of the links between the physical and the social environment (i.e. noise which can bother interpersonal relationships, create isolation).

Integration in the workforce for people with low back pain can also be facilitated by adopting an ecological approach as described in a study by Durand and colleagues (2003). The interdisciplinary team have indeed adopted a model of practice which considers the person, the working environment, and the interaction between both. This model of intervention puts an emphasis on interdisciplinarity and intersector-based intervention to favour the return to work, including interventions on work environment, such as workstation adaptation and adoption of flexible schedules, among others (Durand, Vachon, Loisel, and Berthelette, 2003).

Considering school integration of people with impairments, an ecological assessment was developed by Kellegrew and Kroskmark (1999) by using a method called "time geography methodology". This evaluation is directly performed in the school environment and consists of noticing all moments, places and persons met during a week. It allows understanding how the personal and environmental factors interact to establish better targeted interventions. In the same way, occupational therapists proposed an ecological model called "Synthesis of child, occupational performance and environment in time" (SCOPE-IT Model) for young people having coordination disorders (Poulsen, and Ziviani, 2004). This model has several common characteristics with the MCRO. It emphasizes the time factor in a developmental perspective and favours balance in different activities carried out by the child during a period of time. This model also adopts a positive and preventive perspective, by using activities that are meaningful for the child.

Finally, some authors demonstrated that interactions between contextual and personal factors resulted in significant differences in the prevalence of AIDS (Boerma, Gregson, Nyamukapa, and Urassa, 2004; Drain, Smith, Hughes, Halperin, and Holmes, 2004).

5.4.4. Interactions in the Macrosystem

Governments, climate, industries, and other elements of the macrosystem are associated and influence each other. In a general manner, many authors have identified a relationship between macroenvironment and health (Ashton, and Seymour, 1988; Chu, and Simpson, 1994; Evans, Morris, and Marmor, 1996; Macintyre, and Ellaway, 2000; McLeroy, and Bibeau, Steckler, and Glanz, 1988; Stokols, 1992). The Black Report was one of the first studies to identify a clear and global interaction between socioeconomic level and health (Bartley, Blane, and Smith, 1998; Macintyre, 1997; Marmot, Ryff, Bumpass, Shipley, and Marks, 1997). The precise mechanisms of this interaction are, nevertheless, still unknown and many hypotheses were elaborated in order to explain this association. Disparities in socioeconomic levels or social inequalities seem to affect health more than low income itself. Other studies have also demonstrated this relationship with more specific health problems (Cooper, Kennelly, Durazo-Arvizu, Oh, Kaplan, and Lynch, 2001; Kawachi, 1997; Kawachi, Kennedy, and Glass, 1999; Kawachi, Kennedy, and Wilkinson, 1999; Lynch, Smith, Kaplan, and House, 2000; Rahkonen, Lahelma, and Huuhka, 1997; Syme, 1998).

Many interventions involving interactions in the macrosystem are situated at political and economical levels (laws, rules, resources ...), in values and choices in society. Several ways to act on interactions in the macrosystem are proposed by sciences like sociology, political science, economy or management. For example, in management, Morgan's best seller presents different pictures of organisations which take into account their complexity and their relationship with the environment (Morgan, 1997). Morgan uses metaphors that compare the functioning of an organisation with that of a cell or the brain for example. A part of his book is even dedicated to the most recent theories attempting to conceptualize complexity, such as the theory of chaos. Management principles, ensued from the structuration theory (Giddens, 1984), and presented by Eraly (1986), are other examples of actions targeting interactions in the macrosystem. These authors have demonstrated how any type of organisation is fundamentally based on the interaction between its structure and the people which compose it.

The study of interactions between living species and their environment is the main focus of ecology. After presenting the state of knowledge about interactions in various domains, going back to the roots of ecology, the next section will discuss how some of the fundamental interactions defined in ecology appear to affect human health.

6. FROM HUMAN ECOLOGY TOWARD HUMAN HEALTH

The previous sections made a browsing on ecological thoughts, theories, models, approaches, and many of their applications. A strong convergence supporting this approach is noted on the theoretical plan and from the applications' point of view in various domains, disciplines, and intervention fields. Such synergy is not a coincidence, but rather a consequence of the knowledge evolution and the consideration of the situation's complexity in these different fields of practice. This section brings a different perspective. In the first part, human ecology is discussed and aims at suggesting global research questions, which could help improve life conditions, health, and life quality of populations in general. Having deciphered the human genome and cleared up several mechanisms of brain functioning, the next challenge is probably to study the human being in a more ecological perspective. This explanatory process is necessary because ecological principles, which allowed the evolution of life since its beginning, are not relevant anymore with more than six billions individuals living on this planet (Homer-Dixon, 2001). This analysis is brief and not exhaustive. It leads to improve the understanding of human ecology in order to take better actions to improve human health. The knowledge developments in several domains will be used in this analysis: recent discoveries about humans' origin, genetics, and brain development, among others. Afterward, in the second part of this section, recommendations will be formulated in order to encourage the adoption of ecological approaches in all domains involving human health.

6.1. Some Particularities of Human Ecology

> Inuits have been living in Northern Canada for thousands of years. They sometimes did infanticide in the past. The extent of this practice is not known, but it allowed these peoples to survive in an environment providing few resources, in the absence of other birth control methods. Since they have access to modern medicine, they can use different birth control methods, including the abortion. The white man brought his technologies and he transformed the way of life of Inuits, notably by building houses for them. They thus had to become sedentary and they lost their traditional way of life. These peoples face new major social problems: suicides of young people, violence, alcoholism, apparition of new diseases ...

Ecology is a science studying the characteristics of ecosystems. Populations' growth, mechanisms that ensure the ecosystems stability, biodiversity, and behaviours are some of the main objects of this science (Campbell, 1995; Krebs, 2002; McMichael, 1993). In this section, seven ecology fields will be briefly analyzed according to certain particularities of human health: 1) the balance between resources and populations' needs; 2) populations' growth; 3) mechanisms that ensure the ecosystems' stability; 4) disturbance of ecosystems; 5) biodiversity; 6) behaviours, and 7) human specific regulation mechanisms.

6.1.1. The Balance between Resources and Populations' Needs

The living species need to have access to a minimum of resources to survive and the environment has to provide these resources. For long-term life preservation, a balance is necessary between what the environment can supply and the living species' needs. This general principle applies to all living species, whether they are bacteria, plants, or mammals. The needs of bacteria are naturally relatively simple and vary according to their metabolism. As life becomes more complex, needs are also becoming more complex.

The fundamental human needs were expressed in a known and widespread model: the Maslow Pyramid, published in 1943. Human beings need to respond firstly to their most fundamental needs (food and lodging), but they need additional resources for their development. They have notably social and spiritual needs. Human beings thus live in complex societies providing various resources. Human environments must thus provide elements necessary to the development of all human characteristics: growth, affects, language, cognition, spirituality, etc. A society not providing response to fundamental human needs engenders disease and death.

Besides, human beings can produce resources according to the expressed demand: it is the free market. Human beings are also able to create new needs for others and earn a profit from it when they fulfil this new need. In this context, the Maslow pyramid is no more a reference. Since we live in a material over-abundance in industrialized countries, what is the effect of over-fulfilling some needs – needs that are often not fundamental - on human development and health?

6.1.2. Populations' Growth

Populations' growth obeys to cycles regulated according to available resources. It is possible to observe, for a large number of species, a growth until depletion of resources, followed by a decline of population, and the cycle starts again (Campbell, 1995). The human population has grown for thousands of years. This growth became exponential in the last decades. Human beings can exercise control over the planet's resources, notably by agriculture, breeding, and different technologies in the field of fisheries. Humans also build aqueduct and sewer systems. All these elements allow populations' growth and human beings succeed in living in almost any ecosystems on earth because of their great ingenuity and adaptability. Nevertheless, humans' activities often destroy ecosystems, which were providing at first plenty of resources. The lack of resources leads to disease and death. Facing such problems, we need to know how many humans can live in each ecosystem that provides response to human fundamental needs without destroying irreparably ecosystems. We also need to identify parameters that should be considered in this estimation.

Human beings have the capacity to control birth. Some countries, like China, set up drastic measures to control the population's growth. This control constitutes another means that keeps the balance between the resources and the populations' needs. However, the majority of parents wish to have a boy. A social crisis can be foreseen because the population of young adults will soon count many more men than women. Birth control also provokes numerous religious debates.

Globally, human beings have the power to control the growth of resources and of populations at the same time. The practice of this control is, however, difficult, partial, and is done, most of the time, by trial and error. After determining how many humans could live on earth, which birth control method would be the most ecologic when considering personal, social, and ethical aspects?

6.1.3. Mechanisms that Ensure Survival of Ecosystems

Besides birth control and resources production, several mechanisms keep the ecosystems stable, avoiding over-population and the depletion of resources. Predation, diseases, epidemics, and battles for territory or females are among the most frequent mechanisms.

Considering predation, no big predators really threaten human beings. On the other hand, mankind creates other types of predators like automobile and various type of transportation (plane, train, etc.), and also many kinds of industrial machinery, which kill or hurt thousands of individuals every day. They also provoke environmental disasters which affect health (toxic products spills, nuclear power plants accidents ...). Young adults in wealthy societies love extreme sports, as if life without dangers or without predators was less interesting. Besides, in front of infectious diseases, which can be considered as human predators, human beings have developed treatments like vaccines or antibiotics that prevented numerous epidemics. However, these actions contribute to the development of stronger and more resistant micro-organisms. Consequently, a large amount of the health systems' resources of industrialized countries is spent for the physical rehabilitation of trauma victims and prevent or cure infectious diseases. These facts demonstrate that we do not use the most efficient and sustainable strategies in the fighting of humans' predators.

Because a given environment can only ensure the survival of a limited number of individuals of each species, battles for the territory are other mechanism directly associated to available resources in an ecosystem. For human beings, these battles correspond to organized wars between tribes, nations, or countries. Human beings have invented war machines and atrocious tortures in order to fight their enemies. Nonetheless, human beings have the capacity and the power to negotiate the sharing of territories and resources; thus, avoiding wars and sufferings that ensue from it. Human beings have also developed many forms of competitions, like literature, chess, races, sports, or artistic competitions because of their fighting nature.

Globally, the human species has the capacity to control the resources' production, the populations' growth, and the sharing of resources by using appropriate means. Paradoxically, humans develop powerful technologies in order to cure many diseases and, at the same time, they develop the most infernal destruction machines. Which efficient human specific mechanisms would ensure long-term survival of ecosystems? How can we develop and implement them?

6.1.4. Ecosystems Perturbations

> The miners brought a canary in the mine where they worked so that it warns them of a danger. The canary, indeed, would die quickly if the concentration of poisonous gas increased in the mine and this indicated to the miners that they had to leave, as fast as possible. We live the same situation on the planet; numerous species are in process of extinction and it maybe warning us of a danger for ourselves. However, it is not possible to leave earth ...

Many diseases appearing in modern societies are maybe a warning of a bigger danger for human beings. For example, fibromyalgia, or chronic fatigue, can constitute signs of long-term effects of industrialization and technologies on health. Increased incidence and prevalence of children's developmental delays, children's allergy problems, obesity, diabetes, and cancer constitutes other examples possibly indicating many environmental or way of life problems. These problems should be the results of events or situations occurring many years ago. What is the effect of our current way of life on future generation's health? What are the best indicators of the future generations' health?

Human beings can also control their life cycle: longevity increases; very low weight premature babies or serious accident victims can survive; dysfunctioning organs can be replaced, etc. Among the long-term effects of these curative interventions, there is, for example, an important burden for parents or close relatives of premature children or trauma victims who have to live with severe persevering sequelaes and who will need support for their entire life (Farmer, Marien, Clark, Sherman, and Selva, 2004; Magliano, Fiorillo, De Rosa, Malangone, and Maj, 2005; Wade, Stancin, Taylor, Drotar Yeates, and Minich, 2004). More and more important parts of countries expenses are dedicated to health notably because of ageing populations and technology improvements. A large part of research budgets is also dedicated to improve life expectation and cure diseases. It is the first time in human history that so many resources are dedicated to curative medicine, and these resources are no more available for other purposes (child education, healthy way of life, healthy food, etc.). What is the impact of dedicating so many resources for curative medicine on long term populations' health?

The body possesses defence and regulation mechanisms against disturbances: immune system mechanisms, osseous or nervous regeneration, adaptation process, etc. The body is capable of healing after being affected by changes that seemed irreparable at first. The body is also often able to find a new balance: the person will learn to live with a chronic disease or a disability. These capacities are based on thousands of years of evolution, which has designed it to be efficiently self-regulating. If humans do not let these mechanisms act, a science based on hundreds of thousand years is neglected. How should be designed ecological health care systems emphasizing self-regulation mechanisms?

Humans produce different technologies, always more successful and for various purposes. They also create many new chemical substances. The "life compatible" molecules are those naturally found in the environment; they passed the test of billions of years of evolution. The creation of new molecules in chemistry or in pharmacology might introduce "life incompatible" elements and it is impossible to test these products long enough to know their long-term impacts. It is notably the case of insecticides, herbicides, and medicines that turned out to be harmful after an experiment over long enough periods. Furthermore, the manufacturing of toxic products, their transportation, and their use bring health risks. The presence of such products on earth is incompatible with the long-term life preservation.

Humans are able to modify or control several elements of their environment, but still poorly measure the short and long-term consequences of their activities with current scientific methods. Some interventions can bring short-term profits, but can turn out fatal afterward. How can we evaluate health practices while taking into account their long term effects on health and on the future generations' health? Would it be possible to include a principle of sustainable development in research and practice ethical considerations?

6.1.5. Biodiversity

> Type I diabetes is a disease resulting from the interaction between genetic factors (predispositions) and environmental factors (exposition to a stress affecting cells development during a critical period). Diabetics should not ask themselves if they have the right to procreate or not, with the fear of transmitting the specificity of their genes. From the point of view of biodiversity, elimination of a gene is a loss. Even if these genes seem to have negative effects, in certain environmental conditions, diabetics or people having this genetic factor could be the only ones to survive ...

Density and biodiversity are taken into account when studying ecosystems. Biodiversity is a characteristic that contributes to the preservation of long-term life. Indeed, an ecosystem with a greater biodiversity is less vulnerable to environment fluctuations. Furthermore, biodiversity is desirable because it allows accommodating several species and several individuals in the same ecosystem. With a greater biodiversity, interactions complexity also increases. On the other hand, normalization, bureaucratisation, and organization of the production line work of industrialized societies supply short-term profits, but reduce diversity, and increase risks for diseases.

Besides, many researches concern human genome. The increasing knowledge on genome demonstrates, however, that it will not be as simple as replacing a defective gene. Indeed, we do not know all the interactions implicated and the effects of this kind of change are impossible to predict. Recent discoveries in epigenetic notably demonstrate the high complexity of the genome, its interaction with environmental factors, and the intergenerational transmission of characters or diseases resulting from environmental factors (Crews, and McLachlan, 2006; Whitelaw, and Whitelaw, 2006). In addition, the elimination of seemingly defective genes decreases biodiversity and could make humans more vulnerable. The human being was built from billions of interactions, spaced out over billions of years. In spite of all their competences, humans still cannot understand and master all these subtleties. How can we include elements that favour biodiversity and genome protection in health practices and researches?

6.1.6. Behaviours

Since the 1970s, a branch of ecology is particularly interested in behaviour as a mechanism of maximisation of adaptability (Campbell, 1995). Researchers in this field try to understand why natural selection favoured a particular behaviour over another one. They discovered that animals possess natured and nurtured behaviours. The natured behaviours are stereotypical and are provoked by stimulus. Nurtured behaviours can result from conditioning, observation, and other types of learning, like playing. The most evolved vertebrates, like humans or chimpanzees, would be capable of a sudden understanding, which is to think and find straight off the solution of a problem, without any preceding learning situation. It is also observed that numerous natured behaviours are regulated by elements of the environment, like circadian rhythms or migrations, demonstrating the narrow links between natured and nurtured behaviours. According to current knowledge, it is now generally admitted that most behaviours result from interactions between living species and their environment.

Human beings can base their behaviours on multiple data; they do not only react to stimuli. They can perform a complex analysis of the situation. On the other hand, it is known that human beings also possess stereotypical behaviours, like the young baby's smile. Social life is also an occasion for different interactions that result in various behaviours: cooperation, competition, domination, exploitation, etc. As a new research field, numerous research questions can be formulated to better understand human behaviours. The next paragraphs will present many examples.

A particular aspect of behaviour aims at reproductive success. The capacity of appealing is, notably, on the basis of sexual selection. Birds, flowers, butterflies, insects, fishes, among others, compete in colours and forms to appeal and seduce. Whether it is a moose's panache, a peacock's tail, a bird's song or a trout's coloured stripes, these elements have an unmistakable impact. One of the scientific explanations of these elements is that they can constitute indicators of vigour and health, but numerous situations still remain unexplained in this domain. Human beings also appeal and seduce, but they use more complex mechanisms. They can demonstrate their power and seduce not only with physical appearance, but also with possessions, artistic productions (music, painting, etc.), or certain personal qualities desired, consciously or not, by the "possible partner". Freud explained sexual choices notably by Œdipe's complex. In addition, the capacity of symbolization, associated to the mechanisms which aim at appealing and seducing, can be at the origin of the fondness for various arts (sculpture, painting, music, song, dance, etc.). Again, numerous research questions can be formulated to improve understanding of human sexual behaviours in an ecological perspective.

The cognition was defined as the process by which an individual acquires the consciousness of events and objects of his/her environment. Researchers like Jane Goodall and Donald Griffin consider that some animals like monkeys have behaviours based on a consciousness similar to the human one. Their behaviours demonstrate that they have feelings like fear, jealousy, anger, or sadness. It is possible to seize their feelings because of their body language. Indeed, animals, and young children who do not speak yet, can decode feelings and adjust their behaviour consequently, only by observing the body language of the people around them. The study of the human consciousness in an ecological perspective is certainly a challenge.

Feelings are powerful human behaviour determinants, as they are for numerous animals. On the other hand, only human beings can have feelings on a symbolic basis; that is without really living the events that provoked them; by reading a book, listening to music, or seeing a movie for example. Famous artists are, indeed, those who know how to provoke feelings with their art. The search for pleasant feelings and well-being can explain numerous human behaviours. It seems that the evolution allowed the development of pleasant sensations to favour behaviours that ensure life perpetuation, and vice versa: let us think to the taste, smell, or tactile senses. The pleasure of senses leads to look for sophisticated food (spices, wines, etc.), to listen to music, to dance, and to admire art objects or landscapes. Humans love strong sensations. Speed and adrenalin give them wings... Humans also have good feelings when they use their cognitive skills of reasoning and when they find solutions to problems. Their voluminous brain gives them powerful skills and, in the industrialized societies, they find various ways to use these capacities, like in research and knowledge development, computer gaming, intellectual competitions, etc. On the other hand, if the search for pleasure is not regulated, it can lead to abuses and disease: alcoholism, drug addiction, pathological gaming, obesity, addiction to smoking, sexual deviances, and traumatism, among others.

Besides, some animals seem to demonstrate altruism in their behaviour. It is known, for example, that a mother of one species can raise a baby of another species in some circumstances. Animals can also warn others of a danger, while taking risks for their own life. This behaviour is difficult to explain on a scientific basis, but it seems that the altruistic individual would obtain profits later. Is there any real altruism in human beings or do they only look for later profits? Exceptional persons like Mother Theresa, Jean Vanier, or Santa Clara from Assisi demonstrated such unconditional love for the most rejected people of the society that it is possible, without hesitation, to speak about an altruism which has no equivalent in the animal kingdom. However, this type of altruism is extremely rare. Does it provide exceptional pleasures, specific to humans?

The study of human behaviour, in the perspective of evolution or ecology, is still at its very first steps. It is an emerging field of research that could give us answers to many fundamental questions and contribute, this way, to the improvement of human health.

Globally, human beings can become aware of their behaviours, feelings, and consequences as well, that ensue from them. These skills are strongly associated to complex cognitive functions. The next paragraphs discuss more specifically about human cognitive skills.

6.1.7. Human Specific Regulation Mechanisms

Human communities set up several elements in order to control human behaviour: various religions with their dogma, commands, rules, or rites; governments with their laws, regulations, and justice systems; and, finally, various social structures and organizations with their formal and informal rules (Giddens, 1984). Human beings also have individual self-control mechanisms specific to them.

Cognitive skills are at the base of many human self-control and self-regulation mechanisms. Bandura (2003) clarified the human's particular cognitive skills in his theory and many researches have confirmed these elements. These skills are: 1) humans have the capacity to symbolize, what multiplies tenfold their communications, creativity, possibility of knowledge transmission, and possibility of understanding past and current events; 2) humans can plan the future notably by taking into account past events; 3) humans can learn by observation and not only by their successes and failures. It is not thus necessary to experience a failure to adjust a behaviour; 4) humans have the capacity of insight and self-reflection; they can use self-regulation mechanisms, and can modify by themselves their thoughts and behaviours. For Bandura (2003), this would be the most distinctive human characteristic. Kielhofner (2002; 2004) completed this analysis of humans' characteristics, and defined the volition as the process by which humans are motivated towards and choose what they do.

These skills put humans in front of their individual and collective responsibility. Because humans are conscious of the consequences of their acts, they can control them and thus be their own regulation mechanism. Humans are the only species that can exercise such self-reflection and self-regulation. They do not need mechanisms that regulate other living species. They do not need to wait for resources depletion or epidemics to change their behaviour or their way of life. Humans can plan the future; they have the means to control and to modify their thoughts and behaviour for their well-being and that of future generations. Humans have the choice to apply the solutions that cause least sufferings. Humans certainly have no means to avoid all disasters, but can, at least, not provoke or increase them. For example, birth control can seem preferable than wars, diseases, or epidemics in order to avoid over-population.

To manage self-control or self-regulation, the first condition is above all to **want** it. The will allows mobilizing energies and be goal directed. In addition, to actualise self-control and self-regulation, it is necessary to have the determination and the belief that it is possible to reach there goals.

Self-regulation and self-control mechanisms are specific to human nature. They are the counterparts in powerful cognitive skills; they are the responsibility that accompanies what these skills conferred to humans. They allow exercising notably a control over the populations' growth, the resources exploitation, and the behaviour as well. Self-regulation and self-control could allow avoiding numerous death and diseases. In addition, these human specific regulation mechanisms involve individuals, as well as communities.

Human ecology has numerous specificities if it is compared with animal ecology. It turns out important to understand particular human skills and their consequences. Knowledge about life, its regulation mechanisms, and its evolution is still fragmented. Nevertheless, to exercise self-control, it is necessary to have enough knowledge about life and the consequences of human activities. Due to the lack of knowledge or unawareness, humans cause irreparable harm. A principle of precaution thus turns out essential, until knowledge allows humans to make more enlighten actions. However, often people do not live long enough to see the consequences of their actions and it is a major obstacle to develop the awareness and responsibility taking that are necessary in order to adjust actions.

Human ecology as a science is still at its beginning and numerous disciplines can make a contribution there. This science is at a crossing between biochemistry, genetics, physiology, evolutionism, general ecology, and anthropology among others. Moreover, the study of behaviour, and particularly the social behaviour, makes the link between biology, social sciences, and human sciences (Campbell, 1995). In addition, human beings are probably the only species that can exercise a real conscious choice that leads to philosophy, morality, and to the fundamental debate between Good and Evil, which is also specific to humans. Health disciplines like psychology, occupational therapy, or public health can also enlighten many aspects of human ecology, which will maybe bring new discoveries and have an impact on population health.

After this discussion about the human ecology, the next section investigates intervention strategies ensuing from it and that are applicable today and in the future to improve life conditions, health, and quality of life.

6.2. Ecological Intervention Strategies

> The Masai people are semi-nomadic and live in Kenya and Tanzania. These people kept a large part of their traditional way of life. Even confronted with the modern world, they are proud of their way of life. They still have among their rites of passage to kill a lion with their traditional weapons. The fact of being able to kill lions is an unmistakable source of self-efficacy belief. They seem, in fact, to be afraid of nothing. These people have never known slavery. They are more than one and a half million Masai, what compares advantageously with some thousands of autochthons who still live in North America. The success of Masai peoples seems surprising as they use only very few things to survive. In fact, they have only houses built in ground and straw, a herd of cows and some sheep. The occidental way of life seems much superior to theirs in a lot of consideration: life expectation, child mortality rate, comfort... On the other hand, from the point of view of sustainable development, these people are probably superior to occidentals. They could survive further to events which would have annihilated our way of life, for example the end of petroleum production. With very few resources they could even repopulate the earth ...

The world was recently the theatre of major changes that have significant impacts on life: globalization, climate changes, disturbances of the environment, urbanization, demographic evolution, progress in medical sciences, information technologies, and others. Unfortunately, many of these elements contribute to increase health problems or to create new ones like chronic diseases, cancers, obesity, traumatisms, mental illness, allergies, resistances to antibiotics, pandemics risks, etc. (Barrett, Kuzawa, McDade, and Armelagos, 1998; McMichael, 1993). All these situations have repercussions on the health systems costs. In the industrialized nations, several health systems reforms tried to address these changes, but numerous problems persist and new solutions must be envisaged (WHO, 2005).

The previous sections stated researches demonstrating the relevance of ecological models and approaches in the field of health. The knowledge of human ecology can also serve as a foundation to find solutions to current problems. Ecological models and approaches are centred on life; thus, they can help to protect it, in opposition to traditional curative medical models centred on disease. If the current situation is analyzed with studies results and the previous discussion about human ecology, what concrete recommendations can be made for health professionals in order to improve the life conditions, health, and quality of life? The next paragraphs will propose many suggestions.

6.2.1. Ecological Principles of Intervention in the Field of Health

An ecological perspective can bring new solutions to address current health problems. To reach this goal, at first, it is possible to consider what it means to a health professional to adopt an ecological approach. As described in Section 5, from an individual point of view, ecological principles of intervention are centred on improvement of the individual's natural defence mechanisms, stimulation of self-regulation mechanisms, empowerment, open-mindedness to differences, and respect of diversity. The adoption of the ecological approaches also means to act on environment, occupations, and person-environment-occupation interactions. Targeting the environment and interactions can require networking between the health system resources and those of the community, in an interdisciplinary and intersector-based partnership. Only these elements can constitute an important change in the health professional practices.

The analysis of the populations' needs using ecological approaches can make professionals thinking in a more global and long-term perspective and in a perspective of sustainable development. The sustainable development is defined as: "[...] development that meets the needs of the present without compromising the ability of future generations to meet their own needs" (Brundtland Commission, 1987). This perspective can mean performing individual interventions when keeping in mind a populationist vision and thinking that daily actions do not have to provide, at the same time, an immediate profit for an individual in particular, and damage to others or to environment in a short or long-term period. Professionals must not be aware only of a person's disease, but also of the ecosystem into which he/she is a part of, and the interactions into which he/she is involved. For example, to resuscitate, at all costs, extreme premature babies or severe traumatized people can look like a victory, but the familial and social costs of a child or an adult having severe persistent sequelaes are enormous. But how to refuse survival to someone, while more and more sophisticated technology can make it possible? The biomedical approach fights for survival, but should also consider the interventions' consequences and their costs. Every health intervention should be estimated, not only according to the individual's survival or cure, but also according to the long-term effects on health and the quality of life, while considering the impact on the relatives and the identified elements of the environment. Social parameters should notably be taken into account and also the consideration of ethical aspects.

An ecological perspective also asks to intervene more from the point of view of promotion and prevention, than from the curing diseases. On the other hand, the health systems expenses are mainly made on curative biomedical aspects and infatuation for reductionist biomedical research is still noted. Nevertheless, several causes of many health problems are clearly identified and it would be possible to act at the source by improving the natural defence mechanisms of the individual and by improving healthiness of the environment (providing healthy food, eliminating cigarette, toxic products, etc.). All members of a community could be involved to create an environment that would allow a healthier way of life (bicycle roads, healthy food, universal design, etc.) (Satariano, and McAuley, 2003). These interventions can be more effective than curative treatments for improving population health and could limit the curative health expenses. An example comes from some European countries, notably in Scandinavia, that put the health of unborn or young children foremost by setting up different measures to reach this goal. It is observed in these countries that there are fewer medical interventions surrounding birth, and more mothers who breast-feed and pursuing breast-feeding during a longer period (Direction of the communications of the social Ministry of Health and Service, 2005). These interventions contribute to improve women's self-efficacy beliefs and are done in an empowerment perspective. Medical interventions such as convenient caesarean do exactly the contrary.

On the other hand, the public health and health promotion speech states that fighting poverty is a mean to improve health, because health indicators are better in socio-economically favoured communities (Cooper, Kennelly, Durazo-Arvizu, Oh, Kaplan, and Lynch, 2001; Macintyre, 1997; Marmot, Ryff, Bumpass, Shipley, and Marks, 1997). It is indeed demonstrated that the improvement of socio-economic conditions is the main cause of the increase of life expectation that has occurred in the 20th Century, and not the curative medicine, like antibiotics or vaccines. Nevertheless, this speech can drive to resources over-exploitation for short-term economic profits and improvement of life conditions, but for elements that are not really essentials. Would it not be more relevant in a long-term perspective to speak about sharing resources, wealth distribution and sustainable development?

Besides, considering health systems, the management of biomedical waste is one of the biggest problems regarding the management of waste and recycling. The health sector produces a large amount of waste, and it recycles less than other economical sectors; nevertheless, numerous solutions are available. The application of solutions should be required for this economic sector and for the others. In addition to recycling, it could mean, for example, restricting the use of X-rays, of some types of medicines, or limiting interventions that produce too much waste.

The countries or states, which support at big expense the training of future health professionals, should clearly give the wished orientations. The health professionals must not only be trained to save lives, cure diseases, and apply biomedical techniques, but also to protect life in a perspective of sustainable development. They have to become aware of the long-term consequences of daily choices made in clinical practices and research.

Researches in many fields could improve knowledge in this domain. Satariano and McAuley (2003) suggested, for example, studying the links between social capital and self-efficacy beliefs, the relationships between social groups or the impact of town-planning on health. Other authors suggest using human health as an indicator of the healthiness of the environment, what could allow setting up solutions more quickly than by studying ecosystems (Cook, Jardines, and Weinstein, 2004). As such, indicators must be defined, as well as measurement methods and analysis, which constitutes a vast field of research (Cook, Jardines, and Weinstein, 2004; Mather, White, Langlois, Shorter, Swalm, Shaffer, and Hartley, 2004). To estimate the effects of interventions in an ecological perspective, indicators and methods of evaluation of the environment and interactions will notably have to be developed. Computers and information technologies allow stocking information for future consultation. Maybe, it can help the collective memory for identifying long-term viable solutions, learning from past events, and not repeating the same errors.

Beyond studies and principles, beyond thinking globally, applying a principle of sustainable development, and adopting a promotion and prevention perspective, it is necessary to adopt a new philosophy of life and intervention, new values of solidarity and respect. The adoption of such values can put humans shielded from errors, which the lack of knowledge and desire of short-term earning can provoke. These aspects are developed in the next paragraphs.

6.2.2. Looking for a Balance

The ecological model of Lawton (1986) suggests finding the optimal fit between demands of the environment and capacities of ageing people, to allow them to remain autonomous at home and to improve their quality of life. If this model is applied in a more general way to all human populations, an ecological approach consists in designing environments that correspond to human skills, no more and no less. A too much easy environment is less stimulating and does not allow the development of capacities and mechanisms of self-control and self-regulation, including complex brain development. The environment has to present a reasonable amount of challenges to allow people to develop and become resilient. When designing such environments, human beings must not be considered in a reductionist way, as a series of organs-machines to set up, but as complex living species, including all their dimensions (physical, affective, cognitive, volitional, spiritual, etc.) and their interactions with the environment. The environment does not, either, have to be too much demanding for human beings; it must respect critical periods of development in early life, it does not have to contain life harmful substances, work organization must be conceived in order to respect human characteristics, etc.

Human occupations are among the main health and life quality determinants. One of the priority targets is thus mainly situated from the point of view of our lifestyle, which can voluntarily be modified in order to adopt a more ecologically long-term viable lifestyle. Numerous advices are now widely diffused for the adoption of a healthier lifestyle (food, exercises, recycling, etc.). Each one has to convince him/her of the relevance of this new lifestyle and then take action. Beacons are also in place for communities and populations; for example: laws, town-planning, socially responsible industries, renewable energy, etc.

The objective aimed in the establishment of a new well-balanced lifestyle, which can remain in the long run, in a perspective of sustainable development. To reach such an objective, self-control, self-regulation, and will are essential. Furthermore, humans have to demonstrate as much as determination as they had to go on the moon in order to succeed. It implies every person and every professional individually, associations that represent them, managers, decision-makers, universities, organisms, groups that subsidize research, politicians, etc. All the branches of society and all the disciplines are called in the research for this balance.

The oriental philosophy, placing the collective well-being before the individual one, can serve as a reference (Taylor, 2002). It means, however, a deep transformation because the model based on individual success and productivity is powerful in industrialized societies. Another way of rethinking societies and health systems would be to revise them in the perspective of renewable energies. If life and services were organized as if there was no oil, before the arrival of a possible oil crisis, it would mean a more rational and sustainable resource exploitation, less devastating wars, replacement of all oil by-products (let us think of all the plastic products used in the field of health), a service organization favouring interventions closer if possible to people's homes, etc. Indeed, our way of life would probably disappear with the end of the oil era, and a new era would come. In the current situation, this deadline should come as soon as possible, in a controlled, planned, and willing manner, to avoid wars and disasters. Humans are ingenious and have great adaptation skills; they could even reach a higher quality of life without oil.

Reaching a balance, which can remain for a long time in our way of life, will be, without a doubt, difficult to establish. It is an excicting challenge involving all countries, governments, industries, researchers, professionals, etc. However, if people do not make it voluntarily, with all the wisdom it asks, then maybe the disasters and human suffering will oblige us to make it.

CONCLUSION

After this browsing, what do people have to retain about ecological models and approaches in the field of health? First, that it is more about an emerging science, a philosophy, or a way of thinking than a precise mode of intervention. Second, this approach follows the evolution of knowledge toward a better understanding of the complexity of the world and human beings. In the progressive taming of complexity, other theoretical referents are already in development, notably with the theory of chaos (Grebogi, and Yorke, 1997; Lewin, 2000).

Finally, humans still do not measure the consequences of the presence of so many human beings on planet earth; this situation never occurred before in the known history of humanity. At the same time, it is the first time that humans can have a global awareness. Communications with practically all continents are possible and immediate. Information about what happened almost everywhere on earth is available. Knowledge about the evolution of life, the history of the human species, the place of earth in the universe, as well as the characteristics of other planets (Venus or Mars for example), allow making wiser decisions about the future. Human's behaviour and regulation mechanisms are also better understood. A relative humility also ensues from this knowledge; humans are only a quirk of the evolution in an environment that was, at the origin, favourable for life. Humans become aware of the fragility of the balance and of the exceptional position that allowed the beginning of life on earth and the evolution leading to the human species. Evolution could continue with a little luck and a great determination, if every generation would accept the responsibility for leaving after its passage a planet where it is possible to live. Monkeys or prehistoric men living before Homo sapiens could not imagine the new skills our species would develop (symbolization, self-control, adaptability, etc.). In the same manner, it is impossible for us to conceive the new skills of future species that will appear after the Homo sapiens. Humans have, maybe, the ultimate responsibility for allowing life to continue to evolve toward something that still cannot be imagined exactly ... As the appearance of new skills or new species can take tens of thousands of years and even more, there is a big challenge in front of humanity. On the other hand, human capacities are immense and they can be multiplied tenfold by technical means and communication technologies among others. Humans have awareness, knowledge, and immense means. They now need an individual and collective sense of responsibilities towards life and future generations' health.

REFERENCES

Aitken, S., and Morgan, J. (1999). How Motorola promotes good health. *The Journal for Quality and Participation*, 22(1): 54-57.

Alsaker, S., and Josephsson, S. (2003). Negotiating occupational identities while living with chronic rheumatic disease. *Scandinavian Journal of Occupational Therapy*, 10, 167-176.

Andremont, A., Brun-Buisson, C., and Struenens, M. (2001). Evaluating and predicting the ecologic impact of antibiotics. *Clinical Microbiological Infectious*, 7(Suppl 15): 1-6.

Antoni, M.H., Schneiderman, N., Fletcher, M.A., Goldstein, D.A., Ieronson, G., and Laperriere, A. (1990). Psychoneuroimmunology and HIV-1. *Journal of Consulting and Cllinical Mychology*, 58: 38-49.

Ashton, J., and Seymour, H. (1988). *The new public health*. Buckingham: Open University Press.

Aubier, M., Neukirch, F., and Annesi-Maesano, I. (2005). Epidemiology of asthma and allergies. The prevalence of allergies increases worldwide, and asthma has reached his highest-ever prevalence in Europe: Why? *Bulletin of Academic Natural Medicine*, 189(7): 1419-1434.

Bachman, K.A. (2004). *Drug interactions handbook: The new standard for drug interaction*, 2nd Edition. Ohio: LEXI-COMP.

Bagley, C., and Mallick, K. (2000). Spiralling up and spiralling down: Implications of a long-term study of temperament and conduct disorder for social work with children. *Child and Family Social Work*, 5: 291-301.

Baird, P.A. (1996). Le rôle de la génétique dans la santé des populations. In: R.G. Evans, M.L. Barer, and T.R. Marmor. *Être ou ne pas être en bonne santé*. Chap. 5 (pp. 143-168). Montréal, QC: Presses de l'Université de Montréal.

Bambrick, P., and Bonder, B. (2005). Older adults' perception of work. *Work*, 24: 77-84.

Bandura, A. (1986). *Social foundations of thought and action: A social cognitive theory*. Englewood Cliffs, NJ. : Prentice-Hall.

Bandura, A. (2003). *Auto-efficacité. Le sentiment d'efficacité personnelle*. Traduit de l'anglais par Jacques Lecompte. Paris: De Boeck.

Bandura, A. (2001). Social cognitive theory: An agentic perspective. *Annual Review of Psychology*, 52: 1-26.

Bandura, A. (1991). Self-regulation mechanism in psyiological activation and health-promoting behavior. In: J. Madden IV (Ed.) *Neurobiology of learning, emotion and affect* (pp. 229-270). New York: Raven.

Bandura, A., O' Leary, A., Taylor, C.B., Gauthier, J., and Gossard, D. (1987). Perceived self-efficacy and pain control: Opioid and nonopioid mechanisms. *Journal of Personality and Social Psychology*, 53: 563-571.

Barker, R.G. (1968). *Ecological psychology: Concepts and methods for studying the environment of human behavior.* Stanford, CA: Stanford University.

Barker, D.J. (2004a). Developmental origins of adult health and disease. *Journal of Epidemiological Community Health.* 58(2): 114-115.

Barker, D.J. (2004b). The developmental origins of adult disease. *Journal of the American College of Nutrition*, 23(Suppl 6): 588S-595S.

Barkley, R.A. (2001). The executive functions and self-regulation: An evolutionnary neuropsychological perspective. *Neuropsychological Review*, 11(1): 1-29.

Barnard, S., and Wiles, R. (2001). Evidence-based physiotherapy: Physiotherapists' attitudes and experiences in the Wessex area. *Physiotherapy*, 87(3):115-124.

Barrett, R., Kuzawa, C.W., McDade, T., and Armelagos, G.J. (1998). Emerging and re-emerging infectious diseases: The third epidemiologic transition. *Annual Review of Anthropology*, 27: 247-271.

Bartley, M., Blane, D., and Smith, G.D. (1998). Introduction: Beyond the Black Report. *Sociology of Health and Illness*, 20(5): 563-577.

Baumeister, R.F., DeWall, C.N., Ciarocco, N.J., and Twenge, J.M. (2005). Social exclusion impairs self-regulation. *Journal of Personality Social Psychology*, 88(4): 589-604.

Bayot, A., Capafons, A., and Cardena, E. (1997). Emotional self-regulation therapy: A new and efficacious treatment for smoking. *American Journal of Clinical of Hypnosis*, 40(2): 146-156.

Beauregard, M., Paquette, V., and Levesque, J. (2006). Dysfunction in the neural circuitry of emotional self-regulation in major depressive disorder. *Neuroreport*, 17(8): 843-846.

Begley, S. (1999). Shaped by life in the womb. *Science and Technology*, Newweek September 27: 50-57.

Bélanger, J.P., Sullivan, R., and Sévigny, B. (2000). *Capital social, développement communautaire et santé publique, réflexions sur la santé et le bien-être de la population.* Montréal: Association de santé publique du Québec (ASPQ).

Berrigan, D., and Troiano, R.P. (2002). The association between urban form and physical activity in U.S. adults. *American Journal of Preventive Medicine*, 23(Suppl 2): 74-79.

Best, A., Stokols, D., Green, L.W., Leischow, S., Holmes, B., and Buchholz, K. (2003). An integrative framework for community partnering to translate theory into effective health promotion strategy. *American Journal of Health Promotion*, 18(2): 168-176.

Blanchard, L.T., Gurka, M.J., and Blackman, J.A. (2006). Emotional, developmental, and behavioral health of American children and their families: A report from the 2003 National Survey of Children's Health. *Pediatrics*, 117(6): e1202-e1212.

Boerma, J.T., Gregson, S., Nyamukapa, C., and Urassa, M. (2004). Understanding the uneven spread of HIV within Africa: Comparative study of biologic, behavioural, and contextual factors in rural populations in Tanzania and Zimbabwe. *Sex Transmissible Disease*, 31(6): 365.

Bowlby, J. (1969). *Attachment and loss: Vo.1. Attachment.* New-York: Allyn and Bacon.

Borg, E. (2000). Ecological aspects of auditory rehabilitation. *Acta Oto-Laryngologica*, 120: 234-241.

Bornstein, M.H., Haynes, M.O., and Painter, K.M. (1998). Sources of child vocabulary competence: A multivariate model. *Journal of Child Language*, 25: 367-393.

Bourdieu, P. (1990). *The logic of practice*. CA: Stanford University Press.

Bronfenbrenner, U. (1977). Toward an experimental ecology of human development. *American Psychologist*, 32: 513-530.

Bronfenbrenner, U. (1979). *The ecology of human development: Experiments by nature and design*. Cambridge, MA: Harward.

Brundtland Commission (1987). *Our common future*. Oxford University Press. Retreived 2006-10-15 from http://are.admin.ch/are/en/nachhaltig/international_uno/unterseite02330/).

Buckner, J.C., Mezzacappa, E., and Beardslee, W.R. (2003). Characteristics of resilient youths living in poverty: The role of self-regulatory processes. *Developmental Psychopathology*, 15(1): 139-162.

Bujold, C. (1989). *Choix professionnel et développement de carrière, théorie et recherches*. Gaëtan Morin Éditeur, Editions ESKA.

Byers, J.F. (1997). Holistic acute care units: Partnerships to meet the needs of the chronically ill and their families. *AACN Clinical Issues*, 8(2): 271-279.

Calvert, W.J. (1997). Protective factors within the family, and their role in fostering resiliency in African American adolescents. *Journal of Culture Diversity*, 4(4): 110-117.

Caldwell, P. (1996). Child survival: Physical vulnerability and resilience in adversity in the European past and the contemporary Third World. *Social Science and Medicine*, 43(5): 609-619.

Campbell, N.A. (1995). *Biology*. The Benjamin/Cumming Publishing Company Inc.

Canadian Association of Occupational Therapists (CAOT) (1997; 2002). *Enabling occupation: An occupational therapists perspective*. Ottawa, ON: CAOT Publications ACE.

Canadian Cancer Society (2007). *Prevention*. Retreive 2007-01-20 from: http://www.cancer.ca/ccs/internet/niw_splash/0%2C%2C3172%2C00.html.

Cassidy, J. (1999). The nature of the child's ties. In: J. Cassidy, and P. Shavers (Eds.). *Handbook of attachment: Theory, research and clinical applications* (pp. 3-20). New York: Guilford Press.

Charmaz, K. (1994). Discoveries of self in illness. In : M.L. Dietz, R. Prus, and W. Shaffer. *Doing everyday life. Ethnography as human lived experience* (pp. 226-242). Missisauga, ON: Copp Clark Longman Ltd.

Charmaz, K. (1995). The body, identity and self: Adapting to impairment. *Sociological Quarterly*, 36: 657-680.

Charmaz, K. (2002). The self as habit: The reconstruction of self in chronic illness. *Occupational Therapy Journal of Research*, 22 Suppl: 31S-41S.

Charpak, et al. (2005). Kangaroo mother care: 25 years after. *Acta Paediatric.* 94(5): 514-522.

Christiansen, C., Baum, C.M., and Bass-Haugen, J. (2005). *Occupational therapy: Performance, participation, and well-being*. Thorofare, NJ: Slack, 3rd ed.

Chu, C., and Simpson, R. (1994). *Ecological public health: From vision to practice*. Toronto: University of Toronto Center for Health Promotion.

Cloutier, R. (1996). *Psychologie de l'adolescence*. Québec: Gaëtan Morin Éditeur.

Cnaan, R.A., Blankertz, L., Messinger, K.W., and Gardner, J.R. (1988). Psychosocial rehabilitation: Toward a definition. *Psychosocial Rehabilitation Journal*, 11(4): 61-77.

Cohen, S., Tyrrel, D.A.J., and Smith, A.P. (1991). Psychological stress and susceptibility to the common cold. *New England Journal of Medicine*, 325: 606-612.

Condeluci, A. (1995). *Interdependence: The route to community*. Boca Raton, FL: CRC Press.

Connor, M. (2000). Recreational folk dance: A multicultural exercise component in healthy ageing. *Australian Occupational Therapy Journal*, 47(2): 69-76.

Connor Schisler, A.M., and Polatajko, H.J. (2002). The individual as mediator of the person-occupation-environment interaction: Learning from the experience of refugees. *Journal of Occupational Science*, 9(2): 82:92.

Cook, A., Jardine, A., and Weinstein, P. (2004). Using human disease outbreaks as a guide to multilevel ecosystem interventions. *Environmental Health Perspective*, 112(11): 1143-1146.

Cooper, R.S., Kennelly, J.F., Durazo-Arvizu, R., Oh, J.J., Kaplan, G., and Lynch, J. (2001). Relationship between premature mortality and socioeconomic factors in black and white populations of US metropolitain areas. *Public Health Report*, 116(5): 464-473.

Cope, M.B., and Allison, D.B. (2006). Obesity: Person and population. *Obesity*, 14 (Suppl 4): 156S-159S.

Corcoran, J., Franklin, C., and Bennet, P. (2000). Ecological factors associated with adolescent pregnancy and parenting. *Social Work Research*, 24(1): 29-39.

Cowen, P.S. (2001). Crisis child care: Implications for family interventions. *Journal of the American Psychiatric Nurses Association*, 7(6): 196-204.

Craddock, J. (1996). Responses of the occupational therapy profession to the perspective of the disability movement, Part 2. *British Journal of Occupational Therapy*, 59(2): 73-78.

Crépeau, F., and Scherzer, P. (1993). Predictors and indicators of work status after traumatic brain injury: A meta-analysis. *Neuropsychology and Rehabilitation*, 3: 5-35.

Crews, D., and McLachlan, J.A. (2006). Epigenetics, evolution, endocrine disruption, health, and disease. *Endocrinology*, 147(Suppl 6): S4-S10.

Crisp, R. (1992). Return to work after traumatic brain injury. *Journal of Rehabilitation*, 4: 27-33.

Dahlgren, G., and Whitehead, M. (1991). *Reducing inequalities in health*. Wellington: Ministry of Health.

Day, K., Carreon, D., and Stump, C. (2000). The therapeutic design of environments for people with dementia: A review of the empirical research. *Gerontologist*, 40(4): 397-416.

De Chateau, P. (1988). The interaction between the infant and the environment: The importance of mother-child contact after delivery. *Acta Paediatr Scandinavian Suppl.* 344: 21-30.

De Hope, E., and Finegan, J. (1999). The self determination model: an approach to develop awareness for survivors of traumatic brain injury. *NeuroRehabilitation*, 13: 3-12.

Delgado, M. (1996). Implementing a natural support system AOD Project: Administrative considerations and recommendations. *Alcoholism Treatment Quarterly*, 14(2): 1-14.

Dickie, V.A. (2003). Establishing worker identity: A study of people in craft work. *American Journal of Occupational Therapy*, 57: 250-261.

Direction des communications du ministère de la Santé et des Services sociaux (2005). *Les services intégrés en périnatalité pour la petite enfance à l'intention des familles vivant en contexte de vulnérabilité. Guide pour soutenir le développement de l'attachement sécurisant de la grossesse à un an*. Québec: Ministère de la Santé et des Services sociaux du Québec.

Drain, P.K., Smith, J.S., Hughes, J.P., Halperin, D.T., and Holmes, K.K. (2004). Correlates of national HIV seroprevalence: An ecologic analysis of 122 developing countries. *Journal of Acquire Immune Deficiency Syndrome*, 35(4): 407-420.

Dreiling, D.S., and Bundy, A.C. (2003). A comparison of consultative model and direct-indirect intervention with preschoolers. *American Journal of Occupational Therapy*, 57(5): 566-569.

Dumont, C., Gervais, M., Fougeyrollas, P., and Bertrand, R. (2004). Toward an explanatory model of social participation of adults with traumatic brain injury. *Journal of Head Trauma Rehabilitation*, 19(4): 431-444.

Dumont, C., and Rainville, F. (2006). Self, identity and occupation. In: A.M. Columbus (ed.) *Advances in psychology research*, Vol. 45. Chap. 9 (pp. 181-227). New York: Nova Science Publishers, Inc.

Durand, M., Vachon, B., Loisel, P., and Berthelette, D. (2003). Constructing the program impact theory for an evidence-based work rehabilitation program for workers with low back pain. *WORK: A journal of prevention assessment and rehabilitation*, 21(3): 233-42.

Eckert, J. K., and Murrey, M.I. (1984). Alternative modes of living for the elderly: A critical review. In: I. Altman, P.M. Lawton, and J.F. Wohlwill (Eds), *Elderly people and the environment* (pp. 95-128). New York: Plenum Press.

Effken, J.A. (2001). Nursing theory and concept development or analysis: Information basis for expert intuition. *Journal of Advanced Nursing*, 34(2): 246-255.

Elstad, J.I. (1998). The psycho-social perspective on social inequalities in health. *Sociology of Health and Illness*, 20(5): 598-618.

Eraly, A. (1986). *La structuration de l'entreprise: La rationalité en action*. Bruxelles: Éditions de l'Université de Bruxelles.

Evans, R.W. (1999). Predicting outcomes following traumatic brain injury. *Journal of Rehabilitation Outcomes Measurement*, 3(2): 49-55.

Evans, R.G., Barer, M.L., and Marmor, T.R. (1996). *Etre ou ne pas être en bonne santé. Biologie et déterminants sociaux de la maladie*. Montréal, QC: Presses de l'Université de Montréal.

Evans, R.G., and Stoddard, G.L. (1996). Produire la santé, consommer les soins. In: R.G. Evans, M.L. Barer, and T.R. Marmor. *Etre ou ne pas être en bonne santé. Biologie et déterminants sociaux de la maladie*. Chap. 2 (pp. 37-73). Montréal, QC: Presses de l'Université de Montréal,

Ewing, R., Schmid, T., Killingsworth, R., Zlot, A., and Raudenbush, S. (2003). Relationship between urban sprawl and physical activity, obesity, and morbidity. *American Journal of Health Promotion*, 18(1): 47-57.

Farmer, J.E., Marien, W.E., Clark, M.J., Sherman, A., and Selva, T.J. (2004). Primary care supports for children with chronic health conditions: Identifying and predicting unmet family needs. *Journal of Pediatric Psychology*, 29(5): 355-367.

Felitti, V.J., Anda, R.F., Nordenberg, D., Williamson, D.F., Spitz, A.M., Edwards, V., et al. (1998). Relationship of childhood abuse and household dysfunction to many of the leading causes of death in adults. The adverse childhood experiences (ACE) study. *American Journal of Preventive Medicine,* 14(4): 245-258.

Ferland, F. (1994). *Le modèle ludique: Le jeu, l'enfant avec déficience physique et l'ergothérapie*. Montréal, QC: Presses de l'Université de Montréal.

Finn, P. (2003). Self-regulation and the management of stuttering. *Seminar in Speech Language*, 24(1): 27-32.

Fortune, D.G., Smith, J.V., and Garvey, K. (2005). Perception of psychosis, coping, appraisals, and psychological distress in the relatives of patients with schizophrenia: An exploration using self-regulation theory. *British Journal of Clinical Psychology*, 44(Pt3): 319-331.

Fougeyrollas, P. (1997). Les déterminants environnementaux de la participation sociale des personnes ayant des incapacités: le défi socio-politique de la révision de la CIDIH. *Canadian Journal of Rehabilitation*, 10(2): 147-160.

Fougeyrollas, P. (2001). Le processus de production du handicap : l'expérience québécoise. In : R. DeRiedmatten, *Une nouvelle approche de la différence*. Genève : Médecine et Hygiène.

Fougeyrollas, P., Cloutier, R., Bergeron, H., Côté, J., Côté M., and St-Michel, G. (1996). *Révision de la proposition québécoise de classification: Processus de production du handicap*. Lac St-Charles, Québec: CQCIDIH/SCCIDIH.

Fougeyrollas, P., and Beauregard, L. (2001). Disability: An interactive person-environment social creation. In: G.L. Albrecht, and K.D. Seelman (Eds). *Handbook of Disability Studies*. Michael Burry: Sage.

Fougeyrollas, P., Noreau, L., and Boschen, K.A. (2002). Interaction of environment with individual characteristics and social participation: Theoretical perspectives and applications in persons with spinal cord injury. *Topic in Spinal Cord injury Rehabilitation*, 7(3): 1-16.

Freeman, E.A. (1997). Community-based rehabilitation of the person with a severe brain injury. *Brain Injury*, 11(2): 143-153.

Frentzel-Beyme, R., and Grossarth-Maticek, R. (2001). The interaction between risk factors and self-regulation in the development of chronic diseases. *International Journal of Hygiene and Environmental Health*, 204(1): 81-88.

Frolich, K.L., Corin, E., and Potvin, L. (2001). A theoretical proposal for the relationship between context and disease. *Sociology of Health and Illness*, 23(6): 776-797.

Gadoury, M. (1999). *Cadre de référence clinique pour l'élaboration de programmes de réadaptation pour la clientèle qui a subi un traumatisme cranio-cérébral. Volet adulte*. Direction des politiques et programmes pour les accidentés. Service de la programmation en réadaptation, Société de l'assurance automobile du Québec.

Gagnier, J.P., and Lachapelle, R. (2002). *Pratiques émergentes en déficience intellectuelle. Participation plurielle et nouveaux rapports*. Collection Pratiques et politiques sociales. Québec: Presses de l'Université du Québec.

Gandhi, M., Aweeka, F., Greenblatt, R.M., and Blaschke, T.F. (2004). Sex differences in pharmacokinetics and pharmacodynamics. *Annual Review of Pharmacology and Toxicology*, 44: 499-523.

Germaine, C. (1984). *Social work practice in health care: An ecological perspective*. New York: The Free Press.

Gibson, E. (1988). Exploratory behavior in the development of perceiving, acting, and acquiring of knowledge. *Annual Review Psychology*, 39: 1-41.

Gibson, J. (1977). The theory of affordances. In: R. Shaw, and J. Bransford (Eds.), *Perceiving, acting and knowing* (pp. 67-82). Hillsdale, NJ: Erlbaum.

Giddens, A. (1984). *The constitution of society.* Campbridge: Polity Press.

Gluckman, P., and Hanson, M. (2005). *The fetal matrix: Evolution, development and disease.* Cambridge: Cambridge University Press.

Gluckman, P.D., and Hanson, M.A. (2006). The consequences of being born small- an adaptive perspective. *Homornal Research*, 65 (Suppl 3): 5-14.

Gluckman, P.D., Hanson, M.A., and Pinal, C. (2005). The developmental origins of adult disease. *Maternal Child Nutrition*, 1(3): 130-141.

Goldberg, S., Blokland, K., and Myhal, N. (2000). Le récit de deux histoires: l'attachement, le tempérament et la régulation des émotions. In: G.M. Tarabulsy, S. Larose, D.R. Pederson, and G. Moran (Eds.). *Attachement et développement: le rôle des premières relations dans le développement humain* (pp. 57-90). Québec: Presses de l'Université du Québec.

Gonder-Frederick, L.A., Cox, D.J., and Ritterband, L.M. (2002). Diabetes and behavioral medicine: The second decade. *Journal of Consulting and Clinical Psychology*, 70(3): 611-625.

Goodall, P., and Ghiloni, C.T. (2001). The changing face of publicly funded employment services. *Journal of Head Trauma Rehabilitation*, 16(1): 94-106.

Gould, S.J. (1999). *Rocks of ages: Science and religion in the fullness of life.* U.S.A.: The Ballantine Publishing Group.

Graham, S.F. (2002). Dance: A transformative occupation. *Journal of Occupational Science*, 9(3): 128-134.

Grandjean, E. (1988). *Man-machine systems. Fitting the task to the man: An ergonomic approach.* London: Taylor and Francis.

Grant, W.B. (2002). An ecologic study of dietary and solar ultraviolet-B links to breast carcinoma mortality rates. *Cancer*, 94(1): 272-281.

Grant, W.B. (2004). A multicountry ecologic study of risk and risk reduction factors for prostate cancer mortality. *European Urology*, 45(3): 271-279.

Grebogy, C., and Yorke, J.A. (Eds) (1997). *The impact of chaos on science and society.* Tokyo: United Nations University Press.

Green, A., Payne, S., and Barnitt, R. (2004). Illness representations among people with non-epileptic seizures attending a neuropsychiatry clinic: A qualitative study based on the self-regulation model. *Seizure*, 13(5): 331-339.

Green, L.W., and Kreuter, M.W. (1999). *Health promotion planning an educational and ecological approach* (3rd edition) (pp.xxv-49). Mayfields: Mountain View.

Green, L.W., Richard, L, and Potvin, L. (1996). Ecological foundations of health promotion. *American Journal of Health Promotion*, 16(4): 270-281.

Gross, L.S., Li, L., Ford, E.S., and Liu, S. (2004). Increased consumption of refined carbohydrates and the epidemic of type 2 diabetes in the United States: An ecologic assessment. *American Journal of Clinical Nutritionist*, 79(5): 774-779.

Gruber, B., Hall, N.R., Hersh, S.P., and Dubois, P. (1988). Immune system and psychologic changes in metastatic cancer patients using relaxation and guided imagery: A pilot study. *Scandinavian Journal of Behaviour Therapy*, 17: 25-46.

Gulis, G., Czompolyova, M., and Cerhan, J.R. (2002). An ecologic study of nitrate in municipal drinking water and cancer incidence in Trnava District, Slovakia. *Environmental Research*, 88(3): 182-187.

Gutierrez, R. (2001). Inside the brain, the frontal lobe and social behaviour. *Premier Outlook*, 2(2): 19.

Gutman, S.A. (1997). Enhancing gender role satisfaction in adult males with traumatic brain injury: A set of guidelines for occupational therapy practice. *Occupational Therapy in Mental Health*, 13(4): 25-43.

Harman, G., and Clare, L. (2006). Illness representation and lived experience in early-stage dementia. *Qualitative Health Research*, 16(4): 484-502.

Harvey, M.R. (1996). An ecological view of psychological trauma and trauma recovery. *Journal of Traumatic Stress*, 9(1): 3-23.

Hébert, M., Maheux, B., and Potvin, L. (2002). Théories qui émergent du quotidien de la pratique communautaire de l'ergothérapie. *Journal canadien d'ergothérapie*, 69(1): 31-39.

Hensrud, D.D., and Klein, S. (2006). Extreme obesity: A new medical crisis in the United States. Mayo Clinical Proceeding, 81(Suppl 10): S5-S10.

Herbert, T.B., and Cohen, S. (1993). Stress and immunity in humans: A meta-analytic review. *Psychosomatic Medicine*, 55: 364-379.

Heyn, P., Abreu, B.C., and Ottenbacher, K.J. (2004). The effects of exercice training on elderly persons with cognitive impairment and dementia: A meta-analysis. *Archives of Physical Medicine and Rehabilitation*, 85: 1694-1704.

Hibbards, M.R., et al. (2002). Peer support in the community: Initial findings of a mentoring program for individuals with traumatic brain injury and their families. *Journal of Head Trauma and Rehabilitation*, 17(2): 112-131.

Hocking, C. (2000). Having and using objects in the Western world. *Journal of Occupational Science*, 7(3): 148-157.

Homer-Dixon, T. (2001). *The ingenuity gap: How can we solve the problems of the future?* Toronto: Vintage.

Howie, L. (2003). Ritualising in book clubs: Implications for evolving occupational identities. *Journal of Occupational Science*, 10(3): 130-139.

Huizink, A.C., Mulder, E.J., and Buitelaar, J.K. (2004). Prenatal stress and risk for psychopathology: Specific effect or induction of general susceptibility? *Psychological Bulletin*, 130(1): 115-142.

Jacobs, H.E. (1997). The Clubhouse: Addressing work-related behavioral challenges through a supportive social community. *Journal of Head Trauma and Rehabilitation*, 12(5): 14-27.

Jacqueminet, S., Masseboeuf, N., Rolland, M., Grimaldi, A., and Sachon, C. (2005). Limitation of the so-called "intensified" insulin therapy in type I diabetes mellitus. *Diabetes Meabolism*, 31(4 Pt 2): 4S45-4S50.

Jerrett, M., Burnett, R.T., Willis, A., Krewski, D., Goldberg, M.S., DeLuca, P., and Finkelstein, N. (2003). Spatial analysis of the air pollution-mortality relationship in the context of ecologic confounders. *Journal of Toxicological Environmental Health*, 66(16-19): 1735-1777.

Jirikowic, T., Stika-Monson, R., Knight, A., Hutchinson, S., Washington, K., and Kartin, D. (2001). Contemporary trends and practice strategies in pediatric occupational and physical therapy. *Physical and Occupational Therapy in Pediatrics*, 20(4): 45-62.

Johanson, A., Risberg, J., Tucker, D.M., and Gustafson, L. (2006). Changes in frontal lobe activity with cognitive therapy for spider phobia. *Applied Neuropsychology*, 13(1): 34-41.

Johnston, C.C., et al. (2003). Kangaroo care is effective in diminishing pain response in preterm neonates. *Archives of Pediatric and Adolescence Medicine*, 157: 1084-1088.

Johnson, J.E. (1999). Self-regulation theory and coping with physical illness. *Research in Nursing Health*, 22(6): 435-448.

Johnson, J.E., Fieler, V.K., Wlasowicz, G.S., Mitchell, M.L., and Jones, L.S. (1997). The effects of nursing care guide by self-regulatory theory on coping with radiation therapy. *Oncology Nursing Forum*, 24(6): 1041-1050.

Junien, C., Gallou-Kabani, C., Vige, A., and Gross, M.S. (2005). Nutritional epigenomics of metabolic syndrome. *Medical Science (Paris)*, 21 Spec. No.: 44-52.

Kahana, E. (1982). A congruence model of person-environment interaction. In: M.P. Lawton, P.G. Windley, and T.O. Byerts (Eds.), *Aging and the environment: Theoretical approaches*. Chap. 7 (pp. 97-120), New York: Springer Publishing Company.

Kar, S.B., Pascual, C.A., and Chickering, K.L. (1999). Empowerment of women for health promotion: A meta-analysis. *Social Science and Medicine,* 49: 1431-1460.

Kawachi, I. (1997). Social capital, income inequality and mortality. *American Journal of Public Health*, 87(9): 1491-1497.

Kawachi, I., Kennedy, B.P., and Glass, R. (1999). Social capital and self-rated health: A contextual analysis. *American Journal of Public Health*, 89(8): 1187-1193.

Kawachi, I., Kennedy, B.P., and Wilkinson, R.G. (1999). Crime: Social disorganization and relative deprivation. *Social Science and Medicine*, 48(6): 719-731.

Kellegrew, H. D., and Kroksmark, U. (1999). Examining school routines using time-geography methodology. *Physical and Occupational Therapy in Pediatrics*, 19(2): 79-91.

Kelly, S., Hertzman, C., and Daniels, M. (1997). Searching fort he biological pathways between stress and health. *Annual Review of Public Health*, 18: 437-462.

Kelton, R.W. (2001). Facing up to stigma: Workplace and personal strategies. *Cleft Palate Craniofacial Journal*, 38(3): 245-247.

Kennedy, M.R., and Coelho, C. (2005). Self-regulation after traumatic brain injury: A framework for intervention of memory and problem solving. *Seminar in Speech Language*, 26(4): 242-255.

Kennel, J.H., and Klaus, M.H. (1998). Bonding: recent observations that alter perinatal care. *Pediatric Review,* 19(1): 4-12.

Keysor, J.J., and Jette, A.M. (2001). Have we oversold the benefit of late-life exercise? *Journal of Gerontology: Medical Science*, 56: 412-423.

Kiecolt-Glaser, J.K., and Glaser, R. (1988). Behavioral influence on immune function: Evidence for the iterplay between stress and health. In: T. Field, P. McCabe, and N. Schneiderman (Eds.). *Stress and Coping*. Vol. 2 (pp. 189-206). Hillsdale, NJ: Erlbaum.

Kiecolt-Glaser, J.K., et al. (1985). Psychosocial enhancement of immunocompetence in a geriatric population. *Health Psychology*, 4: 25-41.

Kiecolt-Glaser, J.K., et al. (1986). Modulation of cellular immunity in medical students. *Journal of Behavioral Medicine*, 9: 5-21.

Kielhofner, G. (2002). *Model of human occupation. Theory and application.* 3rd Edition. Baltimore: Lippincott Williams and Wilkins.

Kielhofner, G. (2004). *Conceptual foundations of occupational therapy.* 3rd Edition. Philadelphia: F.A. Davis Company.

Kiernat, J.M. (1983). Environment: The hidden modality. *Physical and Occupational Therapy in Geriatrics,* 2(1): 3-12.

King, G., Tucker, M.A., Baldwin, P., Lowry, K., LaPorta, J., and Matens, L. (2002). A life need model of paediatric service delivery: Services to support community participation and quality of life for children and youth with disabilities. *Physical and Occupational Therapy in Pediatrics,* 22(2): 53-77.

Kitsantas, A., Gilligan, T.D., and Kamata, A. (2003). College women with eating disorders: Self-regulation, life satisfaction, and positive/negative affect. *Journal of Psychology,* 137(4): 381-395.

Klaus, M.H., and Kennell, J.H. (1976). *Maternal-infant bonding.* St. Louis: Mosby.

Koschanska, G., Coy, K.C., and Muray, K.T. (2001). The development of self-regulation in the first four years of life. *Child Development,* 72(4): 1091-1111.

Kondrat, M.E. (2002). Actor-centered social work: Re-visioning "Person-in-environment" through a critical theory lens. *Social Work,* 47(4): 435-448.

Kowalske, K., Plenger, P.M., Lusby, B., and Hayden, M.E. (2000). Vocational reentry following TBI: An enablement model. *Journal of Head Trauma Rehabilitation,* 15(4): 989-999.

Krebs, C.J. (2001). *Ecology.* Fifth edition. San Francisco: Benjamin Cummings.

La Marche, J.A., Reed, L.K., Rich, M.A., Cash, A.W., Lucas, L.H., and Boll, T.J. (1995). The interactive community-based model of vocational rehabilitation. *Journal of Head Trauma Rehabilitation,* 10(4): 81-89.

Last, J.M. (1993). Global change: Ozone depletion, greenhouse warming, and public health. *Annual Review of Public Health,* 14: 115-136.

Law, M. (1991). The environment: A focus for occupational therapy. *Canadian Journal of Occupational Therapy,* 58(4): 171-180.

Law, M. (1998). *Family –centered assessment and intervention in pediatric rehabilitation.* Binghamton, NY: The Haworth Press.

Law, M., Cooper, B., Strong, S., Stewart, D., Rigby, P., and Letts, L. (1996). The Person-Environment-Occupation Model: A transactive approach to occupational performance. *Canadian Journal of Occupational Therapy,* 63(1): 9-23.

Lawton, M.P. (1980). *Environment and aging.* Monterey, CA: Brooks/Cole.

Lawton, M.P. (1982). Competence, environmental press and the adaptation of older people. In: M.P., Lawton, P.G. Windley, and T.O. Byerts (Eds.), *Aging and the environment: Theoretical approaches.* Chap. 3 (pp. 33-59). New York: Springer Publishing Company.

Lawton, M.P. (1986). *Environment and Aging.* Philadelphia Geriatric Center, Classics in Aging Reprinted, Series 1, Volume 1, Center for the study of Aging. New York: Albany.

Lawton, M.P., and Nahemow, L. (1973). Ecology and the aging process. In: C. Eisdorfer, and M.P. Lawton (Eds.). *The psychology of adult development and aging.* Washington, DC: American Psychological Association.

LeBlanc, J.M., Hayden, M.E., and Paulman, R.G. (2000). A comparison of neuropsychological and situational assessment for predicting employability after closed head injury. *Journal of Head Trauma Rehabilitation,* 15(4): 1022-1040.

Letts, L., Rigby, P., and Stewart, D. (2003). Guide has a practice of universal accessibility. In: *Using environments to enable occupational performance.* Thorofare, NJ: Slack Incorporated.

Levine, P. (1997). *Walking the tiger.* Berkeley: North Atlantic Books.

Levine, P. (2005). *Healing trauma: A pioneering program for restoring the wisdom of your body.* Boulder CO: Sounds True.

Levy, A.J., and Wall, J.C. (2000). Children who have witnessed community homicide: Incorporating risk and resilience in clinical work. *Families in Society: The Journal of Contemporary Human Services,* 81(4): 402-411.

Lewin, R. (2000). *Complexity: Life at the edge of chaos.* Second Edition. Chicago ILL: University of Chicago Press.

Lloyd, C., and Chandler, L. (1999). Girrebala and the arts in mental health rehabilitation. *British Journal of Therapy and Rehabilitation,* 6(4): 164, 166-168, 170.

Ludingtioin-Hoe, S.M., and Swinth, J.Y. (1996). Developmental aspects of kangaroo care. *Journal of Obstretical gynecological neonatal nursing,* 25(8): 691-703.

Lynch, J.W., Smith, G.D., Kaplan, G.A., and House, J.S. (2000). Income inequality and mortality: Importance to health of individual income, psychosocial environment, or material conditions. *British Medical Journal,* 320(7243): 1200-1204.

Macintyre, S. (1997). The Black report and beyond what are the issues? *Social Science and Medicine,* 44(6): 723-745.

Macintyre, S., and Ellaway, A. (2000) Ecological approaches: Rediscovering the role of the physical and social environment. In: C.F. Berichan, and I. Kawachi (Eds), *Social Epidemiology* (pp. 332-348). New York: Oxford University Press.

Madrid, A. (1991). Maternal-infant bonding and pediatric asthma: An initial investigation. *Journal of Prenatal and Perinatal Psychology and Health.* 5(4): 346-358.

Madrid, A. (2005). Helping children with asthma by reparing maternal-infant bonding problems. *American Journal Clinical Hypnosis.* 48(2-3): 199-211.

Magliano, L., Fiorillo, A., De Rosa, C., Malangone, C., and Maj, M. (2005). Family burden in long-term diseases: A comparative study in schizophrenia vs. physical disorders. *Social Science and Medicine,* 61(2): 313-322.

Margolin, S. (2001). Interventions for nonaggressive peer-rejected children and adolescents: A review of the literature. *Children and Schools,* 23(3): 143-159.

Marmot, M., Ryff, C.D., Bumpass, L.L., Shipley, M., and Marks, N.F. (1997). Social inequalities in health: Next questions and converging evidence. *Social Science and Medicine,* 44(6): 901-910.

Martins, L.C., Latorre, M.R.D., Saldiva, P.H.N., and Braga, A.L.F. (2002). Air pollution and emergency room visits due to chronic lower respiratory diseases in the elderly: An ecological time-series study in Sao Paulo, Brazil. *Journal of Occupational and Environmental Medicine,* 44(7): 622-627, 639.

Mather, F.J., White, L.E., Langlois, E.C., Shorter, C.F., Swalm, C.M., Shaffer, J.G., and Hartley, W.R. (2004). Statistical methods for linking health, exposure and hazards. *Environmental Health Perspective,* 112(14): 1440-1445.

Maton, K.I. (2000). Making a difference: The social ecology of social transformation. *American Journal of Community Psychology,* 28(1): 25-57.

McCartney, K., and Berry, D. (2005). Gene-environment processes in task persistence. *Trends in Cognitive Sciences,* 9(9): 407-408.

McLeroy, K.R., Bibeau, D., Steckler, A., and Glanz, K. (1988). An ecological perspective on health promotion programs. *Health Education Quarterly*, 15(4): 351-377.

McMichael, A.J. (1993). *Planetary overload. Global environmental change and the health of the human species.* Cambridge: Cambridge University Press.

Mead, V.P. (2004). A new model for understanding the role of environmental factors in the origins of chronic illness: A case study of type 1 diabetes mellitus. *Medical Hypotheses*, 63: 1035-1046.

Mead, V.P. (2006) Timing, bonding, and trauma: Applications from experience-dependent maturation and traumatic stress provide insights for understanding environmental origins of disease. In: D.M Devore, Ed. *New Development in Parent-Child Relations.* (pp. 179-264). New York: Nova Science Publishers.

Meaney, M.J., Weaver, I.C.G., Wu, T., Hellstrom, I., Diorio, J., and McGown, P. (2006). Maternal programming of glucocorticoid receptor expression and HPA responses to stress through DNA methylation in the rat. In: D.M. Hodgson, and C.L. Coe, Eds. *Perinatal programming: Early life determinants of adult health and disease* (pp. 309-324). Abingdon, Oxon: Taylor and Francis.

Meibohm, B., Beierle, I., and Derendorf, H. (2002). How important are gender differences in pharmacokinetics? *Clinical Pharmacokinetic*, 41(5): 329-342.

Minkler, M., and Wallerstein, N. (1997). Improving health through community organisation and community building. In: K. Glanz, F.M. Lewis, and B.K. Rimer (Eds.). *Health behavior and health education. Theory, research and practice* (2nd ed.) (pp. 241-269). San Francisco: Jossey-Bass Publishers.

Mohr, W.K., and Mohr, B.D. (2001). Brain, behaviour, connections and implications: Psychodynamics no more. *Archives of Psychiatric Nursing*, 15(4): 171-181.

Molden, D.C., and Dweck, C.S. (2006). Finding "meaning" in psychology: A lay theories approach to self-regulation, social perception, and social development. *American Psychologist*, 61(3): 192-203.

Morgan, G. (1997). *Images of organization.* Sage Publication Inc.

Nash, J.K., and Bowen, G.L. (1999). Perceived crime and informal social control in the neighbourhood as a context for adolescent behavior: A risk for resilience perspective. *Social Work Research*, 23(3): 171-186.

Nathanielsz, P.W. (1999). *Life in the womb. The origin of health and disease.* Ithaca, NY: Promethean.

Naylor, M.D., and Buhler-Wilkerson, K. (1999). Creating community-based care for the new millennium. *Nursing Outlook*, 47(3): 120-127.

Newes-Adeyi, G., Helitzer, D.L., Caulfield, L.E., and Bronner, Y. (2000) Theory and practice: Applying the ecological model to formative research for a WIC training program in New York State. *Health Education Research*, 15(3): 283-291.

Nightingale, F (1869). *Notes on nursing: What it is and what it is not.* New York, NY: Dover.

Ogden, P., Minton, K., and Pain, C. (2006). *Trauma and the body: A sensorimotor approach to psychotherapy.* New York: W.W. Norton.

Ogden, P., Pain, C., and Fisher, J. (2006). A sensorimotor approach to the treatment of trauma and dissociation. *Psychiatric Clinic of North America*, 29(1): 263-279.

O' Leary, A. (1990). Stress, emotion and human immune function. *Psychological Bulletin*, 108: 363-382.

Ottawa Charter for Health Promotion, (1986). World Health Organisation, Health and Welfare Canada. Ottawa: Canadian Association of Public Health.

Ownsworth, T., and Fleming, J. (2005). The relative importance of metacognitive skills, emotional status, and executive function in psychological adjustment following acquired brain injury. *Journal of Head Trauma Rehabilitation*, 20(4): 315-332.

Pain, K., Magill-Evans, J., Darrah, J., Hagler, P., and Warren, S. (2004). Effects of profession and facility type on research utilization by rehabilitation professionals *Journal of Allied Health*, 33(1): 3-9.

Pajares, F. (2003). *Overview of social cognitive theory and of self-efficacy*. Retreived 2003-01-26 from: *http://www.emory.edu/EDUCATION/mfp/eff.html*.

Passmore, A. (2003). The occupation of leisure: Three typologies and their influence on mental health in adolescence. *OTJR: Occupation, Participation and Health*, 23(2): 76-83.

Pelchat, D., and Lefebvre, H. (2002). *Partenariats familles, professionnels, gestionnaires et appropriation des savoirs: vers une continuité des soins et services répondant aux besoins des familles*. Équipe de recherche interdisciplinaire sur la famille. Rapport de recherche. Université de Montréal.

Peters, M.D., Gluck, M., and McCormick M. (1992). Behaviour rehabilitation of the challenging client in less restrictive settings. *Brain Injury*, 6(4): 299-314.

Peterson, C., and Stunkard, A.J. (1989). Personal control and health promotion. *Social Science and Medicine*, 2: 819-828.

Petronella, S.A., and Conboy-Ellis, K. (2003). Astma epidemiology: Risk factors, case finding, and the role of asthma coalitions. *Nuring Clinic of North America*, 38(4): 725-735.

Pickett, K.E., Kelly, S., Brunner, E., Lobstein, T., and Wilkinson, R.G. (2005). Wider income gaps, wider waistbands? An ecological study of obesity and income inequality. *Journal of Epidemiology and Community Health*, 59(8): 670-674.

Planetree (2006). *The Planetree Model*. Retreived 2006-10-10 from www.planetree.org/about/welcome.htm.

Polatajko, H.J., Mandich, A., and Martini, R. (1999). Dynamic performance analysis: A framework for understanding occupational performance. *The American Journal of Occupational Therapy*, 54(1): 65-72.

Popay, J., Williams, G., Thomas, C., and Gatrell, T. (1998).Theorising inequalities in health: The place of lay knowledge. *Sociology of Health and Illness*, 20(5): 619-644.

Posner, M.I. (2005). Genes and experience shape brain networks of conscious control. *Progress in Brain Research*, 150: 173-183.

Posne, M.I., and Rothbart, M.K. (2000). Developing mechanisms of self-regulation. *Developmental Psychopathology*, 12(3): 427-441.

Potter, M., Gordon, S., and Hamer, P. (2003). The physiotherapy experience in private practice: the patients' perspective. *Australian Journal of Physiotherapy*, 49(3): 195-212.

Poulsen, A.A., and Ziviani, J.M. (2004). Can I play too? Physical activity engagement of children with developmental coordination disorders. *Canadian Journal of Occupational Therapy*, 71(2): 100-107.

Purves, B., and Suto, M. (2004). In limbo: Creating continuity of identity in a discharge planning unit. *Canadian Journal of Occupational Therapy*, 71(3): 173-181.

Racine, L. (1999). Les formes d'action sociale réciproque: dyades et triades. *Sociologie et société*, Vol. XXXI, No. 1.

Rahkonen, O., Lahelma, E., and Huuhka, M. (1997). Past or present? Childhood living conditions and current socioeconomic status as determinants of adult health. *Social Science and Medicine,* 44(3): 327-336.

Ratcliff, E., Farnworth, L., and Lentin, P. (2002). Journey of wholeness: The experience of engaging in physical occupation for women survivors of childhood abuse. *Journal of Occupational Science,* 9(2): 65-71.

Rauch, R.J., and Ferry, S.M. (2001). Social networks as support interventions following traumatic brain injury. *Neurorehabilitation,* 16: 11-16.

Reeves, H., and Levoir, F. (2003). *Mal de terre.* Collection Science ouverte. Paris: Seuil.

Reifsnider, E. (1995). The use of human ecology and epidemiology in nonorganic failure to thrive. *Public Health Nursing,* 12(4): 262-268.

Remondet Wall, J., Rosenthal, M., and Niemczura, J.G. (1998). Community-based training after acquired brain injury: Preliminary findings. *Brain Injury,* 12(3): 215-224.

Resnick, M.D. (2000). Protective factors, resiliency and healthy youth development. *Adolescence Medicine,* 11(1): 157-165.

Reuille, K.M. (2002). Using self-regulation theory to develop an intervention for cancer-related fatigue. *Clinical Nursing Specialist,* 16(6): 312-319.

Reynolds, F. (2003). Reclaiming a positive identity in chronic illness through artistic occupation. *Occupational Therapy Journal of Research,* 23(3): 118-127.

Richard, L., Potvin, L., Kishchuk, N., Prlic, H., and Green, L.W. (1996). Assessment of the integration of the ecological approach in health promotion programs. *American Journal of Health Promotion,* 10(4): 318-328.

Rosen, G. (1979). The evolution of social medicine. In: H. Freeman, et al., *Handbook of Medical Sociology.* 3nd Ed., Englewoods Cliffs: Prentice-Hall Inc.

Rosen, G. (1993). *The history of public health.* Maryland: Johns Hpokins University Press.

Ross, D.M., and Ross, S.A. (1984). Childhood pain: The school-aged child view. *Pain,* 20: 179-191.

Rousseau, N., and Bélanger, S. (2004). *La pédagogie de l'inclusion scolaire.* Collection Éducation Intervention. Québec: Les Presses de l'Université du Québec.

Rowlands, A. (2002). Circles of support building social networks. *British Journal of Therapy and Rehabilitation,* 9(2): 56-65.

Rueda, M.R., Posner, M.I., and Rothbart, M.K. (2005). The development of executive attention: Contributions to the emergence of self-regulation. *Developmental Neuropsychology,* 28(2): 573-594.

Ruffing-Rahal, M.A. (1994). Evaluation of group health promotion with community dwelling older women. *Public Health Nursing,* 11(1): 38-48.

Rule, B.G., Milke, D.L., and Dobbs, A.R. (1992). Design of institutions: Cognitive functioning and social interactions of the aged resident. *Journal of Applied Gerontology,* 11(4): 475-488.

Ryan, R.M., and Deci, E.L. (2000). Self-determination theory and the facilitation of intrinsic motivation, social development, and well-being. *American Psychologist,* 55(1): 68-78.

Saez, M., Figueiras, A., Ballester, F., Perez-Hoyos, S., Ocana, R., and Tobias, A. (2001). Comparing meta-analysis and ecological longitudinal analysis in time-series studies. A case study of the effects of air pollution on mortality in three Spanish cities. *Journal of Epidemiology and Community Health,* 55(6): 423-432.

Salazar, M.K., and Primomo, J. (1994). Taking the lead in environmental health: Defining a model for practice. *American Association of Occupational Health Nurses Journal*, 42(7): 317-324.

Satariano, W.A., and McAuley, E. (2003). Promoting physical activity among older adults. From ecology to the individual. *American Journal of Preventive Medicine,* 25(3) (Suppl 2): 184-192.

Scaer, R. (2001). *The body bears the burden: Trauma, dissociation and disease.* New York: Haworth Medical.

Scaer, R. (2005). *The trauma spectrum: Hidden wounds and human resiliency.* New York: W.W. Norton.

Scherinemachers, D.M. (2003). Birth malformations and other adverse perinatal outcomes in four U.S. wheat-producing states. *Environmental Health Perspective*, 111(9): 1259-1264.

Schneiderman, N., McCabe, P.M., and Baum, A. (Eds.) (1992). *Stress and disease processes: Perspectives in behavioral medicine.* Hillsdale, NJ: Erlbaum.

Schoggen, P. (1989). *Behavior settings: A revision and extension of Roger G. Bakers's ecological psychology.* Standord, CA: Stanford University.

Schore, A.N. (1994). *Affect regulation and the origin of self: The neurobiology of emotional development.* Hillsdale, NJ: Erlbaum.

Schwarzer, R. (Ed.) (1992). *Self-efficacy: Thought control of action.* Washington DC: Hemisphere.

Schwarzer, R. (1994). Optimism, vulnerability and self-beliefs as heath-related cognitions: A systematic overview. *Psychology and Health*, 9: 161-180.

Seigley, L. (1998). The effect of personal and environmental factors on health behaviours of older adults. *Nursing Connections*, 11(4): 47-58.

Servan-Schreiber, D. (2004). *Healing without Freud or Prozac.* London: Roxdale International Ltd.

Sherer, M., Madison, C.F., and Hannay, H.J. (2000). A review of outcome after moderate and severe closed head injury with an introduction to life care planning. *Journal of Head Trauma and Rehabilitation*, 15(2): 767-782.

Sherraden, M.S., and W.A. Ninacs (Editors) (1998). *Community economic development and social work*, Binghamton, NY: The Haworth Press Inc.

Siegel, D. (1999). *The developing mind.* New York: Guilford Press.

Siegert, R.J., McPherson, K.M., and Taylor, W.J. (2004). Toward a cognitive-affective model of goal-setting in rehabilitation: Is self-regulation theory a key step? *Disability and Rehabilitation*, 26(20): 1175-1183.

Simmons, M.R. (2006). *Twilight in the desert: The Saudi oil shock and the world economy.* Hoboken NJ: Wiley.

Specht, J., King, G., Brown, E., and Foris, C. (2002). The importance of leisure in the lives of persons with congenital disabilities. *American Journal of Occupational Therapy*, 56: 436-445.

Sprague, J., and Hayes, J. (2000). Self-determination and empowerment: A feminist standpoint analysis of talk about disability. *American Journal of Community Psychology*, 28(5): 671-695.

Staples, J.A., Ponsonby, A.L., Lim, L.L., and McMichael, A.J. (2003). Ecologic analysis of some immune-related disorders, including type 1 diabetes, in Australia: Latitude, regional ultraviolet radiation, and disease prevalence. *Environmental Health Perspective*, 111(4): 518-523.

Steiner, G.G. (2002). Cancer incidence rates and environmental factors: An ecological study. *Journal of Environmental Pathological Toxicological Oncology*, 21(3): 205-212.

Steinhauer, P. (1997). *Raising a healthy child depends on time and timing. Windows of Opportunity*. Canada: Child and Family.

Stewart, D. (2002). La nouvelle Classification internationale du fonctionnement, du handicap et de la santé (CIH-2): Concepts et conséquences de sa mise en œuvre pour les ergothérapeutes. *Actualités ergothérapiques,* Juillet/août: 17-21.

Stokols D. (1996). Translating social ecological theory into guidelines for community health promotion. *American Journal of Health Promotion*, 10(4): 282-298.

Stokols, D. (1992). Establishing and maintaining healthy environments. Toward a social ecology of health promotion. *American Psychologist*, 47(1): 6-22.

Stokols, D., Allen, J., and Bellingham, R.L. (1996). The social ecology of health promotion: implications for research and practice. *American Journal of Health Promotion*, 10(4): 247-251.

Stokols, D., Grzywacz, J.G., McMahan, S., and Phillips, K. (2003). Increasing the health promotive capacity of human environments. *American Journal of Health Promotion*, 18(1): 4-13.

Stone, A.A., Neale, J.M., Cox, D.S., Napoli, A., Valdimarsdottir, H., and Kennedy-Moore, E. (1994). Daily events are associated with a secretory immune response to an oral antigen in men. *Health Psychology*, 13: 440-446.

Stone, S.D. (2003). Workers without work: Injured workers and well-being. *Journal of Occupational Sciences*, 10(1): 7-13.

Strong, S. (1997). Meaningful work in supportive environments: Experiences with the recovery process. *American Journal of Occupational Therapy*, 52: 31-38.

Struber, J.C. (2003). Physiotherapy in Australia- Where to now? *The Internet Journal of Allied Health Sciences and Practice*, 1(2): 7.

Stuss, D.T., and Levine, B. (2002). Adult clinical neuropsychology: Lessons from studies of the frontal lobes. *Annual Review of Psychology*, 53: 401-433.

Sumsion, T. (1999). A study to determine a British occupational therapy definition of client – centred practice. *British Journal of Occupational Therapy*, 62(2): 52-58.

Sylvestre, A., Cronk, C., St-Cyr Tribble, D., and Payette, H. (2002). Vers un modèle écologique d'intervention orthophonique auprès des enfants. *Journal of Speech Language Pathology and Audiology*, 26(4): 180-196.

Syme, S.L. (1998). Social and economic disparities in health: Thoughts about intervention. *The Milbank Quarterly*, 76(3): 493-505.

Tatro, D.S. Eds (2006). *Drug interaction facts.* Facts and comparisons, St-Louis: MO.

Taylor, C. (2002). *Varieties of religion today. William James revisited*. Cambridge. Mas: Harvard University Press.

Tenhola, S., Rahiala, E., Martikainen, A., Halonen, P., and Voutilainen, R. (2003). Blood pressure, serum lipids, fasting insulin, and adrenal hormones in 12-years-old children born with maternal preeclampsia. *The Journal of Endocrinology and Metabolism*, 88(3): 1217-1222.

Thibeault, R., and Hébert, M. (1997). A congruent model for health promotion in occupational therapy. *Occupational Therapy International*, 4(4): 271-293.

Thorén-Jönsson, A.-L., and Möller, A. (1999). How the conception of occupational self influences everyday life strategies of people with poliomyelitis sequelae. *Scandinavian Journal of Occupational Therapy*, 6: 71-83.

Titus-Ernstoff, L., et al. (2006). Menstrual and reproductive characteristics of women whose mothers were exposed in utero to diethylstilbestrol (DES). *International Journal of Epidemiology*, 35(4): 862-868.

Torrey, W.C., Becker, D.R., and Drake, R.E. (1995). Rehabilitative day treatment vs. supported employment: II. Consumer, family and staff reactions to a program change. *Psychosocial Rehabilitation Journal*, 18(3): 67-75.

Townsend, E. (2003). Reflections on power and justice in enabling occupation. *Canadian Journal of Occupational Therapy*, 70(2): 74-87.

Trickett, E.J. (1994). Human diversity and community psychology: Where ecology and empowerment meet. *American Journal of Community Psychology*, 22(4): 583-592.

UNICEF (2006). *Infant and Young Child Feeding and Care*. Retreived 2006-10-12 from http://www.unicef.org/nutrition/index_breastfeeding.html.

van der Kolk, B. (1996a). Trauma and memory. In: B.A. van der Kolk, A.C. McFarlane, L. Weisaeth (Eds.). *Traumatc stress: The effects of overwhelming experience on mind, body and society* (pp. 279-302). New York: Guilford.

van der Kolk, B. (1996b). The body keep the score: Approaches to the psychobiology of posttraumatic stress disorder. In: B.A. van der Kolk, A.C. McFarlane, L. Weisaeth, Eds. *Traumatc stress: The effects of overwhelming experience on mind, body and society* (pp.214-241). New York: Guilford.

van der Kolk, B. (1996c). The complexity of adaptation to trauma: Self-regulation, stimulus discrimination, and characterological development. In: B.A. van der Kolk, A.C. McFarlane, L. Weisaeth (Eds.). *Traumatc stress: The effects of overwhelming experience on mind, body and society* (pp. 182-213). New York: Guilford.

Wade, S.L., Stancin, T., Taylor, H.G., Drotar, D., Yeates, K.O., and Minich, N.M. (2004). Interpersonal stressors and resources as predictors of parental adaptation following pediatric traumatic injury. *Journal of Consulting and Clinical Psychology*, 72(5): 776-784.

Wagner, A.K. (2001). Functional prognosis in traumatic brain injury. *Physical Medicine and Rehabilitation: State of the Art Reviews*, 15(2): 245-266.

Wehman, P., West, M.D., Kregel, J., Sherron, P., and Kreutzer, J.S. (1995). Return to work for persons with severe traumatic brain injury: A data-based approach to program development. *Journal of Head Trauma and Rehabilitation*, 10(1): 27-39.

Welch, A. (2002). The challenge of evidence-based practice to occupational therapy: A literature review. *Journal of Clinical Governance*, 10(4): 169-176.

Westwood, J. (2003). The impact of adult education for mental health service users. *British Journal of Occupational Therapy*, 66: 505-510.

Whitelaw, N.C., and Whitelaw, E. (2006). How lifetimes shape epigenotype within and across generations. *Human Molecular Genetics*, 15 (Suppl 2): R131-R137.

Whiteneck, G.G., Fougeyrollas, P., and Gerhart, K.A. (1997). Elaborating the Model of Disablement. In: M.J. Fuhrer (Ed.). *Assessing Medical Rehabilitation Practices. The Promise of Outcomes Research*. Baltimore, MD: Paul H. Brookes Publishing Co.

Whitney-Thomas, J., and Moloney, M. (2001). "Who I am and what I want": Adolescents' self-definition and struggles. *Exceptional Children*, 67(3): 375-389.

Wickham, S.E., Hanson, C.S., Shechtman, O., and Ashton, C. (2000). A pilot study: Attitudes toward leisure and leisure motivation in adults with spinal cord injury. *Occupational Therapy in Health Care*, 12(4): 33-50.

Willer, B., and Corrigan, J.D. (1994). Whatever It Takes: A model for community-based services. *Brain Injury*, 8(7): 647-659.

William, S.L., and Kinney, P.J. (1991). Performance and nonperformance strategies for coping with acute pain: The role of perceived self-efficacy, expected outcomes, and attention. *Cognitive Therapy and Research*, 15: 1-19.

Willis, A., Krewski, D., Jerrett, M., Goldberg, M.S., and Burnett, R.T. (2003). Selection of ecologic covariates in the American Cancer Society study. *Journal of Toxicological Environmental Health*, 66(16-19): 1563-1589.

World Health Organisation (WHO) (1980). *ICIDH, International Classification of Impairment, Disability and Handicap*. Geneva: Author.

World Health Organisation (WHO) (2001a). *ICF, International Classification of Functionning, Handicap and Health*. Geneva : Author.

World Health Organisation (WHO) (2001b). *Introduction to the ICIDH-2 (ICF)*. Retrieved 2004-03-18 from *http://www.ncvhs.hhs.gov/010716ap3.htm*.

World Health Organisation (WHO) (2001c). *Publication par l'OMS de nouvelles directives pour mesurer la santé*. Retrieved 2004-03-18 from *http://www.who.int/inf-pr-2001/fr/cp2001-48.html*.

World Health Organisation (WHO) (2005). *The Bangkok Charter for Health Promotion*. Retreived 2006-03-22 from *http://www.who.int/healthpromotion/conferences/6gchp/bangkok_charter/en/index.html*.

Wolkow, K.E., and Ferguson, H.B. (2001). Community factors in the development of resiliency: Considerations and future directions. *Community Mental Health Journal*, 37(6): 489-498.

Yasuda, S., Wehman, P., Targett, P., Cifu, D., and West, M. (2001). Return to work for persons with traumatic brain injury. *American Journal of Physical Medicine and Rehabilitation*, 80(1): 852-864.

Ylvisaker, M., and Feeney, T. (2002). Executive functions, self-regulation, and learned optimism in paediatric rehabilitation: A review and implications for intervention. *Pediatric Rehabilitation*, 5(2): 51-70.

Yody, B.B., et al. (2000). Applied behavior management and acquired brain injury: Approaches and assessment. *Journal of Head Trauma and Rehabilitation*, 15(4): 1041-1060.

Zimmer, M.H., and Panko, L.M. (2006). Developmental status and services use among children in the child welfare system: A national survey. *Archives of Pediatrics and Adolescent Medicine*, 160(2): 183-188.

Zimmerman, B.J., Bonner, S., Evans, D., and Mellins, R.B. (1999). Self-regulating childhood asthma: A developmental model of family change. *Health Education and Behavior*, 26(1): 55-71.

Zlot, A.I., and Schmid, T.L. (2005). Relationships among community characteristics and walking and bicycling for transportation or recreation. *American Journal of Health Promotion*, 19(4): 314-317.

In: Positive Approaches to Health
Editors: C. Dumont, G. Kielhofner, pp. 141-152
ISBN: 978-1-60021-800-2
© 2007 Nova Science Publishers, Inc.

Chapter 6

POSITIVE PSYCHOLOGY AND HEALTH

Renee R. Taylor[*] and Gary Kielhofner
University of Illinois at Chicago
Chicago, IL 60612 USA

ABSTRACT

A question that has been raised with respect to all models of psychotherapy is whether they might overemphasize pathology and underemphasize the importance of recognizing, cultivating, and sustaining positive aspects of thinking and experience. In response to this question, the field of positive psychology was introduced (Seligman and Csikszentmihalyi, 2000). Positive psychology involves the study of positive emotions, such as confidence, hope and trust, positive traits, such as strengths, virtues and abilities, and positive institutions. Other valued emotions, or subjective experiences, include well-being, contentment, and satisfaction with the past, hope and optimism for the future as well as flow and happiness in the present (Seligman, 1998). Valued individual traits include the capacity for love and work, courage, interpersonal aptitude, spirituality, wisdom, high talent aesthetic sensibility, perseverance, forgiveness, originality, and future mindedness (Seligman, 2002). The need for a positive psychological approach to psychotherapy may be more pronounced when treating individuals with chronic medical conditions. Some clients may perceive cognitive therapy strategies, such as Socratic questioning, elicitation of automatic thoughts, and frequent summaries of presenting problems, as overly negativistic, pessimistic, frightening, or otherwise threatening - irrespective of whether alternative approaches to thinking and behaving are introduced. Some clients will have a strong need for reassurance and may request a more optimistic approach on the part of their therapists. In these circumstances, positive psychology approaches to cognitive therapy that emphasize hope and optimism are recommended.

This chapter reviewed the literature on positive psychology and provided a rationale for the need to incorporate positive approaches that emphasize hope and optimism into existing therapy practices. Cognitive behavioral therapy was used as an example of an approach to psychotherapy practice that can naturally accommodate such a complementary approach. However, the potential ways in which health care professionals

---

[*] Corresponding author: Renee Taylor UIC Department of Occupational Therapy, 1919 W Taylor St. (MC 811) Chicago, IL 60611. phone 01-312-996-3412. fax 01-413-0256. E-mail: rtaylor@uic.edu

might incorporate ideas from positive psychology into their everyday clinical practices are probably endless. This chapter should be viewed solely as a launching pad for new practices and research studies that can evaluate the outcomes of a deliberate emphasis on hope and optimism.

POSITIVE PSYCHOLOGY AND HEALTH

When a person faces a traumatic accident, a new diagnosis, or an increase in the severity of an impairment, a number of thoughts are likely to enter into his or her mind. Some of these thoughts may include concerns about physical symptoms (Will I be able to endure this pain?) overall quality of life (Will I be able to keep my job? Can I afford to continue living in my neighborhood? Will I be able to enjoy painting again?), and, sometimes, mortality (How long will I live?). An individual may also wonder how the condition will affect close friends, partners, or family members and worry about who will take care of dependent children or elders. Despite a person's desire to think positively, it is difficult to deny that a certain level of negative thinking, whether realistic or unrealistic, will accompany the experience of chronic illness or disability at some point, particularly if the impairment results in multiple losses for an individual. For these reasons, positive approaches to psychotherapy that emphasize hope and teach optimism have been developed and are in need of further development. This chapter reviews the literature that forms the foundation of existing knowledge in this relatively underdeveloped area of health care practice. It begins with an overview of cognitive behavior therapy and then discusses how positive psychological approaches may be woven into existing approaches to cognitive behavioral therapy in order to promote psychological wellness and improve health-related behaviors.

Professionals from a wide range of disciplines have developed countless approaches to promoting health and supporting individuals in the management of disability. Among these approaches, mental health professionals working in the area of health and rehabilitation have developed specific approaches to psychotherapy that support individuals who are having difficulty maintaining their emotional well-being. Among these, unique applications of cognitive behavioral therapy have generated the most empirical support for efficacy (e.g., Antoni et al., 2001).

What is Cognitive Behavioral Therapy?

Cognitive behavioral therapy is an approach to psychotherapy that can be used by mental health workers and by other medical and rehabilitation professionals to address the thoughts and concerns (i.e., cognitions) that underlie negative emotional states and maladaptive health behaviors (Taylor, 2006; White, 2001; Winterowd, Beck and Gruener, 2003). A variety of approaches to psychotherapy are generally considered to fall within the broader domain of cognitive behavioral therapy (Dobson and Dozios, 2001). These approaches share three assumptions:

- cognition affects behavior
- cognition can be monitored and altered

- behavior change is mediated by cognitive change

Cognitive behavioral therapy always involves cognitive mediation of behavior as the fundamental core of treatment and it emphasizes the way in which systematic errors in thinking and unrealistic appraisals of events can lead to negative emotions and maladaptive behaviors.

According to Dobson (2001), cognitive behavioral therapies can be grouped under three broad categories:

- coping skills methods
- problem-solving methods
- cognitive restructuring methods

These categories reflect differences in the degree of emphasis on cognitive versus behavioral change (Dobson and Dozios, 2001). A more comprehensive analysis of the detailed differences between many approaches to cognitive behavioral therapy can be found in Dobson (2001).

Though at first glance cognitive behavioral approaches may be classified more narrowly as relying primarily on cognitive restructuring methods to correct negative thinking that is unrealistic or distorted, recent applications to individuals with disabilities consider the necessity of working with realistic cognitions that occur as clients face adverse life circumstances associated with their impairments (Moorey, 1996).

Generally, cognitive behavioral therapy is a structured form of therapy guided by the cognitive model. The cognitive model proposes that dysfunctional thinking and unrealistic cognitive appraisals of certain life events can negatively influence feelings and behavior and that this process is reciprocal, generative of further cognitive impairment, and common to all psychological problems (Beck, 1964; 1991; 1996; 1999). The goal of cognitive behavioral therapy is to teach a client to replace distorted thinking and unrealistic cognitive appraisals with more realistic and adaptive appraisals. The initial stages of therapy involve educating clients about the relationships between situational triggers, automatic thoughts, and emotional, behavioral, and physiological reactions according to the cognitive model (Beck, 1995). The initial stages of therapy also involve creating homework assignments, behavioral experiments, and learning experiences that teach clients to identify, monitor, and evaluate the validity of automatic thoughts. This generally leads to a degree of symptom relief. The later stages of therapy involve identifying and modifying the intermediate and core beliefs that underlie the automatic thoughts, cut across situations, and predispose individuals to engage in dysfunctional thinking. The final stages of therapy focus on relapse prevention and on empowering the client to function as his or her own therapist.

Cognitive Behavioral Therapy and Disability

In addition to treating undiagnosed psychiatric disorders or isolated symptoms of anxiety or depression, cognitive behavioral therapy can serve a number of other important functions for clients with disabilities (White, 2001). Cognitive behavioral therapy can address a number of practical issues faced by a client and his or her health care professionals. These include, but are not limited to the following:

- facilitate compliance with medical treatments
- provide emotional support and stability to a newly-diagnosed client in crisis
- prevent or reduce behaviors that have negative consequences for a client's health (eating disorders, overactivity or underactivity, smoking, substance abuse)
- increase clients' access to social, economic, and physical resources
- empower clients to take responsibility for their own health care and decrease reliance on medical providers and family members for care
- facilitate a sense of perceived control over symptoms and teach clients to become their own therapist
- provide clients with health-related education and a framework within which to make decisions about treatment options
- improve health status and immune functioning through stress management
- address non-specific symptoms of chronic conditions that are often difficult to manage and treat with medication or other medical treatments alone
- reduce a client's overall health expenditures due to anxiety-related somatic symptoms or misinterpretation of minor symptoms for serious problems, over-utilization of medication, and excessive doctor-shopping

Positive Psychology and Cognitive Behavioral Therapy

It is sometimes observed that certain approaches to psychotherapy overemphasize pathology and underemphasize the importance of recognizing, cultivating, and sustaining positive aspects of thinking and experience. In response to this observation, the field of positive psychology was introduced (Seligman and Csikszentmihalyi, 2000) and practices derived from positive psychology were blended into existing approaches to cognitive behavioral therapy (Seligman, 1998; 2002; Taylor, 2006). Positive psychology involves the study of:

- positive emotions, such as confidence, hope and trust
- positive traits, such as strengths, virtues and abilities, and
- positive institutions (Seligman, 2002)

Positive psychology attempts to understand valued emotions or subjective experiences including well-being, contentment, and satisfaction with the past, hope and optimism for the future, and flow and happiness in the present (Seligman and Csikszentmihalyi, 2000). It also studies valued individual traits including the capacity for love and work, courage, interpersonal aptitude, spirituality, wisdom, high talent aesthetic sensibility, perseverance, forgiveness, originality, and future mindedness (Seligman and Csikszentmihalyi, 2000).

Positive Psychology and Chronic Conditions

The need for a positive psychological approach to psychotherapy may be more pronounced when treating individuals with chronic conditions. Some clients may perceive cognitive behavioral therapy strategies, such as Socratic questioning, elicitation of automatic thoughts, and frequent summaries of presenting problems, as overly negativistic, pessimistic, frightening, or otherwise threatening. These responses may occur irrespective of whether alternative approaches to thinking and behaving are introduced. Some clients will have a strong need for reassurance and may request a more optimistic approach on the part of their therapists (Moorey and Greer, 2002). In these circumstances, positive psychology approaches to cognitive behavioral therapy that de-emphasizes the focus on identifying and altering negative cognitions and emphasizes the deliberate efforts to instill hope and optimism into a client's thinking may be useful.

Based on a review of the empirical evidence in this area, Salovey, Rothman, Detweiler and Steward (2000) contend that positive emotional states can promote physical health through a number of pathways. These include observations that positive emotion may:

- have direct effects on immunity and illness
- have a salutatory effect on the experience of and emphasis on symptoms and the tendency to over-rely on help-seeking behavior
- be associated with enhanced psychological resources
- inspire health-promoting behavior, and
- lead to social support seeking (Salovey et al., 2000)

Similarly, findings from a study of men with HIV suggest that optimism, personal control, and a sense of meaning may function as health-protective resources in individuals with chronic illness (Taylor, Kemeny, Reed, Bower and Gruenwald, 2000).

Hope Theory

This chapter argues that the practice of cognitive behavioral therapy with individuals with chronic conditions would be enhanced by concepts borrowed from hope theory (Snyder, 1989). Widely embraced by the field of positive psychology, hope theory has been described as a cognitively-based meta-theory that cuts across many approaches to psychotherapy (Taylor, Feldman, Saunders and Ilardi, 2000). Hope theory maintains that hope is rooted in goal-directed thinking and hopeful people engage in two specific forms of goal-directed thinking:

- pathway thinking, and
- agency thinking (Snyder, 1989)

Snyder defines pathway thinking as an individual's active evaluation of his or her ability to achieve a workable means, or "route", to attaining a goal. Pathway thinking involves planning and the consideration of different options. Agency thinking is defined as the mental energy, determination, and motivation toward goal attainment. According to Snyder (1989), the three central components of hope (goal setting, pathway thinking, and agency thinking) are interrelated and synergistic in nature such that each element of hope builds upon the other as a person takes concrete steps toward attaining both short-term (mainly directed toward symptom relief) and long-term goals in psychotherapy.

When considering application of hope theory or any positive psychology approach in cognitive behavioral therapy, caution should be taken to avoid:

- idealizing positive approaches
- using positive psychology as a means of prescribing how people should live, or
- failing to recognize that there are situations and contexts in which an emphasis on strengths or optimism is not appropriate (Aspinwall and Staudinger, 2003)

Moreover, the suggestion that cognitive behavioral therapy might be enhanced by concepts from positive psychology should not be taken to imply that other positive approaches to psychotherapy, such as Buddist approaches (Levine and Levine, 1982), solution-focused therapy (McNeilly, 2000) or humanistic approaches (Rogers, 1951), are not also worthy of consideration.

Cognitive Behavioral Therapy from a Positive Psychology Perspective

Beck (1996) recognized that "positive modes", or activities aimed at increasing needed resources, should be considered in an overall conceptualization of personality and psychopathology. Seligman (1998; 2002) has applied principles of positive psychology, and more specifically, hope theory, to aspects of the practice of cognitive behavioral therapy. Seligman's (2002) orientation involves:

- the promotion of positive emotion, and
- the promotion of positive individual traits

He argues that positive individual traits (e.g., character and other personal strengths) are fundamental to the authentic experience of positive emotion. This argument is valid and important for therapists from any orientation to consider. Because it would be beyond the scope of this chapter to include all aspects of Seligman's approach, readers are referred to Seligman's books, *Learned Optimism* (Seligman, 1998) and *Authentic Happiness* (Seligman, 2002), for more information about the promotion of positive individual traits. In this chapter, the focus will parallel Seligman's approach to positive emotion, with specific emphasis on the promotion of hope and its importance for people with chronic conditions.

Promoting positive emotion is fundamental to effective coping with a chronic condition. Though the primary tradition in cognitive behavioral therapy has been to focus mainly on present circumstances and cognitions (particularly in the initial stages of therapy), Seligman (2002) argues that all time points need to be accounted for in the generation of positive emotional experience. According to Seligman (2002), in order to be hopeful about the future, one must be able to find satisfaction with one's life, which is a historical culmination of past achievements and events, and one must be able to experience pleasure and gratification in the present. Thus, the promotion of positive emotion consists of:

- generating satisfaction about the past
- hope about the future, and
- pleasures and gratifications in the present

Satisfaction about the Past

Being satisfied with past life experiences, life meanings, and the contributions one has made to others is essential in preventing feelings of existential isolation and anger, particularly in circumstances where chronic conditions are highly impairing or terminal. Beck (1996) views meaning from a pragmatic perspective as it is linked to perceived control (Moss, 1992). Beck's view is that life meanings are the product of the meanings we attribute to our life situations (Beck, Rush, Shaw and Emery, 1979). Seligman (2002) capitalizes on this notion and encourages people to reflect upon issues of meaning and satisfaction with life. People are also encouraged to practice gratitude for other people, situations, gifts, and talents that have been part of their life history. Another aspect of past satisfaction that Seligman (2002) emphasizes is forgiveness. Though it is not always possible or appropriate in some circumstances, practicing forgiveness helps to generate positive emotions such as satisfaction, contentment, fulfillment, pride, and serenity.

In addition to supporting positive appraisal of the past within therapy, it can also be useful to provide as tasks in therapy or homework assignments that allow clients to explore their satisfaction with their past. Some clients with chronic conditions may idealize the past because it seems better to them in light of the losses and limitations they are experiencing in the present. A positive psychology approach to cognitive behavioral therapy would not recommend interfering with this idealized perspective of the past (Taylor, Feldman, Saunders and Ilardi, 2000). Other individuals may report that their lives in general, or major aspects of their lives, were not satisfying. They may blame themselves, certain individuals, or life circumstances for negative feelings in the present. Clients having particular difficulty reconciling past experiences and behavior may benefit uniquely from therapy activities and homework assignments that focus on achieving satisfaction with the past.

Instilling Hope

Hope has been found to play a fundamental role in promoting more positive outcomes for individuals with chronic illness (Snyder, Rand and Sigmon, 2002; Taylor, Kemeny, Reed, Bower and Gruenwald, 2000). Research indicates that hope facilitates better adjustment and coping with the pain, impairment, and other stressors involved in a number of chronic conditions. These include burn injuries, spinal chord injuries, severe arthritis, fibromyalgia, and blindness, among others (Affleck and Tennen, 1996; Snyder, Rand and Sigmon, 2002). Hope has also been shown to affect motivation to engage in self-care and health-promoting behaviors among individuals with chronic conditions (Snyder, Rand and Sigmon, 2002).

Those who incorporate hope theory into therapeutic practice (e.g., Lopez, Floyd, Ulven, and Snyder, 2000; Taylor, Kemeny, Reed, Bower and Gruenwald, 2000) recommend that therapists solicit ongoing feedback from clients about both the individual components and overall aspects of hope throughout the therapy process. One means of generating information about the client's degree of hope is the State Hope Scale (Snyder, Sympson, Ybasco, Borders, Babyak and Higgins, 1996). It allows therapists and clients to assess hope as it is reflected in goal setting, pathway thinking and agency thinking.

Taylor, Feldman, Saunders, and Ilardi (2000) have recommended application of the theoretical and clinical aspects of hope theory to cognitive behavioral therapy. They argue that the generation of hope is a central mediator of clinical improvement in cognitive behavioral therapy (Taylor, Feldman, Saunders and Ilardi, 2000). Taylor, and colleagues (2000) discuss hope both as a cause and consequence of cognitive behavioral therapy efficacy. They argue that two aspects of cognitive behavioral therapy, in particular, lead to increased hope. The first is a compelling rationale for change provided by the cognitive behavioral therapist in the initial stages of therapy, and the second is the breakdown of long-range clinical goals into more manageable immediate goals. Both serve to catalyze the client's hope and motivate clients to persist in therapy. Taylor, and colleagues (2000) also argue that cognitive behavioral therapy serves to instill hope because therapists from this orientation take special care in using only the specific techniques that have been demonstrated to be effective in promoting goal attainment through clinical research.

Clients that experience more efficacious outcomes of therapy are more likely to maintain a hopeful attitude over time, and their use of pathway and agency thinking is more likely to be reinforced. According to Taylor and colleagues (2000), many core aspects of the process and practice of cognitive-behavioral therapy are directed toward goal attainment, pathway thinking, and/or agency thinking and in those ways serve to generate and retain hope. These include deconstructing long-range goals into smaller sub-goals, operationally defining goals, and prioritizing goals (all of these processes leading to more frequent experiences of efficacy). In addition, the cognitive behavioral therapy techniques of presenting a clear rationale and model for therapy, teaching self-monitoring, modification of cognitive distortions, and exposure-based strategies, all lead to an increase in motivation, perceived control and a greater sense of efficacy (Taylor, Feldman, Saunders and Ilardi, 2000). Generating hope is arguably the most fundamental goal of cognitive behavioral therapy for individuals with chronic conditions. Seligman (2002) teaches generation of hope using a number of approaches. Two primary approaches are:

- permanence and pervasiveness
- disputation of pessimistic beliefs

Each will be discussed below.

Permanence and Pervasiveness. When interpreting negative events, permanence is defined as a rigid, pessimistic style that defines the timing of events in terms of "always" or "never" (e.g., "My supervisor never gives me the benefit of the doubt"). The converse of a permanent interpretation is the more tentative interpretation of negative events as temporary, or as resulting from ephemeral, situational factors (e.g., "Sometimes my supervisor can be very difficult"). Individuals with a temporary interpretation of negative events consider negative events as occurring "sometimes" and "lately". A positive psychology approach holds that more hopeful people tend to interpret negative events as temporary and positive events as permanent. Similarly, pervasiveness refers to the interpretation of events as either universal or specific. According to this approach, individuals are encouraged to make universal attributions for positive events (e.g., "I am a good worker") and specific attributions for negative events (e.g., "I made a mistake with that client").

Disputation of Pessimistic Beliefs. Another approach to achieving hope and optimism involves disputing pessimistic beliefs with the ABCDE model (Seligman, 2002). Seligman (2002) explains the malleability of beliefs and how to dispute pessimistic beliefs through what he labels as the "ABCDE" model. According to this model:

- A represents adversity or a negative event or circumstance
- B stands for usual beliefs associated with that event
- C represents the usual consequences of having that belief
- D represents one's disputation of the usual belief, and
- E stands for the energy one derives from the successful disputation of a negative belief

This method is similar to methods used in other orientations to cognitive behavioral therapy, such as identifying and evaluating negative automatic thoughts (Beck, 1995) and the disputing of irrational beliefs (ABC method) (Ellis, 1962). The client uses the ABCDE model as a structured means of disputing a pessimistic belief.

In addition to the fact that the successful completion of the ABCDE model can function as a means of generating hope and optimism in itself, Seligman's emphasis on "energization" in the ABCDE model imparts a positive perspective on prior approaches to thought analysis in cognitive behavioral therapy. Training people to focus and reflect upon the positive feelings generated by the effective disputation of a pessimistic belief and on the actual positive outcomes of changing a negative belief serves to reinforce a sense of self efficacy and positive feelings associated with using this approach.

Here and Now Pleasures and Gratifications

Cognitive behavioral therapy can be used to educate clients about the importance of pleasure and gratification in maintaining positive emotion and in managing pain and discomfort. Seligman (2002) presents a complex and sophisticated analysis of the roles of pleasure and gratification in creating and sustaining positive emotion. According to Seligman (2002), positive emotion in the present is a result of two distinct experiences, pleasures and gratifications. Pleasures are defined as immediate and evanescent delights with clear sensory and strong emotional components. They disappear rapidly, habituate easily, and require little thinking. Pleasures can be sub-categorized in terms of bodily pleasures and higher pleasures. Bodily pleasures come through the senses and are usually momentary. They typically involve sensory experiences related to touch, temperature, taste, smell, motion, sight, and hearing, or combinations thereof. Events such as sitting in a whirlpool, listening to one's favorite music, a taste of one's favorite food, or looking at a picturesque landscape are examples of bodily pleasures. Higher pleasures include rapture, bliss, ecstasy, thrill, hilarity, euphoria, kick, buzz, elation, excitement, ebullience, sparkle, vigor, glee, mirth, gladness, good cheer, enthusiasm, attraction, fun, comfort, harmony, amusement, satiation, and relaxation (Seligman, 2002). Sharing a good joke with a friend or enjoying all aspects of a ballet performance might be construed as a higher pleasure. Other examples of bodily and higher pleasures and how to create them with limited physical and economic resources can be found in Louden (1992).

Given that they are often fleeting, taken for granted, or can go relatively unnoticed by some, Seligman (2002) recommends three key strategies for enhancing pleasurable experiences:

- prevention of habituation
- savoring and mindfulness

Each will be discussed below.

Prevention of Habituation. The concept of habituation acknowledges that the human brain is constructed such that repeated indulgence in the same pleasure leads to tolerance, decreased potency of that pleasure, and in some cases, addiction. Habituation can be prevented through plentitude, spacing, surprise, and variation. Seligman (2002) recommends that people aim to experience as many different possible sources of pleasure as are available, that they vary the types of pleasure being experienced, that they spread pleasures out over time, and that they build an element of reciprocal surprise into the experience of pleasure with a friend or lover.

Savoring and Mindfulness. Savoring involves deliberate attention to the experience of pleasure. Savoring can be accomplished through sharing the pleasurable experience with others, maintaining mental and physical reminders (i.e., a souvenir), allowing oneself to be proud of one's actions or accomplishments, choosing to focus on the more pleasurable aspects of an experience to the exclusion of other aspects, and allowing oneself to experience pleasure fully and wholly through the senses (Bryant and Veroff, 1982; Seligman, 2002). Mindfulness can involve heightened awareness of pleasure, immersion in pleasure without thinking about it or evaluating it, and shifting perspectives to make an experience new or fresh (Kabat-Zinn, 1990).

Unlike pleasures, gratifications are comprised of absorbing and enjoyable activities that are not accompanied by a direct sensory or emotional experience. Gratifications are experiences that engage us fully, lead to a loss of self-consciousness, and involve flow (Csikszentmihalyi, 2000; Seligman, 2002). Gratifications comprise flow situations in which we are challenged, forced to concentrate, pursue clear goals, receive immediate feedback, experience deep involvement without perception of effort, have a sense of control, lack a sense of self, and lose a sense of time (Csikszentmihalyi, 2000; Seligman, 2002). Examples of gratifications might involve reading a good book, gardening, catching a fish, or teaching a child to ride a bicycle. Chronic conditions can limit the kinds of gratifications and flow experiences that people are able to have. For this reason, knowledge of volition and the generation of new gratifications are essential elements of behavioral experiments, activity scheduling, or other aspects of therapy that involve the facilitation of engagement in activity.

REFERENCES

Affleck, G., and Tennen, H. (1996). Construing benefits from adversity: Adaptational significance and dispositional underpinnings. *Journal of Personality, 64,* 899-922.

Antoni, M.H., Lehman, J.M., Kilbourn, K.M., Boyers, A.E., Culver, J.L., Alferi, S.M., et al. (2001). Cognitive-behavioral stress management intervention decreases the prevalence of depression and enhances benefit finding among women under treatment for early-stage breast cancer. *Health Psychology, 20*(1), 20-32.

Aspinwall, L.G., and Staudinger, U.M. (Eds.). (2003). *A psychology of human strengths: Fundamental questions and future directions for a positive psychology.* Washington, DC: APA Books.

Beck, A.T. (1964). Thinking and depression: II. Theory and therapy. *Archives of General Psychiatry, 10*, 561-571.

Beck, A.T. (1991). Cognitive therapy as the integrative therapy. *Journal of Psychotherapy Integration, 1*(3), 191-198.

Beck, J. (1995). *Cognitive therapy: Basics and beyond.* New York: Guilford Press.

Beck, A.T. (1996). Beyond belief: A theory of modes, personality, and psychopathology. In: P. Salkovskis (Ed.), *Frontiers of Cognitive Therapy* (pp. 1-25). New York: Guilford Press.

Beck, A.T. (1999). *Prisoners of hate: The cognitive basis of anger, hostility, and violence.* New York: Harper Collins Publishers.

Beck, A.T., Rush, A.J., Shaw, B.F., and Emery, G. (1979). *Cognitive therapy of depression.* New York: Guilford Press.

Csikszentmihalyi, M. (2000). The contribution of flow to positive psychology. In: J.E. Gillham (Ed.). *The science of optimism and hope: Research essays in honor of Martin E.P. Seligman. Laws of life symposia series* (pp. 387-395). Philadelphia, PA: Templeton Foundation Press.

Dobson, K.S. (2001). *Handbook of cognitive-behavioral therapies* (2nd ed.). New York: Guilford Press.

Dobson, K.S., and Dozois, D.J.A. (2001). Historical and philosophical bases of the cognitive-behavioral therapies. In: K.S. Dobson (Ed.), *Handbook of cognitive-behavioral therapies* (2nd ed.) (pp. 3-39). New York: Guilford Press.

Ellis, A. (1962). *Reason and Emotion in Psychotherapy.* Oxford, England: Lyle Stewart.

Kabat-Zinn, J. (1990). *Full catastrophe living: Using the wisdom of your body and mind to face stress, pain, and illness.* New York: Dell.

Levine, S., and Levine, O. (1982). *Who dies? An investigation of conscious living and conscious dying.* New York: Anchor Books.

Louden, J. (1992). The woman's comfort book: A self-nurturing guide for restoring balance in your life. San Francisco: Harper San Francisco.

McNeilly, R.B. (2000). *Healing the whole person: A solution-focused approach to using empowering language, emotions, and actions in therapy.* New York: Wiley.

Moorey, S. (1996). When bad things happen to rational people: Cognitive therapy in adverse life circumstances. In: P. Salkovskis (Ed.), *Frontiers of Cognitive Therapy* (pp. 450-469). New York: Guilford Press.

Moorey, S., and Greer, S. (2002). *Cognitive behavior therapy for people with cancer.* Oxford, England: Oxford University Press.

Moss, D.P. (1992). Cognitive therapy, phenomenology, and the struggle for meaning. *Journal of Phenomenological Psychology, 23*(1), 87-102.

Rogers, C. (1951). *Client-centered therapy.* Boston: Houghton-Mifflin.

Salovey, P., Rothman, A.J., Detweiler, J.B., and Steward, W.T. (2000). Emotional states and physical health. *American Psychologist, 55*(1), 110-121.

Seligman, M.E.P. (1998). *Learned optimism*. New York: Pocket Books.

Seligman, M.E P. (2002). *Authentic happiness: Using the new positive psychology to realize your potential for lasting fulfillment.* New York: Free Press.

Seligman, M.E.P., and Csikszentmihalyi, M. (2000). Positive psychology: An introduction. *American Psychologist, 55*(1), 5-14.

Snyder, C.R. (1989). Reality negotiation: From excuses to hope and beyond. *Journal of Social and Clinical Psychology, 8*, 130-157.

Snyder, C.R., Rand, K.L., and Sigmon, D.R. (2002). Hope theory: A member of the positive psychology family. In: C.R. Snyder and S.J. Lopez (Eds.), *Handbook of positive psychology* (pp. 257-276). London: Oxford University Press.

Snyder, C.R., Sympson, S.C., Ybasco, F.C., Borders, T.F., Babyak, M.A., and Higgins, R.L. (1996). Development and validation of the State Hope Scale. *Journal of Personality and Social Psychology, 70*(2), 321-335.

Taylor, R.R. (2006). *Cognitive behavioral therapy for chronic illness and disability.* New York, NY: Springer.

Taylor, J.D., Feldman, D.B., Saunders, R.S., and Ilardi, S.S. (2000). Hope theory and cognitive behavioral therapies. In: C.R. Snyder (Ed.), *Handbook of hope: Theory, measures, and applications* (pp. 109-122). San Diego, CA: Academic Press.

Taylor, S.E., Kemeny, M.E., Reed, G.M., Bower, J.E., and Gruenewald, T.L. (2000). Psychological resources, positive illusions, and health. *American Psychologist, 55*(1), 99-109.

White, C.A. (2001). *Cognitive behavior therapy for chronic medical problems: A guide to assessment and treatment in practice.* Chichester, England: John Wiley and Sons.

Winterowd, C., Beck, A.T., and Gruener, D. (2003). *Cognitive Therapy with Chronic Pain Patients.* New York: Springer.

In: Positive Approaches to Health
Editors: C. Dumont, G. Kielhofner, pp. 153-168

ISBN: 978-1-60021-800-2
© 2007 Nova Science Publishers, Inc.

Chapter 7

EMPOWERMENT APPROACHES TO IDENTIFYING AND ADDRESSING HEALTH CONCERNS AMONG MINORITIES WITH DISABILITIES

Yolanda Suarez-Balcazar[*] and Fabricio Balcazar
The University of Illinois at Chicago
Chicago, IL 60612 USA

ABSTRACT

Participatory approaches to empowering people with disabilities to increase control over decisions that affect their lives have been suggested in the literature in a variety of disciplines. However, little is known about participatory strategies to promote personal empowerment as it relates to health promotion. This chapter will suggest a contextual framework for participatory and empowerment strategies for health promotion among individuals with disabilities with emphasis on minorities with disabilities. The suggested framework includes the interaction between environmental and person-related variables that can assist individuals in removing barriers to health promotion and strengthening support systems. Examples will be provided to illustrate different empowering strategies. For instance, person-related strategies include peer mentoring. An example of peer mentoring include a peer mentoring approach developed to promote health and prevent secondary conditions among low-income minority individuals with violence-induced spinal cord injuries transitioning in the community after hospital discharge and pursue community integration while maintaining their health and preventing infections or pressure sores. Examples of environmental strategies include advocating for accessible exercise facilities in the community. The implications of empowering approaches to health promotion and the prevention of secondary conditions for individuals with disabilities will be discussed.

---

[*] Yolanda Suarez-Balcazar, Ph.D. Professor and Head, Department of Occupational Therapy, and Fabricio E. Balcazar, Ph.D. Professor, Department of Disability and Human Development (M/C 626), University of Illinois at Chicago1640 West Roosevelt Rd, Chicago IL 60608. Both authors are also part of the Center on Capacity Builidng for Minorities with Disabilities Research. For more information: http://www.uic.edu/orgs/empower; fabricio@uic.edu tel. 312- 413-1646 fax 312- 413-1804. This work was funded, in part, by the National Institute on Disability and Rehabilitation Research (NIDRR).

Chronic illness and disability disproportionately impact members of racial and ethnic minority groups (U.S. Census Bureau, 2002). Research on minority populations estimates that about 16% of all Hispanics, 21% of African Americans, 12% of Asians, and 24% of Native Americans have a disability (National Institutes of Disability and Rehabilitation Research (NIDRR), 2003; Fujiura, Yamaki and Czechowicz, 1998). Nearly 40% of all disabled adults in the U.S. are of Hispanic or African American origin, despite the fact that these groups represent about 25% of the total population (McNeil, 1993). Disability rates also vary by poverty level (Fujiura, et al., 1998). Regardless of age or ethnicity, individuals living in poverty are more likely to have a disability than those who are more affluent.

In addition, positive independent living and health outcomes are less favorable for African Americans, Latinos and other minorities with disabilities than for non-Hispanic Whites (Granados, Puwula, Berman and Dowling, 2001; Lillie-Blanton and Hudman, 2001). Minorities with disabilities experience barriers to independent living and health services, such as lack of culturally appropriate outreach, language, and communication barriers; attitudinal barriers; and the lack of minority or culturally competent service providers (National Council on Disability, 2003). Because of these and other barriers, minorities are often not well integrated into society and the workplace, and are more likely to experience negative health outcomes (Balcazar, Keys and Suarez-Balcazar, 2001; Belgrave and Walker, 1991; Ludwig-Beymer, Blankemeier, Casas-Byots and Suarez-Balcazar, 1996; Suarez-Balcazar, 1998; Zea, Quezada and Belgrave, 1994). As such, they are less likely to take advantage of both formal and informal resources, and the disabling consequences of their impairments are enhanced. According to the National Council on Disability (NCD) (1999) report, minorities with disabilities often view disability not as an individual matter but as the responsibility of the entire family. They are also more likely to experience discrimination on multiple levels, namely due to their disability, racial and ethnic background, gender, and/or class status (Block, Balcazar and Keys, 2002; Bryan, 1999; Roys, 1984; Zea, et al., 1994).

In 1992, the NCD sponsored a national conference entitled "Addressing the unique needs of minorities with disabilities: Setting an Agenda for the future". At this conference, professionals and researchers concluded that minority individuals with disabilities are at a higher risk for being marginalized than non-minorities; have fewer support systems and resources available to them; are less knowledgeable and aware of laws, resources and services; and are at a higher risk for living in poverty and experiencing health problems. The report developed from the conference also highlighted that more research information and data are needed on minority needs, concerns, and ideas for improvement. Additionally, the report states that minorities with disabilities should be encouraged to help identify research issues, interpret findings, and generate ideas to address issues.

In a more recent report by the NCD Cultural Disability Initiative (2003), a similar conclusion was reached: there is a need for more research on outreach, education, and removal of barriers for minority individuals with disabilities. The report concluded that although there is a vast collection of literature available on ethnic and racial health disparities, further research is still needed on outreach efforts and empowerment strategies to involve minorities in improving independent living outcomes.

Latinos, in particular, have great difficulty obtaining employment, gaining access to public accommodations and transportation, and are less likely to have health insurance than other Americans with disabilities (Fujiura, et al., 1998). In addition, they are less likely to know about policies that protect their rights, and often share a sense of distrust of government policies and programs (Zea, et al., 1994). Similarly, other studies have suggested that African Americans with disabilities are more likely to be severely impaired, unemployed, and to have less than a high school education (Alston, Russo and Miles, 1994; Burnett, Silver, Kolakowsky-Hayner and Cifu, 2000; Howard, Anderson, Sorlie, et al., 1994). In short, minorities with disabilities experience multiple oppressions that make it particularly difficult for them to achieve desired rehabilitation, health, and independent living goals (Block, et al., 2002).

Little information is available on participatory empowerment strategies that can assist disadvantaged groups, such as minorities in taking greater control of decisions that impact their lives. In this chapter, we will discuss two Participatory Action Research (PAR) approaches to identifying and addressing health and community issues from the perspective of people with disabilities by involving them in the research process. This entails empowering them to identify the issues of concern, support systems, ideas for improvement, and involving them in action planning or program implementation (Balcazar, et al., 2001). Often, programs and services are developed by service providers and/or experts with little input from consumers themselves. A PAR approach with marginalized populations has been demonstrated to result in increased ownership, self-help, and empowerment (Taylor, et al., 2004). New research methods and strategies within an empowerment approach are needed to enhance the capacity of people with disabilities and service providers in meeting the needs of people with disabilities. The PAR and empowerment research strategies described below enable participants to play an active role in meeting their needs and increasing their degree of control over relevant aspects of their health or rehabilitation process.

EMPOWERMENT APPROACHES

Rappaport (1987) defined empowerment as the process of enhancing people's active control over their lives. He suggested that empowerment is the process by which individuals, communities, or organizations gain mastery over their interactions in such a way that they discover their ability to look for solutions to problems rather than helplessly living with them. Additionally, Fawcett et al. (1994) defined empowerment as the process of gaining control and understanding of relevant aspects that influence one's life, and developing skills to take an active role in improving a particular situation. Furthermore, the use of the term empowerment suggests that people are proactive—rather than reactive—in dealing with contextual and environmental forces that affect one's life (Fawcett, et al., 1994; Israel, Checkoway, Schultz and Zimmerman, 1994; Zimmerman, 2000). Within Fawcett et al.'s contextual model of empowerment, the interaction between support systems available in the community, and the removal of barriers that hinder community integration and independent living, can contribute to empowerment outcomes among minority individuals. Researchers have alluded to the impact of participatory strategies on one's perceived sense of empowerment (see Balcazar, Keys, Kaplan and Suarez-Balcazar, 1998; Sachs, Stocking and Miles, 1992), and in building the capacity of participants to address issues important to them (Balcazar, et al., 2001).

PARTICIPATORY ACTION RESEARCH (PAR) AND PEOPLE WITH DISABILITIES

The amendments to the Rehabilitation Act of 1992 stipulate a policy for promoting the active involvement of individuals with disabilities in research, and improved service delivery (Balcazar, et al., 1998). PAR departs from traditional research by including participants not as passive objects of study but as active contributors to the research process (Jason, Keys, Suarez-Balcazar, Taylor and Davis, 2004). According to researchers (Tewey, 1997), PAR is a research approach which involves a dynamic collaboration between researchers and participants who are empowered to construct and use their own knowledge to increase the relevance of the research process (Whyte, 1991). This is consistent with an empowerment model that encourages individuals to proactively address their self-identified needs (Fawcett, et al., 1994). Most PAR projects tend to focus on solving specific problems, so the research is problem-driven as opposed to hypothesis-driven. This results in a type of research that is socially relevant, and likely to generate or promote change in the community (Selener, 1997).

In 1995, the National Institutes of Disability and Rehabilitation Research (NIDRR) sponsored a conference to discuss the role of PAR in disability and rehabilitation research. Although some raised concerns about granting research power to consumers, others saw the need for even more participatory approaches (Balcazar, 2001; Balcazar, et al., 1998). Researchers have argued that empowerment and participatory approaches to research do not compromise the scientific merit of studies, but enrich the applicability and social relevance of the findings by incorporating the participants' perspective in the process (Jason, et al., 2004; Selener, 1997; Suarez-Balcazar and Harper, 2003). Balcazar et al. (1998) discussed four general principles of PAR with people with disabilities, which are as follows:

1. Individuals with disabilities must independently articulate their concerns, and participate directly in defining, analyzing, and solving them.
2. The direct involvement of people with disabilities in the research process facilitates a more accurate and authentic analysis of their social reality.
3. The PAR process can increase awareness among individuals with disabilities about their own resources and strengths.
4. The ultimate goal of the research endeavor is to improve the quality of life for individuals with disabilities.

A participatory empowerment approach to research can increase the likelihood that services and programs developed will sustain over time (Suarez-Balcazar and Harper, 2003). It also facilitates ownership, adoption of innovations, self-empowerment, and improvement of social conditions (Balcazar, et al., 1998; Selener, 1997). Although PAR approaches have included both qualitative and quantitative methods, neither strategy is more favorable than the other. In this chapter we proposed two PAR approaches that address health issues among minorities with disabilities. These two approaches include a capacity building model for needs assessment and action planning called the Concern Report Method and a peer mentoring program for minority individuals with spinal cord injury.

CAPACITY BUILDING MODEL: THE CONCERNS REPORT METHOD

Based on the principles of PAR and empowerment frameworks, we developed a capacity building model for empowering minorities with disabilities, which is based on the Concerns Report Method (CRM)'s participatory needs assessment strategy developed by Suarez-Balcazar, Bradford, and Fawcett (1988). This is a strategy for identifying the community concerns and brainstorming consumer-centered ideas for institutional and community change. This methodology has been widely utilized by people with disabilities across the country, and it spurred a report disseminated to members of Congress in support of the passage of the American with Disability Act (ADA) (see Fawcett, Suarez-Balcazar, et al., 1988; Suarez-Balcazar, et al., 1988). This report revealed issues of concern related to transportation, employment opportunities, job accommodations and overall accessibility and community integration.

Within the field of occupational therapy, a large body of literature has been published related to needs assessment research strategies (see Black, Grant, Lapsley and Rawson, 1994; Finlayson, 2004; Finlayson, Baker, Rodman and Herzberg, 2002; Freeman and Thompson, 2000). However, few studies have taken a participatory action approach. One such example is the study conducted by Finlayson et al. (2002), in which the findings of the needs assessment evaluation were used to plan and implement changes to improve services at a homelessness shelter, which was monitored for a short period of time.

The CRM also emphasizes the praxis cycle of social action. According to Prilleltensky (2001), this process includes the interaction between reflection, social science and action. This praxis cycle was built upon Freire's (1970) praxis framework, in which an ongoing interaction between reflection and action is achieved through a process of critical awareness within the community. The CRM incorporates the praxis cycle in a process of reflection of values and issues of importance to the community; the identification of community needs; brainstorming for solutions; and planning and taking action (see Suarez-Balcazar, Martinez and Casas-Byots, 2005). In this process, members of the community take an active role in the development of a health concerns survey through focus groups and interviews with leaders and service providers. During this process, a unique concerns survey is developed and distributed. Then, the survey results are analyzed, shared, and discussed with the community in public forums. At these meetings, participants discuss the dimensions of the issues and alternative solutions to address the identified health concerns. This methodology has been used to identify the needs of low-income neighborhoods (Schriner and Fawcett, 1988) people with disabilities (Suarez, et al., 1988), rural villagers (Suarez-Balcazar, Balcazar, Quiros, Chavez and Quiros, 1995), among other groups.

A CASE STUDY TO IDENTIFY HEALTH NEEDS IN A LATINO COMMUNITY

This project was sponsored by a community health center that was interested in reaching out to the Latino community living in a suburb of Chicago. The outreach coordinator of the center approached the researchers to help her organize and conduct the community needs assessment. They wanted to employ a participatory approach in order to increase community involvement and ownership of efforts to promote health and wellbeing (for a detail description of this study see Suarez-Balcazar et al., 2005).

To identify community values and health issues of importance, several steps were undertaken, including conducting focus groups with the community, interviews with leaders and stakeholders, and reviewing pertinent literature. Three focus groups, which lasted about 90 minutes each, were conducted in Spanish with a total of 18 community members. During the focus group, members reflected on issues of importance to them, their values, health-related beliefs, strengths, and needs of the Hispanic community. Values such as respect, dignity and spirituality were identified as strengths. The focus group identified concerns, such as the need for adolescent programming, and Spanish language-based programs that aid recent immigrants with gaining access to affordable housing, education, social support, and medical services (see Ludwig-Beymer, et al., 1996).

Based on the focus groups' results, the team developed a bilingual survey. Input was obtained from local health care providers, including the county health department and health care coalition, and members of the Hispanic community, to ensure clarity of content and word choice. The final survey was pilot tested with eight members of the community, and had a total of 34 items encompassing issues such as dental health, programs for new immigrants, housing, day care, overuse of cigarettes and tobacco, domestic violence, drug use, pediatric care and pre-natal and post-natal care, and services for children with disabilities. Overall, the survey included eight items related to family and culture, 13 items related to health care and prevention and 13 items related to community services for children, adolescents and the family.

A total of 210 households were interviewed. Of the participants included, 52% were female and 48% were male, and ranged from 16 to 81 years of age, with a mean of 35. Seventy-one percent were married. Twenty-five percent had a yearly household income of less than $15,000; 40% had an income between $15,000 and $24,999; 24% had an income between $25,000 and $34,999; and 11% had an income of $35,000 or above. Eighty-two percent of the participants were born in Mexico. Only 33% reported proficient in spoken English. When asked about how they pay for their own health care, 36% of respondents had no insurance and paid for medical services out-of-pocket.

Service Needs: Strengths and Concerns

Respondents identified a few relative strengths, which included items rated by participants as high in importance and high in satisfaction. The most commonly identified strengths were access to friends and families for social support (61%), pre-and post-natal care services (61%), and pediatric care (61%). Although a high number of respondents rated pre-natal and post-natal care services high in satisfaction, it was observed that women were less satisfied than men with such services ($r = -.196$, $p = .007$). Differences between how each gender perceived pre and post-natal care are expected, as women are the direct recipients of such services.

The most common identified service needs were the lack of low-cost bilingual dentists, insufficient social service programs for new immigrants, scarcity of affordable housing, lack of affordable day care, and an absence of youth gang and substance abuse prevention initiatives. Although the availability of programs for new immigrants was rated as a concern for the overall sample, it was observed that the higher the educational level of the respondent, the lesser this concern was rated as important.

The results of the survey were summarized in a brief report and shared at community public forums. The partnership team organized four public forums in which a total of 180 community members participated. One of the forums was conducted at a local community center, and roughly 100 people attended. The other three were conducted in local public schools with an average attendance of 26 people. This is one of the most exciting phases of the process because during these two-hour forums, the Hispanic community was invited to celebrate their strengths, discuss the dimensions of the identified concerns, brainstorm possible solutions, and identify an action plan. Many compelling proposals to address identified service needs emerged in these public forums. Some of the proposed solutions included: developing a directory of bilingual health services for Hispanic families and their children; sponsoring parenting workshops; organizing workshops for parents and adolescents on gang and drug abuse prevention; and creating a resource list of bilingual dental services in the area. A report summarizing the data, the dimensions of the issues, and the ideas suggested during the public forums was developed and presented to several stakeholders, including health center staff and several service providers. This report served as a blueprint for planning new programs.

The committees used a summary of the ideas discussed at the public forum as a blue print for planning and taking action. Members met regularly to plan and implement a series of services and programs including the development of a resource directory of health services in the community with a special section on bilingual dentists and other health professionals. Also, leaders implemented a series of educational workshops for parents, taught by Hispanic professionals in Spanish, on how to prevent and address issues of adolescent drug abuse, as well as a series of educational and recreational activities for adolescents. Additionally, leaders developed a resource directory of facilities that offer English classes for new immigrants in the area. Lastly, the health center began providing preventive health services to Hispanic immigrants.

Conclusion

The CRM as a participatory strategy provided Latino residents an opportunity to identify the issues of concerns to them and participate actively in the implementation of solutions. Emerging community leaders received training on advocacy and leadership development to assist with the implementation of solutions. Community members who participated actively in the process alluded to feeling empowered and feeling positive about themselves by being involved.

A Peer-Mentoring Program for Victims of Gun Violence

In 1999, our research team started a new research initiative to develop and evaluate a hospital-based peer-mentoring program for individuals who had acquired spinal cord injuries due to street violence, usually as a result of a gunshot wound. This population of individuals typically includes young African American or Latino males from inner city, low-income communities who have often had some involvement with gang or drug activities.

The original grant proposal allowed approximately 3 months for program development. Researchers spent a whole year developing the intervention components including familiarizing themselves with the setting by spending time at the hospital, visiting doctors' clinics, and getting to know some of the patients. We hired four young men with violently-acquired injuries to serve as curriculum consultants, and guide us through the program development phase. Furthermore, we met with several relevant groups, including patients who sustained injuries due to violent crime, hospital staff, and rehabilitation professionals, to find out what issues such a program should address. By the end of the year, we had solidified our program model, developed a peer-mentor training curriculum, and had begun training our first cohort of mentors. The "Bullet Project" was born with the full involvement of patients and hospital staff, who from the start acquired a sense of ownership over the intervention.

The focus on full participation continued throughout the implementation of the Bullet Project. Individuals with new disabilities experience a great number of challenges both in the hospital and throughout the community reintegration process. Peer-mentors, who themselves were individuals with violently-acquired spinal cord injuries, played a critical role in supporting these victims of street violence as they struggled to come to terms with their new disabilities. By sharing their own experiences with disability due to violence, and empathizing with their mentees, these peer-mentors became critical components of care for patients with new injuries.

However, mentors' roles expanded well beyond service delivery, as they were viewed by all as an integral piece of the decision-making process. As a formal research framework, we embraced Participatory Action Research because of its alignment with our perception of patients at this hospital as contributors to research and intervention, and not just passive recipients. Peer-mentors actively shaped the project as it evolved, in that they contributed to critical program decision-making, including how to match mentors with mentees. They were involved in training new peer-mentors at new project sites, presenting information at academic and practice-focused conferences, data collection (in addition to serving as a critical data source), and interpreting results from evaluation efforts. This group was a key component of the research process and contributed greatly to the program success (for a further description of project development and project outcomes see Hernandez, Hayes, Balcazar, and Keys, 2001).

As a result of their project involvement, the peer-mentors have embedded themselves in at least three communities. First, at their rehabilitation hospital, the peer-mentors moved from the more passive role of patients and recipients of services, to playing an important role in the rehabilitation service delivery system as members of the hospital staff. Peer-mentors are now called upon by doctors, therapists, and nurses to offer their experiences in an attempt to reach patients in ways that these rehabilitation professionals often cannot. Second, mentors have increased their participation in the disability community, as they have become both role models and advocates for others with disabilities. Many of the mentors serve as exemplars of full, community participation to their mentees, in that they are individuals who work, go to college, participate in sports, and live life to the fullest. Mentors advocate for the disability community by serving as representatives during meetings with local service providers and community groups. They are able to articulate their needs and experiences, as well as the needs and experiences of their mentees, and have become involved in collective social action. In addition to positively affecting mentees by serving as examples and advocates, peer-mentors are contributing to social change by radically altering perceptions of people of color with disabilities held by mainstream society, and even other individuals with disabilities. Greater visibility and participation can foster community changes in terms of garnering more understanding of accessibility needs and broader acceptance of people of color with disabilities.

The following is a summary of information collected from each data source at one of the rehabilitation hospitals that participated in the implementation of the peer-mentoring program.

Peer-Mentors

In order to evaluate how the project was progressing, we conducted qualitative interviews with project mentors, both in the form of tracking interviews, which were conducted amidst the course of the project; and exit interviews, which were given when the mentors departed from the program. During the tracking interviews, mentors reported that the program was going well, and that they were developing positive and effective relationships with their mentees. All the mentors noted that the quality of their relationships with their mentees varied, depending on their natural affinity for one another. In general, these relationships were described as positive. We asked mentors what caused them to view their relationships with such high regard. They reportedly felt this way because of the satisfaction that came from providing their mentees with useful information and advice, watching them succeed, and relating with them on a personal level. The mentors also described some of the issues they addressed with their mentees, which included: medical concerns (e.g., pressures sores); rehabilitation; therapy; sexual functioning; securing financial assistance (e.g., Social Security Income); how to access services (e.g., Department of Rehabilitation Services, transportation); accessibility in general; and housing. We asked the mentors what we could do as program staff to better support them in their role. One mentor commented that we could supply them with more information about resources, as there was a myriad of untapped yet invaluable services in the community. Finally, we asked mentors whether participating in this program has led them to make any changes in their lives. Eighty-three percent of the mentors responded that the program has motivated them to stay off the street and instead concentrate on more worthwhile areas of life. In turn, they reported feeling a heightened sense of responsibility, intellectual achievement, and pride.

Based on the exit interviews conducted with five of the mentors, they appeared to be generally satisfied with their mentor-mentee relationships. However, they found their mentees' decisions not to heed their advice or suggestions frustrating. When asked about supervision, mentors reported feeling content with their supervisors because they managed to supply the mentors with the information needed to aid their mentees; furthermore, these supervisors genuinely cared for the well-being of the mentors. Nevertheless, the mentors were dissatisfied with the supervision meetings. While most of the mentors reported that they gained valuable and necessary information from supervision meetings, one mentor reported feeling unsatisfied because other mentors failed to take their responsibilities seriously including not following up with their mentees consistently. Additionally, one individual felt badgered at the meetings, and another felt that the meetings forced an unnatural structure on the mentor-mentee relationship, in that they forced mentors to contact their mentees the night before in order to have some information to report during the meeting. Finally, when asked about their relationships with other mentors, they responded positively, as they highly prioritized the relationships they cultivated with one another.

Mentees

We also conducted qualitative interviews with project mentees, which included tracking interviews given periodically throughout the project, as well as exit interviews administered when mentees were ready to depart from the mentorship program. A total of 26 tracking interviews were conducted with project mentees. Overall, these revealed that mentees were satisfied with the project's progress, and felt they were gaining useful information from their mentors. Specifically, mentees reported that their relationships with their mentors were fruitful, that they were receiving useful information and advice, and that they could identify with their mentors because of their similar life experiences, age, and levels of injury sustained. When asked what they discussed with their mentors, mentees highlighted topics, such as: transportation; community participation; bowel and bladder programs; searching for employment; family relationships; parenting; and life in general.

During the exit interviews, mentees reported receiving three major sources of support from the mentorship program: social, emotional, and instrumental. Socially, the program offered them opportunities to meet new people and step outside their typical routine. Emotionally, it allowed them to rely on mentors with whom they could easily identify. Finally, instrumentally, the program provided them with the information and advice needed to successfully navigate available community resources. Ultimately, the mentees expressed how gratified they felt because of the strong personal bonds they established with their mentors.

Hospital Staff

Just as with the mentees and mentors, tracking and exit interviews were conducted with staff. During the tracking interviews, staff reported that the program seemed to mutually benefit both mentees and mentors by providing them with education and support. Specifically, staff observed that the program afforded mentees the opportunity to overcome the challenges associated with their newfound disabilities with the help of experienced mentors. Additionally, staff noticed that the mentorship augmented the mentors' self-esteem, sense of responsibility, and leadership skills. Staff reported that the program's efficacy was evidenced by the sense of purpose it instilled in patients with regard to their rehabilitation process. One staff member also noted how relationships developed in light of shared experiences concerning disability, rather than past gang affiliations and background history. The mentor-mentee relationship was strained due to lack of communication as a result of difficulties following through with plans and/or limited access to a telephone.

When the project had come to a close, the staff members interviewed reported once again that the mentorship program was mutually beneficial to mentors and mentees alike. They also discussed some problems with the program, including their impression that weak mentor-mentee relationships could be potentially harmful, specifically if the mentor creates high expectations of assistance and help but doesn't follow through. Participants also thought that the mentorship needed more structure, particularly in terms of mentors and mentees connecting in the community. However, all staff agreed that that the program should continue at the hospital, and provided suggestions for improvement, such as an introductory meeting for mentors and mentees before beginning their relationship in order to clarify expectations and responsibilities. The program continues at that hospital to date and it has been touted by hospital staff as an innovative component of therapy for patients with violently acquired spinal cord injuries.

Conclusion

The participatory peer reviewed program described above provided mentees an opportunity to design a program that despite its challenges empowered participants through a mentor. Mentees were satisfied with the mentors as role models and sources of support and information. Some of the participants revealed that without the mentorship program they would not have had any contact with others outside of a limited number of family members and rehabilitation professionals.

DISCUSSION AND CONCLUSION

Full participation by any group in society is not impossible, and it is, in fact, essential. To avoid marginalization of disadvantaged groups we are called to act in ways that support this value; working in ways that facilitate full participation can be a key first step. As the percentage of minority populations increases, health professionals, researchers, and practitioners need to know about the service needs of minorities, and more importantly, the methodologies required empowering them to contribute to decisions that affect their health and the quality of life. Acceptance and adoption of new programs and services is higher when participants have had an opportunity to identify their own priorities and service needs (Balcazar, et al., 1998; Balcazar, et al., 2001). This chapter provides two examples of participatory action research: the first described a participatory methodology to identify the needs and suggestions for addressing needs from the perspective of Latino immigrants. Participants participated actively in the identification of issues, the development of the survey, and in the discussion of issues of importance to them. The second methodology illustrated a methodology that benefited victims of gun violence with the active involvement of peer-mentors, who had also been victims of gun violence themselves.

Although in neither of the studies described above empowerment was measured as a construct, participants alluded to their feelings of empowerment experienced throughout the intervention and needs assessment process. Participants expressed more control of issues of importance to them, expressed feeling better about their future and about themselves.

The CRM provides a systematic set of PAR strategies aimed at empowering disadvantaged communities by engaging in the praxis cycle of reflection, research and action. Implementing empowering needs assessment methodologies, like the one described in this paper, increases the active role that health professionals and community members themselves can play in health programming and social change. With regards to the peer-mentoring intervention with victims of gun violence, we believe that our research contributed to full participation by providing resources to a population that had few. Our participants had a voice before we began working with them; however, we served as an amplifier by carrying their message to groups that previously had not been listening. The mentors' involvement with this project spurred other endeavors: Mentors returned to school, were encouraged to live independently, and were encouraged to pursue other job opportunities. The point of this case study was not to exalt ourselves, but to showcase the positive and profound results produced when researchers and interventionists alike take into account the needs and desires of the people they serve and seek to collaborate with, while working towards a common goal. As service providers and/or researchers, we have the power to broker resources, and we must do so wisely and altruistically.

We must continue to listen and look for new ways to utilize our skills to build on ideas held by the communities in which we work. As we follow the principles of participation, we all (community members, researchers and/or service providers) come to acknowledge that we hold areas of expertise that can be used together to improve services and create tangible social change. We acknowledge that this type of work is difficult at times; it requires us— particularly researchers and service providers—to relinquish some of our power and to put aside our personal agendas in order to align our goals with the priorities of the people with whom we want to collaborate. This work does not require us to attenuate our knowledge, but rather, it encourages us to keep the spirit of collaboration at the forefront of our research. When undertaking a participatory action research initiative, we take pride in contributing to a project that strengthens and breathes new life into a population that may have at one time seemed so remote and unknown.

Participation plays a key role in research and intervention. In our own area of research with minority individuals with disabilities, studies have demonstrated that having a vital social role contributes to greater satisfaction with life (Chapin and Kewman, 2001; Duggan and Dijkers, 2001, Fuhrer, Rintala, Hart, Clearman and Young, 1992; Kemp and Vash, 1971; Krause, 1996; Krause and Anson, 1997). Yet people with disabilities continue to be one of the most isolated and disenfranchised groups in society. They face a lack of participation in employment, education, and community activities and they are consistently and systematically discriminated against, while efforts to reverse this situation are seen as annoying and cumbersome to the "able-bodied" public (see, for example, Krieger, 2003). We have the opportunity to use our life's work to foster more participation among groups facing multiple marginalization. We are all challenged to continue to do so, and a participatory approach to research serves as a powerful means of achieving this goal.

We have recently received an award to operate a new Center for Capacity Building on Minorities with Disabilities Research. We have chosen to use these resources to promote participatory and empowerment programs like the ones described above intended to give voices to minority individuals with disabilities in the evaluation and design of programs and needed services. The Center will also promote cultural competence among service providers and examine issues of cultural and disability identity, among other research goals. We hope to continue our support for people who not only experience multiple marginalizations but also share our same dreams and aspirations for a higher quality of life.

REFERENCES

Alston, R.J., Russo, C.J., and Miles, A.S. (1994). Brown vs. Board of Education and the Americans with Disabilities Act: Vistas of equal educational opportunities for African Americans. *Journal of Negro Education, 63,* 349-357.

Balcazar, F., Keys, C., Kaplan, M.A., and Suarez-Balcazar, Y. (1998). Participatory action research and people with disabilities: Principles and challenges. *Canadian Journal of Rehabilitation, 12,* 105-112.

Balcazar, F., Keys, C., and Suarez-Balcazar, Y. (2001). Empowering Latinos with disabilities to address issues of independent living and disability rights: A capacity building approach. *Journal of Prevention and Intervention in the Community, 21*(2), 53-70.

Belgrave, F.Z., and Walker, S. (1991). Differences in rehabilitation service utilization patterns of African Americans and White Americans with disabilities. In: S. Walker, F.Z. Belgrave, R. Nicholls, and K. Turner (Eds.). *Future frontiers in the employment of minority persons with disabilities.* Washington DC; Howard University Research and Training Center.

Black, D.A., Grant, C., Lapsley, H.M., and Rawson, G.K. (1994). The services and social needs of people with multiple sclerosis in New South Wales, Australia. *Journal of Rehabilitation, 60*(4), 60-65.

Block, P., Balcazar, F.E., and Keys, C.B. (2002). Race poverty and disability: three strikes and you're out! Or are you? *Social Policy, 33*(1), 34-38.

Bryan, C. (1999) Race and health care. *The Journal of the South Carolina Medical Association, 95(3),* 116-8.

Burnett, D.M., Silver, T.M., Kolakowsky-Hayner, S.A., and Cifu, D.X. (2000). Functional outcome for African Americans and Hispanics treated at a traumatic brain injury model systems centre. *Brain Injury, 14*(8), 713-8.

Chapin, M.H., and Kewman, D.G. (2001). Factors affecting employment following spinal cord injury: A qualitative study. *Rehabilitation Psychology, 46*(4), 400-416.

Duggan, C.H., and Dijkers, M. (2001). Quality of life after spinal cord injury: A qualitative study. *Rehabilitation Psychology, 46*(1), 3-27.

Fawcett, S.B., Suarez-Balcazar, Y., Whang-Ramos, P.L., Seekins, T., Bradford, B., and Matthews, R.M. (1988). The Concerns Report: Involving consumers in planning for rehabilitation and independent living services. *American Rehabilitation, 14,* 17-19.

Fawcett, S.B., White, G.W., Balcazar, F., Suarez-Balcazar, Y., Mathews, M.R., and Paine, A. (1994). A contextual-behavioral model of empowerment: Case studies involving people with disabilities. *American Journal of Community Psychology, 22,* 471-96.

Finlayson, M. (2004). Concerns about the future among older adults with Multiple Sclerosis. *American Journal of Occupational Therapy, 58*(1), 54-63.

Finlayson, M., Baker, M., Rodman, L., and Herzberg, G. (2002). The process and outcomes of a multimethod needs assessment at a homeless shelter. *American Journal of Occupational Therapy, 56*(3), 313-21.

Freeman, J.A., and Thompson, A.J. (2000). Community services in multiple sclerosis: Still a matter of chance. *Journal of Neurology, Neurosurgery and Psychiatry, 69*, 728-732.

Freire, P. (1970). *Pedagogy of the Oppressed*. NY, NY: Continuum International Publishing.

Fuhrer, M.J., Rintala, D.H., Hart, K.A., Clearman, R., and Young, M.E. (1992). Relationship of life satisfaction to impairment, disability, and handicap among persons with spinal cord injury living in the community. *Archives of Physical Medicine and Rehabilitation, 73*, 552-557.

Fujiura, G.T., Yamaki, K., and Czechowicz, S. (1998). Disability among ethnic and racial minorities in the United States: A summary of economic status and family structure. *Journal of Disability Policy Studies, 9*(2), 111-130.

Granados, G., Puwula, J., Berman, N., and Dowling, P. (2001). Health care for Latino children: Impact of Child and Parental birthplace on insurance status and access to health services. *American Journal of Public Health, 91*, 1806-1820.

Hernandez, B., Hayes, E., Balcazar, F., and Keys, C. (2001). Responding to the needs of the underserved: A peer-mentor approach. *The Psychosocial Process, 14*(3), 142-149.

Howard, G., Anderson, R., Sorlie, P., Andrews V., Backlund, E., and Burke, G.L. (1994) Ethnic difference in stroke mortality between non-Hispanic white, Hispanic whites, and blacks. *Stroke, 25*(11), 2120-5.

Israel, B.A., Checkoway, B., Schulz, A., and Zimmerman, M. (1994). Health education and community empowerment: Conceptualizing and measuring perceptions of individual, organization, and community control. *Health Education Quaterly, 21*(2), 149-70.

Jason, L.A., Keys, C.B., Suarez-Balcazar, Y., Taylor, R.R., and Davis, M.I. (Eds.) (2004). *Participatory Community Research*. Washington, DC: American Psychological Association. U.S. Census Bureau (2000). *State and County QuickFacts*. Retrieved March 18, 2004, from *http://quickfacts.census.gov/qfd/index.html*.

Kemp, B.J., and Vash, C.L. (1971). Productivity after injury in a sample of spinal cord injured persons: A pilot study. *Journal of Chronic Diseases, 24*, 259-275.

Krause, J.S. (1996). Employment after spinal cord injury: Transition and adjustment. *Rehabilitation Counseling Bulletin, 40*, 244-255.

Krause, J.S., and Anson, C.A. (1997). Adjustment after spinal cord injury: Relationship to participation in employment or educational activities. *Rehabilitation Counseling Bulletin, 40*(3), 203-214.

Krieger, N. (2003). Does racism harm health? Did child abuse exist before 1962? On explicit questions, critical science, and current controversies: an ecosocialperspective. *American Journal of Public Health*, 93(2), 194-99.

Lillie-Blanton, M., and Hudman, J. (2001). Untangling the web: Race/ethnicity, immigration, and the nation's health. *American Journal of Public Health, 91*, 1736-1739.

Ludwig-Beymer, P., Blankemeier, J., Casas-Byots, C., and Suarez-Balcazar, Y. (1996). Community Assessment in a suburban Hispanic Community: A description of method. *Journal of Transcultural Nursing, 8*, 19-27.

McNeil, J.M. (1993). *Americans with disabilities: 1991-92.* (U.S. Bureau of the Census Current Population Reports, P70-33). Washington DC: U.S. Government Printing Office.

National Council on Disability (1999). *Lift every voice: Modernizing disability policies and programs to serve a diverse nation.* Retrieved February 5, 2004 from www.ncd.gov/newsroom/publications/lift_report.html.

National Council on Disability (2003). *Outreach and people with disabilities from diverse cultures: A review of the literature.* Retrieved November 25, 2003 from http://www.ncd.gov/newsroom/advisory/cultural/cdi_litreview.html

National Institutes of Disability and Rehabilitation Research (NIDRR) (2003). *Long Range Plan.* Retreived November 25 from http://www.ed.gov/rschstat/research/pubs/index.html.

Prilleltensky, I. (2001). Value-based praxis in community psychology: Moving toward social justice and social action. *American Journal of Community Psychology, 29*(5), 747-78.

Rappaport, J. (1987). Terms of empowerment/exemplars of prevention: toward a theory for community psychology. *American Journal of Community Psychology, 15*(2), 121-48.

Roys, P. (1984). Ethnic minorities and the child welfare system. *International Journal of Social Psychiatry, 30,* 102–118.

Sachs, G.A., Stocking, C.B., and Miles, S.H. (1992). Empowerment of the older patient? A randomized controlled trial to increase discussion ad use of advance directives. *Journal of the American Geriatrics Society, 40*(3): 269-73.

Schriner, K.F., and Fawcett, S.B. (1988). Development and validation of a community concerns report method. *Journal of Community Psychology, 16,* 306-316.

Selener, D. (1997). *Participatory Action Research and Social Change.* New York: Cornell Participatory Action Research Network.

Suarez-Balcazar, Y. (1998). Un modelo contextual de incremento de poder comunitario aplicado a una población Hispana en los Estados Unidos. In: A.M. Gonzalez (Ed.), *Psicología Comunitaria: Fundamentos y Aplicaciones.* Madrid, Spain: Universidad Autónoma de Madrid.

Suarez-Balcazar, Y., Balcazar, F.E., Quiros, M., Chavez, M., and Quiros, O. (1995). A case study of international cooperation for community development and primary prevention in Costa Rica. In: R.E. Hess and W. Stark (Eds.), *International approaches to prevention in mental health and human services* (pp. 3-23). New York: The Haworth Press.

Suarez-Balcazar, Y., Bradford, B., and Fawcett, S.B. (1988). Common concerns of disabled Americans: Issues and options. *Social Policy, 19,* 29-35.

Suarez-Balcazar, Y., and Harper, G.W. (Eds.). (2003). *Empowerment and participatory evaluation of community interventions.* New York: the Haworth Press.

Suarez-Balcazar, Matinez, L., and Casas-Byots C. (2005). A participatory action research approach for identifying the health service needs of Hispanic immigrants: Implications for Occupational Therapy. *Occupational Therapy in Health Care, 19,* 145-163. Reprinted with permission in Crist, P. & Kielhofner, G. (2005). The Scholarship of Practice: Academic-Practice Collaborations for Promoting Occupational Therapy. The Haworth Press. NewYork.

Taylor, R.R., Jason, L.A., Keys, C.B., Suarez-Balcazar, Y., Davis, M.I., Durlak, J.A., and Isenberg, D.G. (2004). Capturing Theory and Methodology in Participatory Research. In: L.A. Jason, C.B. Keys, Y. Suarez-Balcazar, R.R. Taylor, and M.I. Davis (Eds.), *Participatory Community Research* (pp. 3-14). Washington, DC: American

Psychological Association. U.S. Census Bureau (2000). *State and County Quick Facts*. Retrieved March 18, 2004, from *http://quickfacts.census.gov/qfd/index.html*.

Tewey, B.P. (1997). *Building participatory action research partnerships in disability and rehabilitation research*. Washington, DC: Office of Special Education and Rehabilitation Services, U.S. Department of Education.

U.S. Census Bureau (2002). *The Hispanic population in the United States*. Retrieved March 15, 2004, from *www.census.gov/population/www/socdemo/hispanic.html*.

Whyte, W.F. (1991). *Participatory Action Research*. Newbury Park, CA: Sage.

Zea, M.C., Quezada, T., and Belgrave, F.Z. (1994). Latino cultural value and their role in adjustment to disability. *Journal of Social Behavior and Personality, 9(2),* 185-200.

Zimmerman, M.A. (2000). Empowerment theory: Psychological, organizational and community level of analysis. In: J. Rappaport and E. Seidman (Eds.), *Handbook of Community Psychology* (pp. 43-63). New York: Plenum.

Chapter 8

INTERSECTORAL ACTION AND EMPOWERMENT: KEYS TO ENSURING COMMUNITY COMPETENCE AND IMPROVING PUBLIC HEALTH

William A. Ninacs and Richard Leroux

ABSTRACT

This chapter is about intersectoral action, individual and community empowerment as keys ensuring community competency in public health. A community is competent when it provides access for its members to the resources required to ensure their health and well-being, and when its members use the accessible resources to their advantage. Intersectoral action is a key to succeeding on the first level while empowerment is a prerequisite to achieving the second. Successful intersectoral action depends on an understanding of the role that each sector plays with regards to a community's diverse functions. The public and private sectors are generally instrumental while the non-profit sector includes an existential component. Concerted action between the sectors can thus result in a broader perspective of health promotion and more comprehensive, partnership-based service delivery. Enabling factors include a win-win approach and realizing that the process takes time and resources. Obstacles include lack of flexibility, especially in government institutions, hidden agendas, and unrealistic expectations. There are at least two simultaneous empowerment processes required for a community to be competent and there exists a dialectical relationship between the two. The individual empowerment process is comprised of four components (participation, technical ability, self-esteem, critical consciousness), each of which evolves along a continuum of its own. Empowerment stems from the interweaving of the four, with each component simultaneously building on and strengthening the others, and thus intervention is needed on all four levels at the same time. The community empowerment process also has four interwoven components: participation, knowledge and ability, communication, and community capital. Intersectoral participation is influenced by the essential interaction of each process' components, since the two processes build upon and strengthen each other. An organisation can be an empowering environment since it is a functional community. The role of organisations in intersectoral participation is thus central. Since the majority of community-based organisations operate in the health arena, either by offering social support to specific — and often at risk — population groups or by providing crisis or specialized interventions on problems such as homelessness, poverty, suicide prevention, prostitution, mental health, food security and nutrition, substance abuse, HIV/aids and domestic violence, ensuring that these organisations support individual and community empowerment can be considered to be a vital public health issue. Finally, an organisation is an entity unto itself and, within the larger community that it is part of, it evolves through an empowerment process similar to that of an individual, but with recognition replacing self-esteem. Intersectoral strategies must take this process into consideration in order to be successful.

INTRODUCTION

Competent communities can play a vital role in public health. Fellin (1995: 5) argues that a community is competent when its different systems provide its members with access to the resources that they need to ensure their health and well-being *and* when its members use these resources efficiently to their advantage. This chapter is based on the premise that both of these actions are essential and that one without the other is ineffective since intersectoral action is a key to succeeding on the first level while empowerment is a prerequisite to achieving the second.

The increasingly complex nature of health determinants and social problems, with human, economic, societal, cultural, and environmental issues intertwined more and more often (Hancock, 2001), calls for a better understanding of the role that each component of a community plays in ensuring its competence. To this end, this chapter will explore a community's main functions as well as the factors that encourage successful intersectoral actions leading to a broader perspective of health promotion and more comprehensive, partnership-based service delivery.

But providing information and services is not enough: individuals must actually use these to improve their situation. In other words, members of a community must be or become empowered and this chapter will show why at least two simultaneous empowerment processes are required in achieving this result, one on an individual level and another involving the community and local organizations. There exists a dialectical and dynamic relationship between the two processes, since each one builds upon and strengthens the other, and this chapter will attempt to explain how this works.

This chapter concludes with a call for an approach that is both community-based and empowerment-oriented when dealing with public health matters.

FOR EXAMPLE...

Numerous studies point to unemployment and poverty as significant determinants of health and well-being (Leroux and Ninacs, 2002a; 2002b). To illustrate our argument in favour of simultaneous intersectoral action and support of empowerment processes, we ask the following question: How might a neighbourhood desirous of reducing poverty proceed to reduce the number of its unemployed members? Our experience leads us to believe that it would most likely have to take into account what might be called "the path to employment":

1) new jobs would have to be created to offer a sufficient number of opportunities to significantly reduce the level of unemployment and poverty in the community;
2) many unemployed individuals would have to undergo some form of training in order to become qualified for available jobs;
3) qualified individuals would have to find some way to overcome obstacles that make it impossible for them to obtain or to maintain a job. These could include lack of adequate transportation, childcare, healthcare, housing or food;
4) some of these same individuals might also need some kind of mentoring in order to correct personal hurdles such as tardiness and resistance to authority.
5) In Figure 1 (Flora, 2000), this process is illustrated with the light blue boxes representing the community's response to the needs of the unemployed (green boxes).

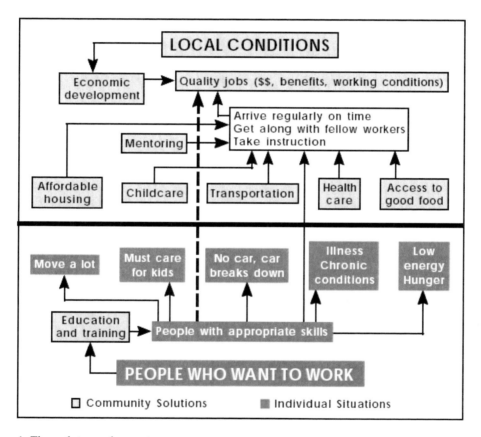

Figure 1. The path to employment.

In order for a community to achieve the intended end result of this process, it must mobilize a considerable number of players both before it begins and at various stages along the way:

- it must ensure that local public and private educational and training establishments can provide unemployed individuals with the skills and knowledge that will enable them to qualify for the available jobs;

- it must ensure that public agencies, private businesses and community organisations will provide the goods and services that unemployed individuals need to overcome barriers that are blocking them from the jobs that they need;
- it must ensure that mentors are available for individuals who require more personalized support;
- it must ensure that the required jobs are indeed available and, if not, it must actively support entrepreneurial efforts to create new ones, and it must see to it that these constitute quality jobs both in terms of working conditions and salaries in order to truly help the unemployed escape from poverty and enhance their well-being.

Making sure that there is a good match between training and available jobs, that services are both available and affordable, that potential mentors understand the challenges faced by individuals integrating the labour market after a prolonged absence or periods of great difficulties marked by homelessness, substance abuse or other problems, that the jobs are indeed "good" jobs, all of this requires some form of co-ordination and planning and all of these efforts can be considered some form of community development.

Our research shows that community development practice is more successful when local strategic planning and control over implementation is exerted by individuals and organisations who will be affected by the outcomes, working in partnership and supported by competent technical assistance and adequate financing (Ninacs, 2003). When issues are complex, such partnerships will almost always include organisations from different sectors and thus, intersectoral action is a key enabling factor for best practice. As illustrated in the path to employment, organisations from the public, private and community sectors would have to come together on many fronts in order to make a dent in the unemployment rate.

However, success from a public health perspective does not rest exclusively on the setting up of relevant programs, no matter how good they may be. Success occurs when the people who need them take advantage of them. In other words, unemployed individuals must be willing and able to undertake the path to employment for the project to succeed. Unfortunately, a number of them are too disempowered to do so. There therefore has to be a conscious effort made to develop the empowerment of those who are unable to act. In our example, this might mean developing alternative forms of empowerment-focussed training that would include a life skills development component (Ninacs and Toye, 2002).

INTERSECTORAL ACTION

Overview

Intersectoral action refers to the adoption of common strategies involving many sectors: it is thus an action that transcends the interests of a single sector. This approach is useful when problems require action by more than one sector or when problems are not well handled by one or more sectors. Generally speaking, the word *sector* refers to a somewhat arbitrary delimitation of society based on the type of governance and objectives pursued:

- public sector:
  - departments and ministries;
  - public authorities and boards;
  - regional and local administrations;
  - cities, boroughs, towns, neighbourhoods;

- private sector:
  - businesses;
  - chambers of commerce;
  - trade associations;

- community sector (also referred to as civil society):
  - non-governmental organisations such as community groups, women's groups, self-help groups;
  - foundations;
  - labour unions and professional associations;
  - churches;
  - intermediary organisations such as roundtables and community development corporations.

Intersectoral action is getting players from two or more sectors to work together towards a goal that each will benefit from reaching. This is not as easy as it sounds given the disparities between players in terms of size, scope and available resources, and given that in the public and private sectors, getting establishments to collaborate within the sector (*intra*sectoral action) is often a feat in itself. Over and above such differences, however, is a more fundamental one: simply put, each sector plays distinct roles in ensuring a community's health and well-being and, to that end, each one has developed different types of networks to pursue the goals stemming from their respective roles. Understanding these networks and their functions is therefore vital to ensuring thriving intersectoral action.

THE COMMUNITY AND ITS FUNCTIONS

A community is basically a group of people having something in common and, while the focus of this chapter will be on the geographical one, other types exist as well, notably those centered on a common identity or interest. It follows that individuals can be members of several communities at the same time and that certain communities can exist within a greater community — for example, neighbourhoods within a borough and boroughs within a city. Sociologists and political scientists insist on other aspects of the community, such as the relationships between individuals, the psychological bonds with the place where they live, and a common culture. The *Centre for Disease Control and Prevention* has referred to communities as living organisms (CDC/ATSDR, 1997: 8), an idea that seems to coincide with the holistic perspective put forward by the *National Cooperative Extension System's Denver Team* that considers a community to be "a system of interdependent components [...] comprised of a dynamic interaction between individuals, groups, organizations and institutions that are both internal and external to the community"[1].

For the purposes of this chapter, when we refer to a community we will be talking about a territorial unit small enough to be considered one's home and to instil a sense of belonging but also large enough to have its own institutions and a certain level of governance: a neighbourhood, a town, a village. We will consider it to be a tangled web of interdependent individuals, groups, organizations and institutions that interact constantly with each other as well as with others from the outside and that are ever-evolving.

Scholarly works dealing with communities generally build upon Tönnies seminal studies of groups in the late 19th century, notably his opposition of *Gemeinschaft*, seen as groupings of interdependent individuals linked by bonds of solidarity stemming from common values, with *Gesellschaft*, where formal rules prevail over emotional ties. Studies usually insist on the harmonious character of *Gemeinschaft*, which appears naturally, in contrast to the believed alienating nature of *Gesellschaft*, more transitory and superficial, and blame modern communities for not offering the congenial environment of the first and thus for contributing to the decline of interpersonal relations.

Tönnies' idea of duality seems to be the basis for a distinction made by Deena White between: a) the existential community, that she sees as a moral space serving as a rampart against rationality, exclusion and isolation because it makes it possible for groups to express who they are and how they are different; and b) the instrumental community, that she believes is defined by what it does rather than by its moral significance for its members (White, 1994: 40-45). This does not mean that the instrumental community is not significant. The opposite is in fact true since a community accomplishes major functions in ensuring the wellbeing of its members. White, in fact, does not see the two ways of conceiving a community as incompatible and neither do we.

However, we believe that White's analysis in fact describes the two main dimensions of a single community rather than two different types of communities. These dimensions are:

1. an instrumental dimension that has to do with both managing local resources through the production of goods and services, making these available to the community's members and ensuring members' security, health care, education, employment, cultural development and leisure activities within a clean environment;
2. an existential dimension that instils a community's members with a sense of belonging, trust and self-esteem on both individual and collective levels.

Both dimensions rely on members' solidarity to one another to achieve their respective functions, but the instrumental dimension rests upon a more mechanical operation whereas the way the existential dimension builds solidarity can be deemed to be organic. The efficient working of both of these dimensions is required to produce health and wellbeing.

---

[1] The National Cooperative Extension System, a publicly-funded linkage of thousands of educational institutions, municipal services and rural development organizations in the United States. See: http://www.ncrcrd.iastate.edu/projects/corecomp/fop.pdf, downloaded on January 4, 2007.

Over the years, we have observed that both dimensions rely on organizations grouped together in networks to accomplish their functions but that the types of networks generally present in each dimension are quite distinct. Generally speaking, the instrumental side of a community is made up of institutions, businesses, foundations, and similar organizations that most often work together in formal arrangements. We refer to these as normative networks wherein roles and responsibilities are well-defined within a hierarchical framework of some kind. As for the existential dimension, it is most often comprised of community organizations, self-help groups and various membership-based associations whose ties are much looser and much less hierarchical if at all but all remain interconnected just the same. We call these free networks. There are, of course, networks that overlap both of these extremes but the point is that normative and free networks work differently, mainly because they pursue different goals and because they are based on a different set of core values (Figure 2).

We have also observed that institutions of the public and private sectors most often operate within normative networks because of their basic instrumental functions while the non-governmental organisations of the community sector frequently gather together within free networks when they incorporate an important existential component. There are numerous exceptions to this rule such as when small businesses play a significant existential role, but the point is that getting normative and free networks to work together is a major challenge.

	normative networks	free networks
Mission	do for	do with
Objectives	results	processes
Activities	planning, co-ordination, execution, evaluation	supporting mutual help and co-operation
Management	hierarchy (weak organizational autonomy)	consensus (strong organizational autonomy)
Ties	formal	informal
Focus of Work	complementary (institutional systems)	collaboration (value systems)

Figure 2. Characteristics of normative and free networks.

In reality, these different networks are increasingly being called upon to work together at the community level in order to enhance local capacity to address issues related to health determinants. Here in Québec, public hospitals, chronic care facilities, and homes for the elderly have recently been merged into one health and social service agency. The avowed public health strategy is to build a health and social service network of public, private, municipal and community organisations and institutions with the new agency at its core. Unfortunately, this is being met with strong resistance, especially from community-based organisations and self-help groups. One of the reasons is that public sector health officials and government planners, who generally deal with normative networks, seem not to have taken into account that their future community-based partners are used to operating collectively within free networks and that these latter organisations have no desire to change the way their collective structures operate since their role in maintaining their community's existential dimension requires more flexibility and less hierarchy than what is generally the case in normative networks.

CONCERTED ACTION AND PARTNERSHIPS

So how can different networks work together? Sadan and Churchman (1997) distinguish between task-focussed community development work and process-focussed endeavours. As noted in Figure 2, normative networks are generally results-oriented whereas free networks are more concerned with process. In both cases, however, even when the goals are opposed, the authors indicate that the first step is inevitably one of **developing relationships and establishing dialogue (Figure 3). There is no doubt that intersectoral action must begin in this way since it requires the development of a common vision both in terms of the initial identification of the situation to be** improved and of how this will be accomplished.

TASK FOCUS STAGES	PROCESS FOCUS STAGES
Developing relationships and establishing dialogue	Developing relationships and establishing dialogue
Building co-operation	Creating participatory system
Clarifying planner's roles	Defining planner's roles
Maintaining contact with public	Developing organization
On-going feedback from public	Developing strategy
Presentation of plan – feedback	Presentation of joint plan
IMPLEMENTATION	**IMPLEMENTATION**
Evaluation	Evaluation

Figure 3. Community planning stages.

An examination of best intersectoral practices makes it possible to distinguish the two successive but distinct stages of this approach (Ninacs, 2002a):

1) consensus-building stage

This initial phase is basically a voluntary and more or less formal decision-making process that brings together organisations and institutions to seek a consensus on the problem or situation that they are concerned with. Basically, they pool their analyses and information in order to develop a common vision of what is or is not working and of what must be done to address the issue. The dynamics of this stage are simultaneously co-operative and conflictual because each participant, outside of this gathering, often pursues objectives that are at odds with those of other participants. Enabling factors include a win-win approach and realizing that the process takes time and resources. Obstacles include lack of flexibility, especially in government institutions, hidden agendas and unrealistic expectations.

2) partnership stage

A partnership is a contract between specific actors that includes a specific mission, objectives, responsibilities and time frame. It is through partnerships that strategies, policies and practices are actually implemented. Each partner's responsibilities, mandates and contributions are precisely laid out with penalty clauses compelling each partner to follow through on his or her commitment.

Here in Québec, a large number of organisations have been set up over the past twenty years whose sole purpose is to ensure consensus-building among all of the players concerned with specific issues (e.g., domestic violence, homelessness) or population groups (e.g., women, youth). Projects often emerge from the work of these organisations but the main objective is ensuring that each participant understands the role and point of view of each other participant. From what we have seen and heard, this has resulted in better communications, less duplication, improved interventions and less turf wars – although the latter can never be completely eliminated since all concerted action involves power-based relationships to some degree (Gagnon and Klein, 1991).

Other such organisations have also emerged here that combine both consensus building and partnership development activities, often around community economic development (Ninacs, 1995) but also targeting broader social and health issues. A good example of these are the thirty neighbourhood roundtables in Montréal funded via a partnership between the City of Montréal, the Public Health Department of the Regional Health and Social Services Board of Montréal-Centre and Centraide of Greater Montréal. The purpose of the partnership is to support intersectoral action to enhance social development (Ninacs and Gareau, 2003). While results vary considerably, some of these organisations have made remarkable progress in obtaining consensus around complex, poverty-related issues that have resulted in concrete projects, many of which are partnership-based [2].

EMPOWERMENT

Beyond the BuzzWord

For initiatives stemming from intersectoral action to succeed, the individuals who make up targeted population groups must be able to access and take advantage of them. We have observed that this does not happen as frequently as it should. One of the reasons is that some individuals are disempowered, in the sense that they do not have the capacity to act in a way that should normally be beneficial for them, and few projects and programs seem to be aware

---

[2] A good example of this is the *Vivre Saint-Michel en santé* initiative profiled by the Tamarack Institute at http://tamarackcommunity.ca/g2s25.html.

of the complexity of the processes that lead to empowerment. We have thus developed a conceptual framework to explain these and we present an overview of our findings here[3].

To be empowered is being able to exert power. We define power from a social intervention perspective, not from a sociological or political one. For the sake of this discussion, power is the capacity to do three things: 1) to voluntarily choose a course of action; 2) then to decide to actually see the choice through; 3) and finally, to act accordingly, including taking responsibility for the consequences. We believe that power is acquired and developed progressively, and that it cannot be given or received: only authority can be transferred, not the capacity to use it. Being empowered is thus being able to act autonomously and to take a calculated risk.

Our construct of empowerment is based upon the idea that individuals and communities have the right to participate in decisions that concern them and that the knowledge and skills required to participate in such decisions are already present within the individuals or communities concerned (or the potential to acquire them exists). An empowerment process begins by voluntary participation and rests upon it: becoming empowered cannot be forced nor can a person go through someone else's empowerment process.

There are at least two simultaneous empowerment processes required for a community to be competent (Figure 4). Most writings on empowerment target one or the other (and quite often subsets of each) but do not take into consideration the essential interaction of each process' components nor the dialectical relationship between the two. We have thus developed a conceptual framework to explain the links between them as well as the specific roles that each one plays.

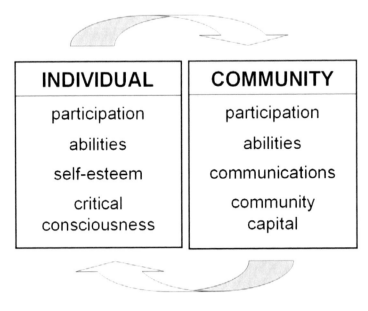

Figure 4. Basic empowerment processes.

---

[3] Much of this section stems from William A. Ninacs' Ph.D. dissertation (Ninacs, 2002b). Obviously, several of the ideas and conceptualizations presented here were not his at the outset and, in the dissertation, are provided the complete references to the works from which they are drawn. The complete dissertation is available online free of charge at http://www.lacle.coop/publications.htm.

INDIVIDUAL EMPOWERMENT

The individual empowerment process is comprised of four components (participation, technical ability, self-esteem, critical consciousness), each of which evolves along a continuum of its own. Empowerment stems from the interweaving of the four, with each component simultaneously building on and strengthening the others, and thus intervention is needed on all four levels at the same time.

Each component is multidimensional:

- *participation* has two dimensions: 1) one that is psychological wherein the individual progresses from simple attendance (often silent) to participating in simple discussions (right to speak), and then to participating in debates (right to be heard) and finally to participating in decisions, because the true exercise of power is expressed in decisions, either positively when agreement is given or negatively when consent is refused; and 2) the other on the practical level that includes a capacity to contribute and to assume the consequences of one's participation, which implies being able to act in a rational way and a propensity to commit oneself;
- *abilities* are progressively acquired (and sometimes simply acknowledged or refreshed) with the individual learning the technical and practical knowledge and skills required for participation in both discussions and the actions that result from the decisions taken;
- the development of *self-esteem* refers to a psychological transformation by which an individual arrives at recognizing the legitimacy of his or her identity and being (love of oneself), and then at recognizing his or her capacity (vision of oneself), and finally, at having his or her capacity recognized by others (self-confidence). An individual thus perceives himself or herself as being able to achieve personal or collective goals as long as his or her contribution to reaching the objectives, no matter how small, is acknowledged by other people;
- *critical consciousness* is developed through a four-phase process: 1) becoming aware of one's own problem (individual consciousness); 2) realizing that others have a similar or an identical problem (collective consciousness); 3) becoming aware that the way that society is organised or functions has an effect on the problem (social consciousness); and 4) recognizing that solving structural problems requires collective action and thus accepting some personal responsibility for change (political consciousness). The third phase helps reduce the burden of guilt that a disempowered individual feels towards the problem as well as any stigma attached to being part of a particular population group.

The components of the individual empowerment process are intertwined like a cable made up of four cords, with each one both supporting and applying pressure on the others. This reciprocal reinforcement is carried out gradually on a continuum which varies according to a considerable number of variables. Although it is not clear how each component affects the others, it would seem that it is the interaction of the components that produces empowerment, since each one plays a precise part in the process (Figure 5). This means that the absence of a component would reduce if not cancel the empowerment process. Moreover, since various dimensions are in constant interaction and change, the individual empowerment process would be one of perpetual renewal.

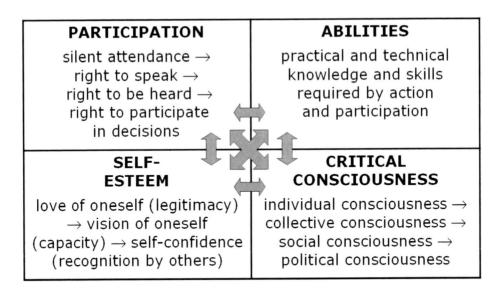

Figure 5. Components of the individual empowerment process.

The development of a critical conscience is necessary to surmount psychological barriers because it makes it possible to understand that problems are not the sole responsibility of an individual, neither regarding their causes nor their solutions. In practice, developing critical consciousness can prove to be a psychological step forward towards socio-economic or political structural changes. Empowerment must, indeed, lead to problem-solving action and a change in the environment, notably for those who have been disempowered because of structural or societal impediments. For many authors, empowerment is above all about structural change and a more equitable distribution of power.

We have also noted that a capacity to act on one level of one's life is not automatically transferred to other levels. Here again, the development of a critical conscience can be useful since it enables some individuals to understand how forces beyond their control affect their capacity to act and reduces the guilt and stigma of being associated with a maligned population group.

COMMUNITY EMPOWERMENT

Community empowerment is the means by which communities increase their collective capacity. This capacity rests upon that of the individuals and organisations that make up the community. It follows that community empowerment can be seen as the community's ability to encourage, strengthen and maintain the empowerment of its individual and organisational members.

The characteristics of community empowerment can be classified as follows:

- participation: Since empowerment requires participation in making decisions, an empowered community has to ensure that spaces are available for its constituents to take part in making decisions that are significant to them. This is not as easy as it sounds and a number of issues have to be spoken to in order to accomplish efficient participation:

    - there must be an equitable redistribution of power within the spaces which means that they should usually be democratically-structured;
    - individuals not perceived as natural leaders must be included and encouraged;
    - the spaces must be open to change, to new ideas, to diverse and divergent views in order to allow individuals to use their rights to speak and to be heard, but without setting aside the need for shared values and a common vision in order to ensure peer support;
    - a learning environment must exist in order to allow individuals to acquire the skills and knowledge that they need but there must also be opportunities for them to contribute so that their capacity can be seen and acknowledged;
    - a consensus-oriented, supportive and motivational leadership is required, one that is able to focus on both process (to ensure empowerment) and results (to ensure credibility and sustainability);
    - resources must be available for participants who require them and these can include: material resources such as basic goods and services (food, clothing, shelter), those required for action (equipment, tools) and those to remove situational obstacles (health care, transportation, childcare); information resources including specific facts and contacts; financial resources (generally to acquire other resources or to ensure participation).

- abilities: A community's strengths begin with those of its members and an empowered community will both know and recognize these while allowing its disempowered members to develop the skills and knowledge to fully participate in its life and take advantage of its systems. This means that it must also see to it that there exist networks of both professional and non-institutional support for its most disenfranchised members. But the community must also the capacity to get local resources to work together, to see them cooperate and develop partnerships, and to benefit from synergies which result from all of this collective action which is often called social capital (Putnam, 2001). An empowered community must thus possess consensual and decisional skills, know how to resolve conflicts, be able to manage change and transitions, and uphold high standards of accountability.
- communication: An empowered community seeks positive interaction between its members and encourages the expression of divergent points of view anchored in trust and thus transparency in decision-making processes. It generally ensures both the broad, free and effective circulation of general information and the access to the specific information needed for the success of its members' projects.
- community capital: In our model, community capital is comprised of two interwoven elements: 1) the feeling of belonging that its members have to both the community and the larger environment; and 2) their sense of citizenship, of their rights and their

responsibilities. The development of community capital helps to ensure mutual assistance and self-help on the individual level and allows for broader action on societal issues.

Taken separately, each element of community empowerment contributes to the reversal of an individual's state of disempowerment, and combined, they allow the community or one of its parts to build its overall capacity to fix objectives and to act in accordingly.

ORGANIZATIONAL EMPOWERMENT

The systems of a community consist of formal mechanisms which are, in fact, the tools that the community uses to carry out its mission. These mechanisms are places where community members work, provide, and receive services, advocate for themselves and for others, and have all sorts of leisure activities. We call them organisations and they become communities unto themselves, functional communities in fact because the people that they bring together share an interest and a common function and because each organisation responds in some way to the needs of its members (Fellin, 1995: 121-132). It follows that community empowerment is played out on two levels: first, on the level of the functional community, i.e. the organization; and second, on the level of the broader community (Figure 6).

This means that organisations have a community empowerment function with regards to their members and to other individuals that take part in their activities. In the path to employment, for example, this means that when the community responds to training or other needs of individuals seeking the jobs that they require by setting up organisations or mobilizing existing ones, the organisations should have the characteristics of community empowerment outlined above to develop and maintain the empowerment of its members. This is why programs that provide job and life skills development — for example, training businesses (Ninacs and Toye, 2002) – can often produce more satisfactory results than conventional ones when dealing with people who are victims of social exclusion.

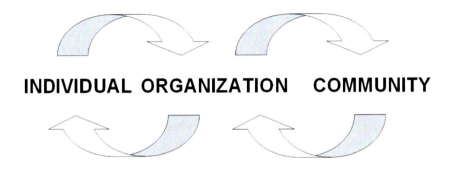

Figure 6. Ties between the empowerment processes.

However, an organisation is an entity unto itself and it has its own strengths and weaknesses, its own history, its own capacity to make choices, to take decisions and to act on its own. But because it is more than the sum of its members, it evolves through an empowerment process similar to that of an individual within the larger community that it is a part of:

- *participation:* an organization can take part in decisions taken by those organizations that it is member of as well as in the broader community;
- *abilities:* these are the knowledge and skills shared by an organisation's members, its committees, its management and its personnel, and there is a transfer of knowledge between these people, which ensures continuity when one of them leaves;
- *recognition* (which replaces self-esteem): which refers to the process by which an organization arrives at recognizing its own legitimacy and its capacity, and that is initially fashioned by the way that its members see it and then by the way that the broader community accepts and supports it;
- *critical consciousness:* that is the capacity of the organisation to clarify situations and analyze issues by identifying what the stakes are for both its members and the general population.

These four components of organizational empowerment are interrelated in the same way that those of the individual empowerment process are (Figure 7). The interaction of the components, i.e. the support that each one brings to the others as well as the pressure that each one exerts on the others, is not less essential in the case of organizations than it is in the case of individuals. Intersectoral strategies must take this into consideration in order to be successful.

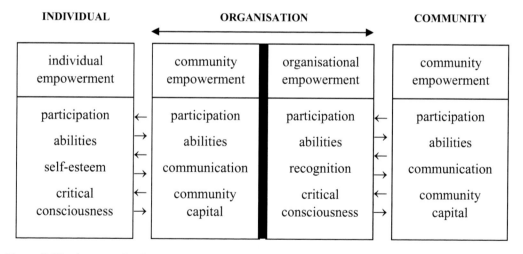

Figure 7. Ties between the three empowerment processes.

CONCLUSION

In an empowered community, people, either individually or collectively through organisations and networks, share their abilities and their resources, and ultimately, this builds the community's capacity. This suggests that the ultimate objective of both intersectoral action and empowerment is the development of the community since it is through communities that individuals ensure their well-being.

The *National Cooperative Extension System* recently developed a *Community Development Foundation of Practice*, a framework that maps out core competencies required by professionals who, notwithstanding a dazzling variety of job titles and settings, all strive to build strong, vibrant and sustainable communities. This document stresses the complex and inherently interdisciplinary nature of such work and of the challenges that these professionals face in addressing issues such as ecological integrity, social cohesion, effective decision-making and taking advantage of relevant economic opportunities. Some of these core competencies such as "ensuring broad based participation and bringing people to the table", "engages residents in determining their own future" and "building community engages residents in determining their own future" and "building community collaborations and partnerships" fall clearly within the realm of the topics discussed in this chapter.

We believe that such community development work aims at transforming targeted individuals, organisations and communities into players who will take an active part in their own development. The people and the communities concerned must thus have, acquire or reacquire the capacity for taking action generally associated with the concept of empowerment, the capacity that they need to ensure their health and well-being.

REFERENCES

CDC/ATSDR Committee on Community Engagement (1997). *Principles of Community Engagement*, Atlanta (Georgia), Centre for Disease Control and Prevention, Website visited on February 19, 2007: http://www.cdc.gov/phppo/pce/.

Fellin, P. (1995). *The Community and the Social Worker, Second Edition*, Itasca (Illinois), P.E. Peacock Publishers, Inc., 292 pages.

Flora, C.B. (2000). Poverty Reduction and Rural Development. *Rural Development News*, 24(4), 3.

Gagnon, C., and Klein, J.L. (1991). Le partenariat dans le développement local, *Cahiers de géographie du Québec*, 35(95), 239-256.

Hancock, T. (2001). People, partnerships and human progress: building community capital. *Health Promotion International*, 16(3), 275-280.

Leroux, R., and Ninacs, W.A. (2002a). *La santé des communautés : perspectives pour la contribution de la santé publique au développement social et au développement des communautés*, Montréal, Institut national de santé publique du Québec [http://www.inspq.qc.ca/pdf/publications/082_SanteCommunautes.pdf].

Leroux, R., and Ninacs, W.A., with assistance from M. Croteau, F. Gareau, and M. Toye (2002b). *Revue de littérature sur le développement social et le développement des communautés*, Montréal, Institut national de santé publique du Québec, 42 pages.

Ninacs, W.A. (1995). Initiatives de développement économique communautaire au Québec : typologie et pratiques. In : C. Mercier, C. Gendreau, J.-A. Dostie, and L. Fontaine (sous la direction), *Au cœur des changements sociaux : les communautés et leurs pouvoirs*,

Sherbrooke (Québec), Regroupement québécois des intervenants et intervenantes en action communautaire en CLSC et en Centre de santé, 55-77.

Ninacs, W.A. (2002a). Le pouvoir dans la participation au développement local dans un contexte de mondialisation. In : M. Tremblay, P.-A. Tremblay, and S. Tremblay, *Développement local, économie sociale et démocratie*, Sainte-Foy, Presses de l'Université du Québec, 15-40.

Ninacs, W.A. (2002b). *Types et processus d'empowerment dans les initiatives de développement économique communautaire au Québec*, doctoral dissertation, Sainte-Foy (Québec), École de service social, Université Laval, 332 pages.

Ninacs, W.A., and Toye, M. (2002). Overview of Integration-through-Work Practices in Canada. *Économie et Solidarités*, 33(1), 74-92.

Ninacs, W.A., with the collaboration of F. Gareau (2003). *Centraide of Greater Montreal: Case Study,* Ottawa, Caledon Institute of Social Policy, 17 pages

Ninacs, W.A., with assistance from F. Gareau, and R. Downing (2003). *Financing Community-Based Rural Development: Profiles of the Prevalent Instruments Used to Finance Community-Based Rural Development in Various Industrialised Countries*, Ottawa, Rural Secretariat, Agriculture and Agri-Food Canada, 85 pages.

Putnam, R. (2001). Social capital: measurement and consequences, *Isuma*, 2(1), 41-51.

Sadan, E., and Churchman, A. (1997). Process-Focused and Product-Focused Community Planning: Two Variations of Empowering Professional Practice, *Community Development Journal*, 32(1), 3-16.

White, D. (1994). La gestion communautaire de l'exclusion, *LSP-RIAC [Revue internationale d'action communautaire]*, 32, 37-51.

In: Positive Approaches to Health
Editors: C. Dumont, G. Kielhofner, pp. 187-201

ISBN: 978-1-60021-800-2
© 2007 Nova Science Publishers, Inc.

Chapter 9

LITERATURE AND MEDICINE: POSSIBLE AMALGAM?

Jean Désy
Faculty of Medicine, Laval University
Quebec, Canada

On blue summer evenings, I shall go down the paths,
Prickled by stalks of wheat, crushing the short grass:
Dreaming, I shall feel its coolness on my feet.
I shall let the wind bathe my bare head.

I shall not speak, I shall think about nothing:
But endless love will grow into my soul,
And I shall travel far, very far, like a gipsy
By the Nature – as happy as if I were with a woman [1].

Arthur Rimbaud, *Sensation*.

I am a physician. A physician working on the fringes, it is true, but working all the same. I make my living and that of my family. I treat people. Or I attempt to treat them. I suffer. I use my own suffering to remain compassionate.

The other day, when I visited a friend who had agreed to read one of my texts, I realized that he was coughing a lot. He had been coughing for a week. Bronchitis, clearly. Contracted from his flatmate, who had been coughing for almost a month. It was probably mycoplasmal bronchitis, easily cured if one agrees to be treated with the appropriate antibiotics. I was happy to help this friend, to be there with him to question him better; to better "smell" the sickness that was giving him so much trouble. He was coughing every ten seconds, completely breathless, even though he does not smoke, and is not even thirty years old. While he sat on a small table in the lounge, his sweater pulled up, I put my ear to his back, as physicians used to do before the invention of the stethoscope. I had no instrument with me. I was nevertheless able to listen to his lungs very well. I listened for crackles, placing my ear firmly against the skin of his back on several different quadrants, changing position in a logical way to listen to all the lobes. It is not usual to examine someone this way! In spite of this, my friend was glad to have me give this attention to his cough. When I had finished, and had heard what he had to say, I prescribed an inexpensive antibiotic for him, one I know to be effective against this kind of infection. As if to overcome the mild embarrassment I was feeling at having examined him this way, I told him that the stethoscope had been invented because in the olden days, physicians visiting large women at home, had grown tired of having to place their heads under enormous bosoms, in constant fear of being suffocated! My friend smiled. It did not even occur to him to get out his health card. As a friend, one doesn't think of paying for a service performed in such an unusual fashion. He told me that he would go for the medicine straight away. He was in a hurry to feel some relief. I left his home in a cheerful mood. I had once again been able to provide care, happy not to have really been a physician, while being one all the same.

It is necessary to believe in values which go beyond the powers of science, although science is useful, often quite extraordinary, in fact. Of these values, the most essential one is still love, however obvious that statement may seem. At the end of the road, as at the very beginning of every road, at all the points along our common roads, only love counts. Without love, love for others, as well as love for the poor, it is quite possible that nothing is worthwhile. But to love, to really love, to love others as ourselves, turns out to be one of the most difficult tasks there can be. In my own life, health professionals have often given me the worst problems, worse than the patients themselves, as if the world of sickness had the power to contaminate health professionals by making them sickly or arrogant, and difficult to love.

We become doctors of medicine by learning an enormous number of things, by acquiring knowledge which allows us, among other things, to juggle with more and more powerful and extremely effective medicines. All my life, I have felt myself to be an intellectual, even when this has involved cutting myself off from my emotional source and from my soul, which is capable of crying at the sight of a lilac in bloom, and even though I often rage thinking about the misery of the world (and sometimes the extreme misery of others). Nevertheless, one day, I said to myself that the poetic universe was better than the scientific one, because in poetry lay the essence of the world and its Truth. Ever since then, I have had to face the difficulty of making science and poetry coincides, as if both were destined to be eternally in opposition to one another. The modern world does not expect the poet who has succeeded in expressing truths about our essential feelings (Saint-Denys Garneau or Arthur Rimbaud, for example) to explain or to think. We believe that the poet has only to sing, to juggle or to dance, and that it is up to the exegete or the professor to make understandable the poetic magma that flows from the lips of this speaker, this beautiful madman stimulated by the Muses. This world is in a dreadful state of split, a split which has lasted for too many centuries, and which has always been unacceptable to me. The fact that the poet can sing of the world with as much "intelligence" as emotion delights me, reassures me, gives me wings, and restores meaning to my existence, which has so often been grazed by the sharpness of human suffering.

That suffering is the lot of marching humanity, this I am willing to accept! But that the absurd should render suffering obsolete, and lead to all forms of suicide, I say no, I mean no, I wish to rebel, I rebel, although it requires a powerful energy which must be renewed daily. Without the presence of certain exceptional human beings (virtual, sometimes, in the case of authors whom I shall never know personally, such as Hermann Hesse, Albert Camus, Carl

Gustav Jung, Jacques Ferron or Théodore Monod), I would perhaps have admitted my impotence, and be satisfied by travelling in the forests or the tundra in search of what I have always found in nature, that is: peace and the feeling of belonging, of being in the right place at the right time, at my best, giving my best, for those close to me and for the crazy people who agree to follow me.

Literature and poetry remain anomalous, a kind of pain, a beauty shouted in the face of the universe. It is maybe why, having touched the poetic essence, Rimbaud felt the intense need to approach the other hillside of his life, rougher, more prosaic, more mortal, but simpler also. In state of "apoetry", we know why a crushed finger hurts. In the poetic state, a shattered soul leaves the one suffering in the most total fog:

"Je suis le saint, en prière sur la terrasse, -- comme les bêtes pacifiques paissent jusqu'à la mer de Palestine.

Je suis le savant au fauteuil sombre. Les branches et la pluie se jettent à la croisée de la bibliothèque.

Je suis le piéton de la grand'route par les bois nains; la rumeur des écluses couvre mes pas. Je vois longtemps la mélancolique lessive d'or du couchant.

Je serais bien l'enfant abandonné sur la jetée partie en haute mer, le petit valet suivant l'allée dont le front touche le ciel.

Les sentiers sont âpres. Les monticules se couvrent de genêts. L'air est immobile. Que les oiseaux et les sources sont loin! Ce ne peut être que la fin du monde, en avançant [2] "

"I am the saint praying on the terrace, as the peaceful herds graze as far as the sea of Palestine.

I am the savant in a dark armchair. Branches and rain flail the window of my library.

I am the way farer on the highway through the dwarf woods. The roar of sluice-gates drowns out my steps. I see for a long time the melancholy gold wet wash in the west.

I could be the child forgotten on the pier drifting toward the high gear, the little page going along the tree-lined walk whose top touches the sky.

The paths are rough. Broom is covering the hills. The air is motionless. How far away the words and springs are! It can only be the end of the world ahead [3]"

One day, I was bewitched by *The Illuminations* of Rimbaud. I had no means to analyse this text. Nevertheless, I saw taking place, page after page, portions of the abyss in which the young man had fallen. It was written in ways more complex than those of the logical and understandable language. It was registered in the material itself of language, any language, THE language, the *Ur-sprache* [4] It was more my instinct than my rational understanding which participated in the poetry of Rimbaud. When I had ended my reading, when I knew that the poet had finished the main part of his work at nineteen years old, then had begun running his adventure around the world, I said to myself that this man had probably felt the obligation to pass in other acts of reality to survive, not to have to face anymore the state of hell into which he had sunk. Rimbaud had dreaded that his task of clairvoyant would end very early in his life. It was necessary for him to leave for a journey from which he would not come back, or from which he would come back bloodless, lethally hurt, of one of these Abyssinia so necessary to the adventurers. Did Rimbaud simply wish to reinstate the world of the small mysteries of man's life, to feed on game as on the wind which whips the face and makes understanding that the essential part is somewhere else? More than anybody else, he put his feet in the anteroom of the after-life. In a sense, the poetry almost was his abyss. Living to express the world and then flop, here was what I retained of my reading of Rimbaud. The poet had the flash of genius to show that the Christianity had roamed, since European Enlightenment, and that human beings had made of it a machine of war. Rimbaud showed all his dignity when he asserted that the key of any work of life was the charity, but not any charity: the charity to spit, to bite, to run away. He then chose the exile and stopped writing.

Maybe we allow ourselves to engage with literature in order to sense that doubts can fade in certain privileged moments of our existence, and that the transcendent truth, the one which exceeds by far our small individual life, does exist, though always in a fog.

And what a fog! The most determining masterpieces of the universal corpus always seem the most inaccessible, because founded on the most imperceptible aspects of human soul. It so goes this way for *Hamlet*, written by Shakespeare. Can a man, even prince, be saved from the lucid madness which makes him so much procrastinate, but which pushes him nevertheless to murder, to "parricide" a criminal uncle who killed his true father, then married his mother?

The conflict is deep. Hamlet listens to spectral voices which have all the appearances of psychotic voices. Hamlet is crazy, but from now, it is not visible. Could an irrational being, listening to his drives and suffering from certain madness, look nevertheless completely reasonable? And what is the madness truly? For sure, we know that the total and uncontrollable mental distress which tangles all thoughts and feelings cannot support normal life. But do not exist some madnesses, more subtle and more perverse? Certain characters close to Hamlet in Shakespeare's masterpiece, hear the spectre's voice too. Is not the madness contagious? Are not we humans eminently influenced by the madness of others or the madness of one "Other", when he knows how to be devilish? We only have to think of Hitler, Stalin, Pol Pot, Ceaucescu ... Mad or not, Hamlet hears the avenging and passionate voice, he listens to it and follows its directives. Blinded, he only has one idea: to take revenge. He even has to "mime madness" to pursue his goals. Hamlet becomes inhabited by a real avenging madness, but intelligent and lucid at the same time. Hamlet wants to kill, and he shall kill. The will eventually keeps silent any other sort of "healthier", wiser or more loving emotion. Hamlet leads his fate with a determination which would make anyone shivers. Hamlet, as Oedipus in Sophocles' masterpiece, possesses an extreme intelligence, although this intelligence depends mostly on "insipid thought", as said in Oedipus the King. A morbid fate leads Hamlet towards tragedy. Nevertheless, Hamlet loved Ophelia when he wrote:

> "Thus in her excellent white bosom (...)
> Doubt thou the stars are fire,
> Doubt that the sun doth move,
> Doubt truth to be a liar
> But never doubt I love.
> O dear Ophelia, I am ill at these numbers, I have not art to reckon my groans. But that I love the best. O most best, believe it. Adieu [5]."

Despite this love, full of rage, believing that Claudius spies on him, Hamlet cries out: "A rat, a rat!". With his sword, he strikes the person hidden behind a curtain, in his mother's room. Ophelia's father Polonius falls down. Hamlet has no regret. Guilt is not the concern of the avenger. Could Ophelia prevent this abominable act? We would not say so. Ophelia has no means to react, because of her frail love, of her past of well-bred girl. To save Hamlet, she would have been a fury, an "egeria" or Mother Teresa! When her brother dies from Hamlet's hand once again, Ophelia cannot survive. In the sea of her tears, she lets herself go. Was Hamlet's fate too intense, too much ordered beforehand, i.e. directed by tragic forces (in which believed the Greeks of the Antiquity), so that Ophelia's simple love can change anything there? Hamlet had really proclaimed: "In her excellent white bosom..." Nevertheless, the suicide of his lover becomes almost anecdotal for him. The masterpiece ends in a total tragedy.

What about redemption. Was Hamlet's redemption possible? Did he have the capacity not to kill? The force? The courage? The will? Where is love when fate leads somebody towards his biggest evil? To read Hamlet, to study it and understand it, and to read it again, does it protect to be pulled towards our strongest fate, even if this one is going to be despicable? To read, to write, to create and to play drama, does it prevent Evil? Does literature make us better? And what is to be "better"? To be more affectionate, more compassionate, more upright, stronger in front of others' weakness and one's own weakness, while remaining a loving person? Yes, a little, obviously. This obvious fact is so easy when it is a question of expressing it in words, and so difficult to put it into practice in everyday life! Does art help us to live better, or is it only a simple diversion, a way to express what could be "better" with humans, but always and eternally places of pure representation? The implacable ordinary of life does not seem to expect masterpieces, neither art nor poetry? The reality itself leads to a merciless fate: death. Believing in humanity's "progress", is it having been blind, deaf and idiotic during all the XXth century? Who would now dare to claim that the XXIth century announces so much "progress"?

Nevertheless, it remains that poetry touches our soul, as much as music and this emotion is capable of generating good. Music is certainly what brings every "reader-listener" closer to the essence of the world. By reading, writing, looking, and listening, we are sometimes made serene again, touched by the truth, in spite of visible chaos, and powers of fate. Music is probably the supreme outcome of human life. But the question remains complete: do arts make us better? At this moment of the "big collective walk forward", as so many scientific discoveries add up hundreds of million pages on the Web, is it still possible to prevent the catastrophic robotization into which the humanity appears to rush?

Kafka was a real prophet when he sensed that bureaucratism was going to throw hundreds of million individuals in situations worse than those of the Middle Ages. Did literature contribute to delay the decay, the shamefulnesses of mechanization and contemporary robotization? Will seven billion human beings be happy tomorrow with transmitting their enjoyments and fate to small screens, in a world where people are paid to invent the worst insignificances which have never been created since the beginning of the world? If I was Hamlet, called to scuttle myself by a force that exceeds me, which Ophelia of literature, poetry, music and love could even, during a few seconds, think of changing my fate?

In short, do arts, any kind of art, possess an ethical function? Is the humanity thrown in a hysteric, aesthetic and brilliant race, both scientific and artistic, but which leads it at top speed towards the abyss, either is there hope? Where does this hope come from?

Devoting ourselves to literature allows us unquestionably to build our own vision of the world (the *Weltanschauung*). So, by reading some fundamental texts, an attentive reader achieves probably to protect himself from totalitarian commands imposed by most, otherwise all, societies. As some "elected members", certain dictators, allow themselves to impose visions which eventually are only malpractice of simplest laws of human life, and of life itself. In literature, it is the sweet madness as well as the creation of impossible realities - absolutely insolvable tragedies- that allow tolerating life itself, as it is, a mix of joy and sadness, sorrow and jubilation, birth and death, being part of the same existential whirlwind, until the supreme test from which nobody went out alive, test which generate so much writings, test that a character as Faust wished to win, even at the price of what was most precious to him, his soul.

To try to understand the conflict existing between aesthetics and ethics, there are many good reasons to read *Faust*, from Goethe, *Tao-Tö-King* from Lao-Tseu, and *Glances and Games in the Space* from Saint-Denys Garneau. Understand, yes, although we anticipate that it remains completely vain trying to understand everything. It is in poetry, in Rimbaud's poetry in particular, as well as in some famous Russian novels, that are certain elements of answer to the human condition, in the deep irrationality of *A Season in Hell*, or in the boiling souls of the *Brothers Karamazov*, outside any logical thought. In the dive towards a poetic state commanded by the reading of Rimbaud, the senses, all the senses are made use of, but without the exclusive control of rationality. Ultimately, it is by poetry that literature becomes useful in the quest of "the best of ourselves", although a better understanding of others and their soul can become an abominable trap for whoever acquires some skills to understand others, because then, there is possibility to manipulate them while stopping to love them. And the power is constantly the opposite extreme of love.

In the essay entitled *Prométhée, Faust, Frankenstein*, Dominique Lecourt mentions Pico della Mirandola who, with Giordano Bruno and Paracelsus during the Middle Ages, had grasped what we have stopped considering today, but that certain poets try desperately not to let people forget about: it is inside the most sacred mixture of gathered rational and irrational functions that humanity can hope not being destroyed:

> "After thinking a long time, I have figured out why man is the most fortunate of all creatures and as a result, worthy of the highest admiration and earning his rank on the chair of being, a rank to be envied not only by the beasts but the stars themselves and by the spiritual natures beyond and above this world" (Translated by Richard Hoocker). This reason belongs by no means to the eminent place that the creator would have attributed to him, on the scale of living beings according to the classic explanation. It is not thus associated to a particular perfection of his nature. On the contrary, it refers to the fact that paradoxically, the man does not have a nature in the sense that one was attributed to other living beings. (...) God having finished building "the house of the world" as we know it, He wished "that there would be somebody to consider the reason of such a work, to like its beauty, to like its greatness. (...) Everything was already fulfilled: everything had been distributed to the superior, intermediate and lower beings. (...) God addresses the man in these terms: "if we have created you neither celestial nor terrestrial, neither mortal nor immortal, it is so that, endowed with the honorary power to model and to shape yourself, you give yourself the shape which would have had your preference"[6].

In the universe of gathered rational and irrational functions, the human maybe has only one reason for being and acting on earth: demonstrating its Beauty. Staying on the look-out, grasping the beauty of the world requires however a large amount of energy, as well as lucidity which is "the wound closest to the sun ", to resume René Char's word.

What can I say to a woman who presents herself at the emergency doubled up with the terrible pains of acute pancreatitis? Shall I recite poems to her or do I rather have to take all possible measures to relieve her of her pain? I inject a painkiller (medical science produces good analgesics), I hydrate her, then I transfer her somewhere else, to a hospital where there are specialists (as I practice medicine in the Quebec's Great North, I often have to use planes. Even when they're knocked to pieces, these machines prove that they are infinitely faster than dog sleds!). In this day and age, with all the risks but also all the positive effects of science and technology, it is necessary to admit that the Nordic "poetry" remains quite relative, even if we wish to believe in poetry, even if we have faith in the archaic, essential and Hyperborean shamanism which accompanies any injection of painkiller.

My belief in value of literature is not a matter of choice. I feel it from deep down in my gut and from my rational consciousness at the same time, although I remain fundamentally a prisoner of an extremely down-to-earth existence, particularly regarding my professional practice. It appears extremely difficult for me to conciliate the ideals of poetry and the inescapable reality of abdominal pains that bring on vomiting, this particular suffering being combined with a thousand other difficulties of all kinds: social, economic, psychic, or metaphysical. What honest poet could hope to change the world in order to really reduce the suffering in it? And yet, every poet feels that outside of the world of art, nothing really makes sense, and human suffering, which has the potential for total non-sense, remains essential in its intimate relation with happiness, essential to the creation of happiness itself. Every poet senses that the mystery of life can be solved, and *is* solved, though usually only fleetingly, with all the suffering that it implies, solved with words and through words, in a flash, like autumn light possesses the extraordinary capacity to set fire to the foliage of birches of the North.

How I suffer sometimes as physician! The dilemma is a major one. I need poetry, and when my poetic sensibility is kindled, I become unable to tolerate disease and death. Then, it becomes necessary for me to fall again into the "*a*poetry" of the world, even though contact with this "*a*poetry" produces violent reactions inside of me. Poetry is a vital necessity for me. But any exaggeration of poetic ecstasy can lead to death or self-destruction, the body asking for, above all, simple things, such as water, songs, or cries of joy. Young children know about this instinctively. They do not need poetic words, being themselves "poetry", which is the explanation for Christ's important affirmation: "Nobody shall enter the kingdom of Heaven unless he first becomes like these little children."

Animal of the spirit, similar to a child, revolutionary and unbearable for anybody who did not follow him, Vincent van Gogh explored the world through colours. His everyday life did not have much importance. Was it changed into what his spirit wished it to be, e.g. a "more-than-life"? I believe that the dilemma introduced by poetry turns out to be most of the time impossible to resolve during one's life. Consequently, this explains the lack of realism of poetry, although its origins remain firmly rooted in a fundamental reality. It is necessary to accept the irreconcilable adventure of life based on this precept expressed by Kenneth White: "Poetry begins with a radical rejection of the world. It looks like religion which has its "realm of spirit" and its "realm high above us which is not a part of this world"[7].

Poetry depends on a horrible paradox: it is necessary to accept the unacceptable, and to accept radical rejection as the cornerstone of a life which cannot be lived without suffering and rejection. To lose one's life in order to gain it: the idea is a religious one, even before being poetic.

To love, as physician or health professional, means listening and trying to help. As a friend who likes to take inspiration from Paulo Coelho confided in me: "We must never forget that spiritual experience is, above all, an experience of love. And, in love, there are no rules. However hard we try to follow textbooks, to control our heart, to have behaviour strategies, in the end it is useless. It is the heart that decides, and what it decides becomes law." This friend is one of the best physicians I have ever met.

A few weeks ago, I visited a friend. She sleeps twenty hours a day nowadays. Her boyfriend works when she rests. He is almost as tired as she is, but he is not sick, far from it. He profoundly loves his girlfriend. He works to be with her, to take care of her, to earn money which makes them survive. They love each other. She is very slow, with blue eyes, so intense blue eyes; and her face is swelled up because of cortisone. Nevertheless, medicines are useful for her. Her legs are like blocks, she suffers from phlebitis in calves. She laughs if we make jokes, but she laughs weakly. What is remarkable is that she is still capable of being tender and welcoming. She "is" love. It seems to me that we see the best of her. She loves her boyfriend. She simply loves. She looks at the world with delicacy, although she is really suffering. A powerful painkiller is pushed every hour in one of her veins by a small pump attached to her belt. It is what makes her groggy. Otherwise, her pain could be unbearable. She has been hospitalized recently during several days because she had too much pain. The monster has spread itself in her spine during the last months. It invades cell by cell ganglions, blood vessels, and nerves. The metastases of her cancer eat away nerves and bones of her pelvis. The pain could become again at any time completely horrible.

My friend is emaciated. Her arms are nothing but skin and bones. Her body drifts away. Her boyfriend is still in love with her, more than ever. He loves his soul, he cannot love his destroyed body, but they love each other. My friend is going to die. I gulp only by saying that. I would like to embrace my friend, to reassure her, to swear to her that life after death is better, but I am as much atheist as believer. Indeed, I do not believe in anything as soon as I am not close to the tundra or to the rivers of the North, as soon as I move away from telluric or heavenly sources. If I am a cloud in the tundra, if I am a flake of snow in the taiga, if I am twig of aspen on the banks of a Laurentian lake, then, yes, my belief allows me to tolerate suffering, the suffering of others and my suffering. Otherwise, I am lost.

I write about my difficulty to be happy as a physician in a society which I find, often, greatly insignificant, but a society which feeds me well, which has not only defects, but a society which is agonizing, cynic, agnostic and happy to be like that, although the worst individuals, the most dangerous, remain God's fools. I understand that humanity needed atheism to survive the profound madness of all fundamentalisms. Nevertheless, without the Absolute, without the absolute of God or Poetry, how would it be possible to tolerate human existence?

I thus write. But the task of writing as an art is horribly complex. Sometimes, I would prefer to give up. I say to myself that artistic work requires too much effort. And then, two hours or two days later, I say to myself: art is challenging, but that is why it makes sense. Rilke was a lover as great as Mother Teresa. Saint-Denys Garneau loved the world as Jean Vanier still loves it. One has funded "L'Arche" to take care of others. The other has written:

"Je ne suis pas bien du tout assis sur cette chaise
Et mon pire malaise est un fauteuil où l'on reste
Immanquablement je m'endors et j'y meurs.

Mais laissez-moi traverser le torrent sur les roches
Par bonds quitter cette chose pour celle-là
Je trouve l'équilibre impondérable entre les deux
C'est là sans appui que je me repose [8]"

"I am far from easy sitting on this chair
And the clasp of an armchair is the worst of all
There I am bound to drowse and die
But let me cross the torrent by the rocks
Pass bounding from one thing to another
I find my buoyant balance between the two
It is in suspension that I am at rest [9]"

I cooked a meal for my dying friend and her boyfriend. They did not suspect that I would come home with fresh caribou. They did not expect to eat my food. A few weeks earlier, I had shot down a caribou in the Great North. We laughed a lot during the meal. Then the time came for me to go. My friend waved to me through the window. She showed me that kindness and beauty are still possible when the body is disintegrated. This Death like a sword of Damocles above us is challenging, it remains the most catastrophic and the most fundamental event that can happen to us.

The contemporary world judges severely acts of faith as well as intuitions about the relevance of a life other than the one we get nowadays. But we only have to believe in life after death so that it exists. Everything is about faith. Without faith, there is only reality, which is sometimes funny, and too often dramatic. We have to believe in redemption, in beauty of souls, even dead souls. Believing means not considering the rational thoughts which say that it is stupid to believe in life after death.

Last Friday, my sick friend lived, as she will live the Sunday preceding her funeral. My friend will live as long as we shall cherish her memory. I would like to add that even after her death, she will still live. I believe it.

"Rationality, common sense, and science embodying it in a concentrated manner, are convenient for a while and for a serious stage, but never go beyond the borders of the most commonplace reality and the average human normality. In fact, they give no solution to the problem of psychic suffering and its underlying signification. Psychoneurosis, in last analysis, is a suffering of the soul which did not find its sense. From the suffering of the soul emerges every spiritual creation and from it originates every progress of the man as a spirit; yet, the motive of this suffering is spiritual stagnation, infertility of the soul."

"The perfect adaptation is certainly an ideal. Nevertheless, it is not always possible; in some situations, the only adaptation is a patient resignation."

"Beyond that orderly world, a nature controlled by rationality waits, eager for revenge, for the moment when the fragile barrier will collapse to spread itself, destroyer, in the conscious existence. From the early phases of humanity, man has been conscious of this danger, the danger of the soul; that is why religious and magic rites had been created, to protect from this threat or to cure psychic devastations. That is why the medicine-man has always been a priest, a saviour of the body and the soul, and why religions have always been systems that cure the sufferings of the soul. It is true at least for two of the most important religions of humanity, Christianity and Buddhism. What relieves the suffering man, it is never what he imagines, but only truth which he believes supra-human, revealed, and that extracts him from the state of suffering"[10], as Carl Gustav Jung writes in *The Soul and the life*.

This reminds me of good doctor Rieux, in *The Plague* written by Albert Camus. I shall never have his tenacious courage in front of adversity, a humanist courage but as a total "stranger" to any form of mystic spirituality. I believe in life after death, but with my heart aching to have any logical or coherent explanation, facing nothingness presented by modern thought, by so many philosophers, by good friends also, who live the agnostic existentialism in the most true way, a way of living which I share in everyday life, I know it, but which I reject, in my heart, for irrational reasons.

One day, I met at the emergency ward of an Inuit hospital a fifteen-month-old child who was in coma having fallen on the head. I ventilated him, he had difficulty to breathe, and his right lung was full of vomit. I prepared his transfer to the South. His mother and father were there, attentive, present, but quiet, very quiet. The mother often came to speak to her child who did not answer. She took his hand. A machine was sending air into the child's lungs. The mother was hot in her *amauti* [11]. She left to the cafeteria of the hospital with her husband. I joined them to eat. We had supper together. These Inuits were grateful for my work, with dignity and without submission. This baby in coma was their seventh child. They asked me if he would survive. I said yes. He was going to leave soon with the air-ambulance. The mother was smiling, the father was affectionate. He was so affectionate at this time, attentive, and kind. He thanked me. I found him and his wife beautiful. It gave me the desire to continue working, still a little, while in spite of another physician who had come to help me intubating the child. Extremely nervous, she had taken all responsibility of the situation and the working atmosphere returned unbreathable. My God! How it is difficult to cure dying people! How a father and a mother can contribute to the quiet beauty of the world! We left urgently because the air-ambulance was going to arrive at the airport. The child hardly breathed. I manually sent air into his lungs with a rubber balloon. The emergency truck did not start up at the first attempt; the door of the garage refused to open. There was no more electricity in the village: generalized breakdown. The baby tossed restlessly; he tried to take away the tube out of his trachea. We finally took seats into another emergency truck, in the cold, by 30 degrees Celsius below zero. The baby stopped moving when I sent him to sleep more profoundly by using an appropriate medicine. We moved slowly on the road to the airport, the baby still alive. It was pitch-dark. The air-ambulance was there. A physician, aboard the plane, took responsibility of the child. I told him his entire story. Outside, it was snowing and storming. I was tired. I had to work another ten hours.

Until today, I ran away in front of death, by fear, I admit it, immense and terrible fear. I am not really afraid of falling into a ravine. I am not afraid of the possible delight which reigns beyond this life. I am afraid of the disappearance, the ghostly state. I made death mine when I went through the continent in snowmobile between Hudson Bay and Ungava Bay. It is rather the hideous condition of the degraded body and the absent soul that frightens me, more than death itself. I am never afraid in the forest or in the tundra. I like what I am when I know how to face my possible death, by cold days or in high mountains, whereas, in front of disease, decay of the body, suffering of organs and cells, I crash. There is here subject to nausea.

I liked challenges when I was twenty years old. I thus leapt into life by approaching the impossible: being physician while facing what had given me so many shudders. Every day, I still have to learn to tame disease. A sadness reigns in me and I cannot get rid of it in front of the possible death of loved ones. It is not death that frightens me; it is nothingness, possible nonsense. It is my countless doubts that give me shudders in front of incurable disease. And these eyes that ask me for something. Doctor, doctor ... But I cannot do anything about it. I am an incompetent. I still have humour, and love of humour and jokes; to be able to do more than making bearable the unbearable. To laugh thinking of my mother who danced with her feet full of corns, herself and the way she said everything with tenderness in silence, never asking her son to be there or to visit her, still wishing him "have a good trip", waving to him while she was standing on the doorstep, because love asks for nothing, because love forgives, because love is a body in a state of decomposition, because if I had to die now, I would not have gone yet where I have to go, because death always arrives too soon for some, for others and for us. But for all of us, patient which are reprieved, all this has to make sense, because otherwise ... The only honour which is worth while is to die having let love reign. When a dying person knows that love he or she has sown will survive, in the grave, in the sky or in the dust, he or she can be happy, a little.

Who am I? An adventurer. An explorer. A lover of trees and rivers, ice, and space. I first love living beings of nature. The human beings, sometimes, discourage me. A few days ago, a young man was brought to the hospital because he had a head injury, his facial bones were broken down, and he had an extracted eye. He was extremely agitated. He had gulped down too much drugs. Besides, a subdural haematoma was killing him. A companion of unworthiness had stricken him several times with a dumbbell. We had to send the patient immediately to a surgeon, in the South. Humans sometimes want to kill other people. I thus like the spruces which fight against winter; they do not hate each other. They hate nothing. They have other fish to fry. The young and lost Inuit inhaling gasoline or propane have a burned soul, all this because of a long chain of resentful perversions. But so many Inuits are beautiful, deserving, charming, strong, and magnificently healthy.

In the Great North, we often eat in a friendly way; we swallow and taste with serenity the finest flesh which is offered to us. Then comes a time when it is no more food that we touch, it is beings and true people loving what they are and hoping that their country of happiness will not be too much plundered, or despoiled, or destroyed by some force coming from somewhere else. They are afraid, deep down in their soul, the sensible Inuits, they remain patient, they go fishing or they sing, they look at, crying slowly, their weakest people dying hanged, and they say to themselves that between two cultures, two moments, two civilizations, two places of globalizing technology, two visions of the world, they have to work as hard as they did ten thousand years ago, to prevent their universe from being annihilated by a negative trend which reigns almost everywhere, this trend not being natural at all, but essentially human. "Human, all too human", would say Friedrich Nietzsche.

But Inuit festivities remain magnificent to live. One day, both sexes will get together, and women will be able to exult with their men, and vice versa, men knowing that it is possible to work with women. This day will come; then, the partridges will fly low, graceful, white and black along the ice fields, secure about their future.

One night, I had to go urgently by plane in a small and isolated village of the south coast of Hudson Bay; an old woman was dying, victim of a spontaneous pneumothorax. Once we got back to Puvirnituq hospital, I inserted a big plastic tube into her rib cage, on the right side of the body. When she began breathing a little better – a few hours later a tension pneumothorax would have crushed her heart and her other lung -, she appreciated the treatment. She thanked me, in her language, by stopping to pant like a small dog. I was tired, but pleased with myself.

Who am I? A lover of ice fields and fishing. One day of February, by 35 degree Celsius below zero, on the ice of Povungnituq river, big winds were blowing, the sun was shining- a sun to take one's breath away-, we were five persons to dig a two-metre hole in the ice of the river, using a *tuuk* [12]. It took us more than one hour. Then, using three fishing lines, we caught sixteen beautiful cods. They gave us their life. We made fillets out of them. In the evening, we ate the best fish and chips ever made. It was more than cold on the ices of this edge of the world in the Great North. The next day, we explored some of the islands beyond the embouchure of the river, in Hudson Bay, just to fill us up with landscape. The magnificence exists, I swear! If our snowmobile had broken down during this trip, it would have been very cold. But it is worth risking freezing our buttocks and our heart. In the coldness of February or March, we were five people to love each other. I love the human race when I am fishing and that nothing is easy. I hate so much not loving. This weekend full of big shudders had reminded me of what I am: a small boy sensitive to the cold who, without appropriate clothes, could die in a few minutes. Ah, true life, always within the realms of possibility!

Reality as well as everyday life can be perfect destroyers of communication soul to soul. Friendship, literature, love, great passions, here are reasons to remain in contact with each other. And then, there is fishing, this supreme state of contact with ourselves and with other's strength, this brother, this sister, close to nirvana, maybe better than nirvana itself, especially when the fish bites and when that the sun goes down greeting us cheerfully.

I am thus a nature-lover. I say aloud that humans have to love their nature and the Nature otherwise, it is only a matter of time and hatred: the human planet will soon be destroyed!

I am a suicidal person although the many times I have come within a hair's breath of death have given sense to my life. Without death touching me so often, who would I be? I consider myself as an *ignitor,* a creator of projects, an *inebriator*, a being, and a survivor. I am sometimes a dangerous man who, if he had not possessed a sixth sense, would have been able to fall several times into the abyss. When I practice medicine, particularly at the hospital, I touch the worst part of the world. But I also touch its essential part. And I often fell happy, although I am still on the brink of ruin. I find there strengths which I did not consider holding; I try not to throw a tantrum. Some patients live total shamefulness. One night, a fourteen-year-old girl came to the emergency because she had been raped by her father. She confided me that this man raped her regularly. She had wanted to kill herself by swallowing all the pills she could find at home.

This is the world into which I have fallen, like a lost child, from the first days of my arrival in the medical reality. Since, I have tried to go back up from the deep well into which I had sunk. I held on, I made a thousand small falls, but without ever falling that low again. I broke fingers and bones against the walls of this well, but now, I see the light, there is some silt on the walls, I can see a pulley supported by a beam, there is a bucket and a small rope hanging, I am going to hold out the hand, soon, it will be finished, my ascent will be completed. I shall be born finally and I shall shout for joy. I shall say that snobbery and middle-class capitalism everywhere are not at all forgivable, that this planet suffers partly because of rich people egocentrism and that it is necessary to react or to die. I choose reaction and then death, because the hysteric rot which surrounds me, in this zone of power of extreme consumption where I wade, can only lead to hatred of miserable men.

I did my best cures as physician when I believed not to be curing. Without literature, I believe that I would not have been capable of living with this paradox in the head and in the heart. But this paradox will eventually kill me, or will drive me crazy (but no, I shall not die crazy. I shall always have the forest, the happy coldness of taiga and tundra. There will always be a small snow bank to sink into, as in an igloo, and to love this nice coldness which reminds me that it is necessary to warm us up, always, at all costs, by sticking together).

Who am I? A writer. A teacher. For me, it goes hand in hand. I am a quiet madman. But I stop being quiet when a person's life is put in my hands. In general, I like to love humans, even if these humans are billions of times harder to love than all other entities of the galaxy. I would sometimes parachute if I could take refuge far from any form of humanity.

I like meeting myself in places where the Spirit reigns. I have the firm conviction that certain places are more convenient than others for the Spirit's blossoming. I like the university campus, the atmosphere of numerous schools where I had the privilege to be invited as a speaker. Often, I felt the inspiration which animated these places. I like the students' presence, their dynamism, and their enthusiasm. Teaching always delights me, although I still feel this necessity of pursuing my exploration of the world, and the world of the Great North in particular. Writing allows me to be a little bit of everything at the same time, doctor, teacher, animator, intellectual, artist, poet, adventurer, father, lover, friend, anarchist and madman. When I write, I place my knowledge in a small bag, and I mix it. To create, we need silence, silence and time, more than for any other activity. We need a lot of time to let poetry express itself.

I write to say that love and harmony are better than cynicism and nihilism. I write to speak about caribous and their dance in the tundra, to say that Inuits have a whole universe to reveal to the South. I write to express my moods when I observe a flight of Canada geese in the sky of the Great North. I write on the art to be transformed into small game or into dwarfish birch. I write to deliver to the world and to me a less unfinished portion of my heart, to express, oh, sometimes by small awkward touches, what, otherwise, could never be expressed.

I like to tangle everything, literature, philosophy, anthropology, poetry, geography, languages, medicine, music, *northness*, and quantic physics. I love. I love to have this feeling that poetic contact established itself from soul to soul between two human beings, between several human beings, as in a text. I write to say this. Each day the madness of writing comes to feed my runs-up, my comings and goings in this world, my crushes, my way of leading my work.

Literature and medicine are only excuses. Maybe everything is only an excuse to reach the soul, mine as well as others'. Words as well as human diseases are only excuses to love better. Nevertheless, launched in the world anyhow, words can prevent from loving with harmony. The words also have the power to be simple and empty images. "The language which can form Socrates' ethics, Christ's parables, Shakespeare or Hölderlin's masterful constructions of human, is capable of, in accordance with its unlimited potentialities, organizing death camps and making the chronicle of torture chambers. The linguistic virtuosity peculiar to the quack, which was also characteristic of Hitler, is antimatter, it gives shape to anti-logos, which conceptualizes, then carries out, the deconstruction of human being"[13], writes George Steiner.

But rushing into literature remains for me a vital necessity, like burying myself in *The Idiot* written by Dostoïevski for example, without knowing what value this crazy (and even sickly) enterprise which is literature can have. Without the Word, the Logos, without words and poetry revealed by these words, life could be only vain, cruel and aimless. But what is this force of faith and hope which drives the poet to forge ahead forward, despite all opposition? Is it the force of music of the world which continues its eternal reassurance, which sings, from the extreme limit of the Universe, while bringing its song to the smallest soul, the most flighty and the most scatterbrained one?

To become acquainted with prince Mychkine, in *The Idiot*, allows us to become aware of what is compassion. Lucidity is useful, even necessary. But does the art of living ask for such an enterprise of lucidity that it is necessary to associate literature to daily activities, or even to the study of medicine, mechanical engineering or philosophy? Where is the Quality (in Pirsig's opinion, in his book *Zen and the Art of Motorcycles Maintenance: an Inquiry into Values*) when we consider the immense work necessary to go through certain literary works while there is so much to do in so many domains, while such a mass of knowledge must now be crammed assimilated to somehow understand a little piece of the modern world? Why literature, so many words and written pages? To fight. What? Maybe the total robotization of the world and spirits.

There is at the same time a strange and terrifying combination of good and evil in every human being, the greatest good being often associated to what looks like the greatest evil. The romantic complexity in which every reader is buried can only be beneficial. We become more lucid when we realize that the murderer, the madman, the jealous person, or the hysteric, are complex beings in whom the capacity to love is never withdrawn totally.

I only wish to continue to believe in humanity. But sometimes, I am afraid that nothing makes sense, that human is only the result of an unfortunate fate which arose one day in the galaxy. A career is nothing. One hundred masterpieces are nothing compared to the song of a white- throated sparrow, in the evening, when we camp near a lake of the North.

When I walk in the tundra or when I paddle down a river in my canoe, the living poetry of nature refrain me from losing faith in myself and in humanity. Then, I know that love exists.

REFERENCES

[1] Arthur Rimbaud, *Sensation*, poem translated by Claire Dumont and Anne Martineau.
[2] Arthur Rimbaud, *Poésies/Une saison en enfer/Illuminations*, Paris, Gallimard, 1988, p. 158-159.
[3] Translation by John Porter Houston, New Haven and London, Yale University Press, 1963, p.255.
[4] *The Ur-sprache*, it is the idioma that exists before the multiplication of all languages, this original form that so many mystics looked for and that the passionates of language are still looking for, that is about in the first pages of *Faust,* from Goethe, and which could, possibly, constitute the "Truth" behind all the others announced truths, that cement which make possible, in spite of all impossibilities, the traduction.
[5] William Shakespeare, *Hamlet*, Paris, Gallimard (bilingual edition), 2004, p. 126.

[6] Dominique Lecourt, *Prométhée, Faust, Frankenstein/Fondements imaginaires de l'éthique*, Paris, Livre de Poche, 1996, p. 186-187. Translation by Claire Dumont and Anne Martineau.
[7] Kenneth White, *La figure du dehors*, Paris, Grasset, 1978, p. 47.
[8] Hector de Saint-Denys Garneau, *Regards et jeux dans l'espace*, Montréal, Boréal, 1993, p. 10.
[9] Translated by John Glassco, *Complete poems of Saint-Denys Garneau*, Oberon Press, 1984, p. 20.
[10] C.G. Jung, *L'Âme et la vie*, Paris, Buchet/Chastel, 1963, p. 329-330. Translation by Claire Dumont and Anne Martineau.
[11] Coat worn by Inuit women.
[12] Inuit tool to make holes in the ice composed of a band of steel and of a long handle.
[13] George Steiner, *Réelles présences*, Paris, Gallimard, 1988, p. 83. Translation by Claire Dumont and Anne Martineau.

INDEX

A

abortion, 111
academic performance, 16
access, x, 50, 96, 97, 107, 111, 144, 154, 158, 161, 163, 166, 169, 170, 177, 181
accessibility, 133, 157, 161
accidents, 113
accommodation, 26, 97
accountability, 181
accuracy, 8, 9, 29, 73
achievement, viii, 161
action research, 163, 164, 165, 167, 168
activation, 123
adaptability, 112, 115, 122
adaptation, viii, xiii, 2, 4, 16, 17, 18, 70, 72, 74, 80, 83, 86, 88, 89, 91, 109, 114, 122, 132, 139, 195
adaptive functioning, 4
addiction, 94, 95, 116, 150
adjustment, 4, 135, 147, 166, 168
adolescence, 19, 80, 82, 125, 135
adolescent behavior, 134
adolescents, xiv, 125, 133, 158, 159
adult education, 139
adulthood, 81
adults, 36, 70, 79, 101, 103, 105, 113, 123, 124, 127, 140, 154
advocacy, 95, 159
aesthetics, 192
Africa, 42, 124
African American(s), 125, 154, 155, 160, 165
age, viii, 1, 3, 5, 7, 8, 9, 19, 21, 44, 68, 75, 78, 82, 84, 95, 105, 154, 158, 162, 193
ageing, 69, 71, 72, 93, 94, 99, 114, 121, 126
ageing population, 114
aging, 132
aging process, 132
agriculture, 66, 112

AIDS, 69, 70, 100, 110
air pollution, 130, 136
alcohol, 7
alcohol use, 7
alcoholism, 93, 111, 116
alienation, 23
allergy, 113
alternative(s), x, 38, 40, 42, 43, 45, 50, 72, 73, 141, 145, 157, 172
altruism, 116
ambiguity, 54
ambivalence, 49
amendment(s), 53, 156
American Psychological Association, xi, xiv, 132, 166, 168
Americans with Disabilities Act, 165
amniocentesis, 81, 105
anger, 91, 116, 147, 151
animals, 9, 68, 115, 116
anoxia, 7
antagonism, 87
anthropology, 78, 85, 103, 118, 199
antibiotic, 188
antibody, 93
antigen, 138
antimatter, 199
anxiety, 16, 91, 93, 143, 144
appraisals, 128, 143
aptitude, ix, 3, 15, 141, 144
argument, 39, 57, 146, 170
Aristotle, 39, 57
arousal, 24, 35
arthritis, 104, 147
assessment, viii, 1, 3, 6, 7, 9, 19, 25, 26, 30, 32, 94, 109, 127, 129, 132, 140, 152, 156, 157, 158, 164, 166
assimilation, 83
assumptions, 142

asthma, 80, 95, 104, 106, 123, 133, 135, 140
athletes, 102
attachment, 125
attention, viii, 1, 7, 8, 10, 12, 13, 14, 17, 38, 50, 53, 55, 103, 136, 140, 150, 188
attitudes, iv, 51, 71, 79, 101, 124
attribution, 15, 16
Australia, 60, 137, 138, 165
authenticity, 55
authority, 171, 178
autoimmune disease(s), 69, 83, 104
automobiles, 68
autonomy, 71, 95, 99, 102, 107, 175
availability, 80, 96, 97, 159
awareness, 35, 60, 66, 118, 122, 126, 150, 156, 157

B

bacillus, 67
bacteria, 69, 84, 88, 111
banks, 194
barriers, x, 41, 60, 108, 109, 153, 154, 155, 172, 180
behavior, 3, 18, 23, 24, 26, 34, 79, 123, 128, 134, 140, 142, 143, 145, 147, 151, 152
behavior therapy, 142, 151, 152
behavioral change, 143
behavioral medicine, 129, 137
beliefs, 30, 48, 57, 61, 74, 79, 86, 93, 120, 137, 143, 148, 149, 158
beneficial effect, 94, 98, 101
bias, 38, 55
biochemistry, 118
biodiversity, 111, 114, 115
bioethics, 57
birth, 7, 68, 81, 104, 105, 106, 111, 112, 117, 120, 192
birth control, 68, 111, 112, 117
birth weight, 20, 104
bladder, 162
blame, 147, 174
blind spot, 59
blindness, 147
blocks, 194
blood, 83, 93, 104, 194
blood pressure, 104
blood vessels, 194
bonding, 80, 81, 105, 106, 132, 133, 134
bonds, 162, 173, 174, 195
bowel, 162
boys, 6
brain, 3, 7, 20, 70, 80, 90, 91, 95, 104, 110, 111, 116, 121, 128, 130, 135, 136, 140
brain damage, 3, 7

brain development, 20, 80, 111, 121
brain functioning, 111
brainstorming, 157
Brazil, 133
breaches, 40, 42, 44
breakdown, 148, 196
breast cancer, 151
breast carcinoma, 129
breastfeeding, 139
breathing, 197
breeding, 112
bronchitis, 187
browsing, 110, 122
Buddhism, 195
burn, 147
by-products, 68, 122

C

caesarean section, 81, 105
Canada, 1, 7, 18, 19, 21, 47, 65, 111, 135, 138, 185, 187, 199
cancer, xii, 38, 44, 113, 125, 130, 136, 151, 194
capacity building, 156, 157, 165
capitalism, 198
carbohydrates, 129
carcinogenesis, 69
career development, xi
case study, 134, 136, 164, 167
casting, 41
catecholamines, 93
categorization, 46
causal relationship, 86
causality, 68, 70, 76, 86, 90
causation, 24, 29, 33, 34, 35, 78
cell, 70, 110, 194
cellular immunity, 131
Census, 154, 166, 167, 168
central nervous system, 93
cerebral cortex, 91
chaos, 110, 122, 129, 133, 191
child abuse, 18, 166
child development, 19, 20, 107, 108
child maltreatment, 5
child mortality, 98, 118
child protection, 5
childcare, 171, 181
childhood, 19, 82, 102, 127, 136, 140
children, viii, xiii, 1, 2, 3, 4, 5, 6, 7, 8, 9, 10, 12, 13, 14, 15, 16, 17, 18, 19, 20, 21, 26, 42, 69, 70, 79, 81, 89, 91, 95, 97, 99, 104, 105, 106, 113, 116, 120, 123, 124, 127, 132, 133, 135, 138, 140, 142, 158, 159, 166, 193

China, 112
cholera, 67
Christianity, 190, 195
chronic diseases, 69, 75, 76, 78, 92, 94, 95, 100, 105, 107, 119, 128
chronic fatigue syndrome, xiv
chronic illness, 25, 26, 30, 31, 38, 60, 80, 81, 101, 105, 125, 134, 136, 142, 145, 147, 152
chronic pain, 105
circadian rhythm(s), 115
circulation, 181
citizenship, 181
civil society, 173
classes, 21, 159
classification, 13, 15, 76, 77, 84, 128
clients, ix, xiii, 26, 29, 30, 31, 32, 33, 34, 35, 38, 41, 42, 48, 141, 143, 144, 145, 147, 148, 149
climate change, 66, 118
clinical assessment, viii, 23
close relationships, 102
clusters, 8
cognition, 3, 15, 26, 79, 86, 95, 112, 116, 142
cognitive abilities, 5, 17
cognitive capacities, 96
cognitive deficit(s), viii, 1, 2, 3, 13, 19
cognitive development, 7, 18
cognitive flexibility, 17
cognitive function, viii, 2, 3, 14, 16, 17, 102, 117
cognitive impairment, 99, 130, 143
cognitive performance, 13, 17
cognitive perspective, 73
cognitive profile, viii, 1, 14, 15, 17
cognitive therapy, ix, 131, 141
cohesion, 97, 98
cohort, 14, 160
colds, 93
collaboration, xiv, 156, 164, 175, 185
coma, 196
commensalism, 87
commerce, 173
communication, x, 40, 43, 45, 58, 70, 84, 86, 92, 106, 123, 154, 163, 169, 181, 183, 198
communication technologies, 123
community, x, xiii, xiv, 78, 79, 82, 83, 87, 89, 90, 97, 98, 101, 106, 107, 108, 109, 119, 120, 124, 126, 130, 132, 133, 134, 136, 138, 139, 140, 153, 155, 156, 157, 158, 159, 160, 161, 162, 163, 164, 166, 167, 168, 169, 170, 171, 172, 173, 174, 175, 176, 177, 178, 180, 181, 182, 183, 184
community psychology, xiv, 106, 139, 167
community service, 158
community support, 98
community-based services, 107, 140
compassion, 200
competence, viii, ix, xi, 9, 25, 33, 36, 37, 48, 54, 56, 57, 58, 72, 93, 102, 125, 165, 170
competency, x, 30, 169
competition, 89, 115
complement, 38
complexity, 15, 17, 39, 70, 72, 84, 87, 98, 105, 110, 111, 115, 122, 139, 178, 200
compliance, 23, 144
complications, 105
components, viii, ix, x, 2, 3, 15, 31, 51, 65, 66, 75, 77, 78, 79, 81, 82, 83, 84, 85, 86, 87, 88, 89, 90, 91, 96, 98, 100, 105, 146, 147, 149, 160, 169, 174, 178, 179, 183
comprehension, 4
concentration, 4, 16, 30, 83, 113
conception, 54, 67, 68, 105, 139
conceptual model, 78
conceptualization, 24, 48, 71, 72, 79, 84, 86, 87, 146
concrete, ix, 26, 37, 42, 43, 52, 53, 72, 101, 107, 119, 146, 177
concussion, 7
conditioning, 24, 115
conduct disorder, 123
confidence, ix, 17, 33, 94, 95, 97, 141, 144
conflict, 69, 190, 192
confounders, 130
Congress, iv, 157
congruence, 72, 131
consciousness, x, 50, 116, 169, 179, 180, 183, 193
consensus, 3, 84, 175, 176, 177, 181
consent, 7, 179
conservation, 36
constraints, 79
construction, ix, 37, 39, 50, 52, 70
consultants, 160
consumers, 155, 156, 165
consumption, 90, 91, 94, 102, 129, 198
continuity, 135, 183
control, viii, x, 1, 2, 4, 5, 9, 10, 13, 14, 15, 16, 17, 18, 24, 31, 34, 46, 68, 79, 91, 93, 94, 95, 98, 111, 112, 113, 114, 117, 124, 135, 137, 150, 153, 155, 164, 166, 172, 180, 192, 194
control group, viii, 1, 2, 10, 13
convergence, 110
conviction, 199
coping strategies, 86
corporations, 173
correlation(s), 10, 12, 52, 53
cortisol, 104
Costa Rica, 167
costs, 108, 109, 119, 199
cough, 188

coughing, 187
covering, 93, 189
creative process, 42
creativity, xii, 3, 16, 19, 38, 39, 45, 58, 117
credibility, 181
crime, 134
critical period, 80, 84, 87, 114, 121
crying, 188, 197
cultural norms, 79
culture, 55, 61, 71, 84, 158, 173
curing, 75, 120, 199
curiosity, 33, 35
curriculum, 160
cycles, 112

D

daily living, 29
danger, 69, 113, 116, 195
data collection, 160
database, 48
death(s), xi, 53, 67, 83, 89, 112, 118, 127, 191, 192, 193, 194, 195, 196, 197, 198, 199
decay, 191, 196
decision making, 25, 66
decision-making process, 160, 176, 181
decisions, viii, x, 25, 41, 94, 107, 109, 122, 144, 153, 155, 161, 163, 178, 179, 181, 182, 183
decomposition, 197
deconstruction, 199
defects, 194
definition, 3, 48, 57, 77, 94, 126, 138
deforestation, 68
delivery, x, xi, 80, 107, 126, 132, 156, 160, 169, 170
demand, 72, 112
dementia, 126, 130
demographic change, 66
demographic characteristics, 72, 75
Denmark, xii, 37
density, 97
dentists, 158, 159
deontology, 56
Department of Health and Human Services, 20
dependent variable, 10
depression, 5, 89, 93, 94, 95, 105, 143, 151
deprivation, 19, 131
desensitization, 106
desire(s), viii, 24, 74, 91, 121, 142, 164, 175, 196
destruction, 91, 92, 113
developing countries, 127
developmental delay, 69, 113
developmental psychopathology, 18
diabetes, 69, 70, 80, 83, 95, 104, 105, 113, 114, 130

diabetes mellitus, 130
dignity, 158, 190, 196
dilation, 91
directives, 70, 140, 167, 190
disability, viii, x, xii, 29, 31, 38, 45, 52, 53, 54, 60, 61, 62, 77, 101, 114, 126, 137, 142, 152, 154, 156, 160, 161, 163, 165, 166, 167, 168
discipline, 47, 55, 65, 78, 105
discomfort, 48, 51, 149
discourse, 23, 48
discriminant analysis, 10, 13, 15
discrimination, 88, 100, 139, 154
disorder, 91, 139
dissociation, 91, 96, 102, 134, 137
distortions, 30, 148
distress, 4, 190
distribution, 13, 68, 180
diversity, 68, 95, 115, 119, 139
division, 50
divorce, 49
DNA, 68, 134
doctors, 160, 188
domestic violence, xi, 158, 170, 177
dramatic narrative, 39
drinking water, 67, 96, 130
drug abuse, 159
drug addict, 93, 116
drug addiction, 93, 116
drug interaction, 123
drug use, 7, 158
drugs, 68, 87, 96, 197
duplication, 177

E

earth, 66, 67, 68, 112, 113, 114, 118, 122, 192, 193
eating, 93, 95, 132, 144
eating disorders, 93, 95, 132, 144
ecological models, ix, 65, 66
ecology, ix, 66, 68, 70, 87, 110, 111, 115, 117, 118, 119, 125, 133, 136, 137, 138, 139
economic development, 137, 177
economic resources, 150
economic status, 3, 19, 98, 166
economic systems, 71
ecosystem, 88, 112, 113, 114, 119, 126
ecstasy, 149, 193
Education, xiii, 2, 3, 66, 93, 94, 97, 98, 100, 114, 134, 140, 144, 154, 155, 158, 162, 164, 165, 166, 168, 174
educational institutions, 174
ego, 18, 36, 55, 57, 59
egocentrism, 198

elaboration, xiii
elderly, ix, 36, 37, 45, 101, 102, 103, 127, 130, 133, 175
elders, 142
electricity, 196
elementary school, 19
email, 23
emergence, 136
emotion(s), xi 16, 70, 86, 123, 134, 141, 144, 145, 146, 149, 151, 188, 190, 191
emotional experience, 146, 150
emotional responses, 91
emotional stability, 4
emotional state, 142, 145
emotional well-being, 142
employability, 132
employees, 88, 98
employment, xi, 90, 101, 109, 129, 139, 154, 157, 162, 164, 165, 166, 170, 171, 172, 174, 182
empowerment, viii, x, xi, xiii, 31, 65, 83, 92, 94, 95, 103, 106, 107, 108, 119, 120, 137, 139, 153, 154, 155, 156, 157, 164, 165, 166, 167, 169, 170, 172, 178, 179, 180, 181, 182, 183, 184, 185
encephalitis, 7
encouragement, 34
endocrine, 126
energy, 29, 30, 33, 36, 50, 69, 149, 188, 192
engagement, xii, 24, 25, 33, 37, 41, 43, 44, 135, 150
England, 45, 94, 151, 152
Enlightenment, 190
enthusiasm, 149, 199
environment, vii, ix, xi, xiii, 4, 14, 15, 16, 17, 26, 31, 33, 34, 35, 65, 66, 67, 68, 69, 70, 71, 72, 73, 74, 76, 78, 79, 80, 81, 82, 83, 84, 85, 86, 87, 88, 89, 90, 91, 92, 94, 95, 96, 97, 98, 99, 100, 102, 103, 104, 105, 106, 107, 108, 109, 110, 111, 113, 114, 115, 116, 118, 119, 120, 121, 122, 124, 126, 127, 128, 131, 132, 133, 169, 174, 180, 181
environmental change, 134
environmental conditions, 78, 79, 83, 109, 114
environmental context, 34
environmental factors, xii, 16, 67, 69, 70, 75, 77, 79, 87, 91, 94, 95, 98, 100, 104, 109, 114, 115, 134, 137, 138
environmental influences, 73
environmental issues, 170
environmental protection, 91
environmental resources, 34, 91
epidemic, 67, 129
epidemiology, 135, 136
epigenetics, 104
epilepsy, 7
epileptic seizures, 129

epistemology, xiv, 58
equipment, 181
equity, 97
ergonomics, 98, 106
ethics, xiii, 7, 50, 56, 57, 59, 192, 199
ethnic background, 154
ethnic minority, 154
ethnicity, 55, 154, 166
euphoria, 149
Europe, 75, 123
evening, 198, 200
evil, 191, 200
evolution, ix, 65, 66, 67, 69, 70, 74, 75, 77, 80, 83, 101, 111, 114, 116, 117, 118, 122, 126, 136
evolutionism, 118
exaggeration, 193
exclusion, 89, 91, 97, 124, 150, 174, 185
excuse, 152, 199
execution, 175
executive function(s), viii, 1, 7, 124, 135
exercise, x, 48, 53, 57, 99, 112, 117, 118, 126, 131, 153, 179
expertise, xiii, 164
exploitation, 68, 69, 89, 90, 91, 115, 117, 120, 122
exposure, 80, 81, 93, 104, 133, 148
external environment, 80, 86
external locus of control, 5
extinction, 68, 113
eye movement, 106
eyes, 194, 197

F

facial expression, 9
facilitators, 74, 75, 89, 91, 95, 97
failure, 2, 42, 80, 117, 136
failure to thrive, 136
faith, 51, 193, 195, 200
family, xiii, 2, 3, 6, 7, 33, 42, 43, 70, 75, 77, 81, 86, 87, 95, 98, 99, 100, 102, 105, 106, 107, 108, 125, 126, 127, 139, 140, 142, 144, 152, 154, 158, 162, 163, 166, 187
family environment, 105, 108
family income, 3
family interactions, 106
family members, 33, 81, 106, 107, 142, 144, 163
family relationships, 162
family support, 98
family system, 106
family structure, 3, 166
famine, 68
far right, 15
fasting, 138

fat, 69
fatigue, xiv, 29, 42, 105, 113, 136
fear(s), 41, 62, 114, 116, 188, 196
feedback, 31, 147, 150
feelings, 24, 25, 30, 31, 32, 40, 73, 78, 95, 96, 101, 102, 116, 117, 143, 147, 149, 164, 188, 190
feet, 187, 189, 197
females, 89, 112
fibromyalgia, 105, 113, 147
financial resources, 181
financing, 172
fish, 83, 150, 197, 198
fisheries, 112
fishing, 197, 198
flexibility, x, 14, 16, 100, 101, 109, 169, 176, 177
flight, 91, 199
fluctuations, 115
fluid, 39
focus groups, 157, 158
focusing, xiii, 30, 32, 66, 82, 92, 98, 101
food, xi, 66, 68, 69, 83, 96, 98, 100, 112, 114, 116, 120, 121, 149, 170, 171, 181, 195, 197
food production, 66, 69
Football, 28
Ford, 69, 129
forest management, 90
forests, 90, 189
forgiveness, ix, 141, 144, 147
fossil, 68
fossil fuels, 68
fractures, 105
fragility, 122
free recall, 8
freedom, vii, 39
freezing, 83, 198
friends, 33, 42, 43, 87, 142, 158, 196
friendship, 4
frontal lobe, 95, 130, 131, 138
fulfillment, 25, 26, 101, 102, 147, 152
full employment, 100
funds, 56
fusion, xi
futures, 42, 44

G

gasoline, 197
gender, viii, 1, 6, 75, 84, 87, 103, 130, 134, 154, 158
gender differences, 134
gender role, 130
gene(s), 70, 80, 83, 86, 114, 115
generation, 113, 122, 146, 148, 150
genetic factors, 114

genetics, 69, 70, 111, 118
genome, 83, 115
genotype, 104
geography, 55, 85, 109, 131, 199
Georgia, 184
gift, 9, 44
girls, 6
globalization, 118
glucocorticoid receptor, 134
goal attainment, 74, 145, 148
goal setting, 146, 148
goals, 26, 30, 33, 34, 54, 57, 59, 73, 94, 117, 146, 148, 150, 155, 164, 165, 173, 175, 176, 179, 190
goal-setting, 137
God, 49, 50, 58, 59, 192, 194, 196
gold, 189
goods and services, 172, 174, 181
governance, 172, 174
government, x, 66, 86, 117, 122, 155, 169, 175, 177
grants, xiv
grass, 187
greed, 68, 69
GRIN, xiii
group membership, 10, 12, 13
groups, viii, 6, 7, 10, 13, 14, 38, 77, 79, 95, 98, 121, 154, 155, 157, 158, 160, 161, 163, 164, 173, 174, 175
growth, 52, 68, 75, 80, 111, 112, 113, 117
guidelines, 60, 130, 138
guilt, 179, 180
gut, 193

H

habituation, 78, 150
hands, 199
happiness, ix, 141, 144, 152, 193, 197
harm, 70, 108, 118, 149, 166, 199
harmony, 70, 149, 199
hate, 151, 197, 198
hazards, 133
head injury, 132, 137, 197
healing, viii, 54, 89, 114
health, iv, vii, viii, ix, x, xi, xii, xiv, 2, 6, 7, 23, 25, 38, 40, 41, 42, 47, 48, 50, 51, 54, 56, 57, 59, 62, 65, 66, 67, 68, 69, 70, 71, 72, 74, 75, 77, 79, 80, 81, 82, 83, 84, 85, 86, 90, 91, 92, 93, 94, 95, 96, 97, 98, 99, 100, 101, 102, 103, 104, 105, 107, 108, 110, 111, 112, 113, 114, 115, 117, 118, 119, 120, 121, 122, 123, 124, 126, 127, 128, 129, 131, 133, 134, 135, 136, 137, 138, 141, 142, 144, 145, 147, 152, 153, 154, 155, 156, 157, 158, 159, 163,

164, 165, 166, 167, 169, 170, 173, 174, 175, 177, 181, 184, 188, 193
health care, ix, 38, 41, 42, 47, 50, 51, 54, 57, 59, 62, 66, 81, 114, 128, 141, 142, 144, 158, 165, 174, 181
health care professionals, 51, 141, 144
health care system, 41, 66, 114
health education, 68, 134
health expenditure, 144
health insurance, 154
health problems, 42, 47, 68, 69, 74, 75, 80, 84, 95, 96, 98, 99, 104, 110, 118, 119, 120, 154
health services, ix, 47, 93, 154, 159, 166
health status, 144
health-promoting behaviors, 147
heart disease, 94
height, 84
heredity, 78
heterogeneity, viii, 1
high blood pressure, 91
high school, 155
higher quality, 122, 165
Hispanic population, 168
Hispanics, 154, 165
HIV, xi, 123, 124, 127, 145, 170
HIV-1, 123
homelessness, xi, 157, 170, 172, 177
homeostasis, 107
homework, 143, 147
homicide, 133
hospitals, 65, 66, 83, 96, 99, 161, 175
hostility, 151
House, 98, 110, 133
household income, 158
households, 158
housing, 72, 99, 158, 161, 171
human behavior, 124
human brain, 95, 150
human condition, 50, 192
human development, 71, 81, 95, 105, 112, 125
human experience, vii, 51
human genome, 70, 83, 104, 111, 115
human motivation, 74
human nature, 117
human sciences, 118
human values, 36
humanity, xi, 52, 68, 122, 188, 191, 192, 194, 195, 199, 200
humility, 122
hunting, 83, 89
hurricanes, 68
husband, 94, 196
hygiene, 2, 67, 69, 98

hypercholesterolemia, 104
hypertension, 69, 104
hypnosis, 106
hypothesis, 48, 93, 156

I

ICD, 76
identification, xiii, 30, 102, 157, 163, 176
identity, 35, 49, 75, 86, 101, 102, 103, 125, 126, 127, 135, 136, 165, 173, 179
idiosyncratic, 80
illusion(s), 57, 59, 152
imagery, 129
images, 8, 38, 96, 199
imitation, 39, 58
immersion, 150
immigrants, 158, 159, 163, 167
immigration, 166
immune function, 131, 134, 144
immune regulation, 93
immune response, 138
immune system, 69, 93, 114
immunity, 4, 130, 145
impairments, vii, viii, 23, 30, 32, 38, 72, 74, 76, 77, 82, 92, 97, 106, 107, 108, 109, 143, 154
implementation, xiii, 155, 159, 160, 161, 172
impotence, 189
in situ, 191
in transition, 103
in utero, 107, 139
incentives, 73, 109
incidence, 69, 113, 130, 138
inclusion, 89, 91, 97, 102, 108, 136
income, x, 3, 6, 110, 131, 133, 135, 153, 157, 158, 160
income inequality, 131, 135
independence, 77, 109
independent variable, 10
indicators, 77, 113, 115, 120, 121, 126
individual character, 4, 87, 128
individual characteristics, 4, 87, 128
induction, 130
industrialisation, 69
industrialized countries, 69, 92, 112, 113
industrialized societies, 115, 116, 122
industry, 66, 72
inequality, 133
infancy, 80
infection, xiv, 188
infectious disease, 69, 113, 124
infertility, 195
inflammatory bowel disease, 80, 105

influenza a, 69
inhibition, 9, 10
injuries, x, 90, 147, 153, 160, 163
input, 155
insects, 84, 115
insight, 29, 102, 117
inspiration, 44, 193, 199
instinct, 189
institutions, ix, x, 56, 65, 71, 75, 84, 107, 108, 136, 141, 144, 169, 174, 175, 176
instruction, 9
instruments, 3, 29, 57
insulin, 68, 83, 130, 138
insurance, 66, 108, 158, 166
integration, viii, x, 1, 7, 8, 10, 13, 55, 61, 82, 97, 99, 107, 108, 109, 136, 153, 155, 157
integrity, 75, 76, 184
intellectual development, 3
intellectual disabilities, 75
intelligence, 2, 3, 14, 188, 190
intensity, 14, 80
intentions, 38
interaction(s), ix, x, xii, 15, 16, 17, 65, 66, 67, 70, 71, 74, 75, 78, 79, 80, 81, 82, 83, 84, 86, 87, 90, 91, 92, 96, 103, 104, 105, 106, 107, 108, 109, 110, 114, 115, 119, 121, 123, 126, 128, 131, 136, 138, 153, 155, 157, 169, 174, 178, 179, 181, 183
interaction effect(s), 15
interdependence, 108
interference, 8
International Classification of Diseases, 76
internet, 68, 125
interpersonal relations, 109, 174
interpersonal relationships, 109
interpretation, 15, 39, 55, 78, 148
interrelations, 71
interrelationships, 78
intervention, x, xii, xiii, 5, 6, 19, 32, 36, 38, 48, 51, 54, 57, 58, 59, 66, 71, 74, 78, 79, 86, 90, 92, 93, 94, 95, 98, 99, 100, 103, 104, 106, 107, 108, 109, 111, 118, 119, 121, 122, 127, 131, 132, 136, 138, 140, 151, 160, 164, 169, 178, 179
intervention strategies, 38, 118
interview, 30
intrinsic motivation, 136
intrinsic value, 94
intuition, 98, 127
inversion, 53
investment, 33
isolation, 109, 147, 174
Israel, 155, 166

J

jobs, 100, 109, 171, 172, 182
judges, 195
justice, 117, 139

K

Kenya, 118
killer cells, 93
killing, 197
knowledge transfer, 90

L

labour, 80, 99, 107, 172, 173
labour force, 107
labour market, 172
landscapes, 116
language, viii, xii, xiii, xiv, 1, 2, 3, 7, 9, 10, 12, 13, 14, 17, 18, 49, 55, 56, 57, 58, 59, 70, 75, 98, 112, 116, 151, 154, 158, 189, 198, 199, 200
language impairment, xii, xiii
language skills, 70
Latinos, xi, 154, 165
laws, 77, 86, 88, 100, 106, 109, 110, 117, 121, 154, 191
leadership, 159, 162, 181
learning, viii, xiii, 1, 4, 5, 7, 8, 10, 12, 13, 14, 16, 17, 24, 32, 34, 75, 80, 115, 121, 123, 143, 179, 181, 188
learning environment, 181
learning process, 5, 16, 80
leisure, 29, 68, 79, 97, 101, 102, 135, 137, 140, 174, 182
lens, 132
life changes, 32
life course, 84
life cycle, 113
life expectancy, 70, 98
life experiences, 5, 80, 81, 96, 104, 147, 162
life quality, 111, 121
life satisfaction, 36, 132, 166
lifespan, 79
lifestyle, 34, 78, 121
lifetime, 104, 108
likelihood, 156
linkage, 174
links, 42, 54, 93, 96, 104, 109, 115, 120, 129, 178
lipids, 85
listening, 116, 149, 164, 190, 191, 193
liver, 105

liver disease, 105
living conditions, 16, 136
living environment, 83
lobbying, 100
local community, 159
locus, 4, 5
logging, 31
long run, 121
longevity, 113
longitudinal study, 3
long-term impact, 114
love, ix, 86, 113, 116, 141, 144, 179, 187, 188, 190, 191, 192, 193, 194, 197, 198, 199, 200
low back pain, 109, 127
LSD, 10, 11
lung disease, 104
lymphocytes, 93

M

machinery, 68, 112
mainstream society, 161
major depressive disorder, 124
malaise, 194
males, 130, 160
malnutrition, 99
maltreatment, 2, 3, 6, 14, 19, 20
management, vii, xiii, 16, 23, 31, 38, 66, 85, 93, 98, 99, 110, 120, 128, 140, 142, 144, 151, 183
mandates, 62, 177
manners, 55, 86
MANOVA, 10
manufacturing, 68, 114
marginalization, 163, 164
market, 112
Mars, 122
mastery, viii, 33, 155
material resources, 181
matrix, 129
maturation, 80, 87, 95, 134
meals, 17
meanings, 39, 40, 44, 67, 102, 147
measurement, 121, 185
measures, viii, 6, 23, 26, 30, 109, 112, 120, 152, 193
meat, 83, 96
media, 71, 105
mediation, 55, 56, 143
medication, 106, 144
membership, 13, 101, 103, 175
memory, viii, xiii, 1, 7, 8, 10, 14, 15, 16, 17, 96, 121, 131, 139, 195
men, 43, 82, 112, 122, 138, 145, 158, 197, 198
meningitis, 7

mental energy, 145
mental health, xi, xiv, 20, 75, 93, 101, 102, 104, 133, 135, 139, 142, 167, 170
mental health professionals, 142
mental illness, 23, 63, 119
mental retardation, 7
mentor, 160, 161, 163, 166
mentoring, x, 130, 153, 156, 160, 161, 164, 171
mentoring program, 130, 156, 160, 161
mentorship, 162, 163
messages, 31, 32, 92
meta-analysis, 126, 130, 131, 136
metabolic syndrome, 131
metabolism, 83, 111
metacognitive skills, 135
metastatic cancer, 129
methylation, 134
Mexico, 158
mimesis, 39, 40, 58
minerals, 90
minorities, x, xi, xiv, 153, 154, 155, 156, 157, 163, 167
minority, x, xi, 153, 154, 155, 156, 163, 164, 165
missions, 68
misunderstanding, 53
model system, 165
models, ix, 58, 65, 66, 67, 70, 71, 74, 77, 78, 79, 81, 82, 83, 84, 87, 92, 94, 98, 104, 106, 107, 108, 110, 119, 122, 141, 161, 163
modules, 34
molecules, 81, 82, 114
money, 194
mood, 99, 188
morale, 62
morality, 61, 118
morbidity, 76, 127
morphology, 106
mortality, 77, 126, 129, 131, 133, 136, 142, 166
mortality rate, 77, 129
mosaic, 85
mothers, 89, 104, 106, 120, 139
motion, 149
motivation, vii, viii, 23, 24, 25, 26, 32, 33, 34, 36, 93, 101, 102, 109, 140, 145, 147, 148
motives, 24, 25, 78
motor skills, 8, 72
moulding, 42
mountains, 196
movement, 38, 45, 74, 78, 101, 126
multidimensional, 17, 179
multiple factors, 70
multiple interpretations, 39
multiple sclerosis, 69, 80, 104, 165, 166

multiplication, 200
murder, 190
music, 28, 116, 149, 191, 199, 200

N

narratives, ix, 37, 39, 43, 44, 58
nation, 166, 167
National Council on Disability, 154, 167
Native Americans, 154
natural environment, 65, 83, 107
natural selection, 115
nausea, 196
negative consequences, 144
negative emotions, 143
neglect, viii, xiii, 1, 2, 3, 5, 6, 13, 15, 16, 17, 18, 19
negotiating, 41, 42, 94
negotiation, 39, 152
neonates, 131
nerves, 194
nervous system, 24, 70, 80, 81, 93, 104, 107
network, 99, 175
networking, 119
neurobiology, 80, 137
neuroendocrine, 93
neuronal circuits, 105
neuropsychiatry, 129
neuropsychological assessment, viii, xiii, 1, 3, 13, 14
neuropsychological tests, viii, 1, 3, 9, 12, 13
neuropsychology, xii, xiii, 1, 2, 3, 7, 10, 17, 138
New England, 126
New South Wales, 165
New Zealand, 20
next generation, 105
Nietzsche, 197
nitrate, 130
noise, 109
North America, 3, 118, 134, 135
Norway, xii
nurses, 51, 62, 98, 160
nursing, 41, 62, 67, 71, 85, 95, 98, 131, 133, 134
nursing care, 131
nursing home, 41
nutrition, xi, 104, 139, 170

O

obesity, 69, 99, 104, 113, 116, 119, 127, 130, 135
objectivity, 57, 58
obligation, 189
observations, 45, 131, 145

occupational therapy, ix, xii, xiv, 36, 47, 48, 50, 51, 52, 53, 54, 55, 56, 58, 59, 60, 61, 62, 71, 78, 85, 94, 118, 126, 130, 132, 138, 139, 157
oceans, 90
oil, 68, 122, 137
older adults, 137, 166
older people, 132
open-mindedness, 74, 119
oppression, 31
optimism, ix, 16, 93, 140, 141, 142, 144, 145, 146, 149, 151, 152
organ, 104
organism, 80, 91
organization(s), xiii, 8, 18, 66, 68, 79, 96, 98, 107, 109, 115, 117, 121, 122, 134, 155, 166, 170, 174, 175, 182, 183
orientation, 50, 52, 54, 55, 93, 94, 99, 106, 146, 148
originality, ix, 141, 144
overload, 134
ownership, 102, 155, 156, 158, 160
ozone, 68

P

pain, 25, 29, 40, 42, 93, 94, 124, 131, 136, 140, 142, 147, 149, 151, 189, 193, 194
palliative, 38, 40, 41, 45, 46
palliative care, 38, 40, 45, 46
pancreatitis, 192
parental care, 105
parental support, 80
parenting, 6, 77, 103, 104, 126, 159, 162
parenting behaviours, 104
parents, 2, 6, 7, 16, 17, 80, 85, 99, 104, 105, 106, 107, 112, 113, 159
particles, 85
partnership(s), x, 86, 94, 119, 159, 168, 169, 170, 172, 177, 181, 184,
passive, 34, 44, 72, 156, 160
pathology, ix, 31, 141, 144
pathways, 131, 145
patterning, 84
pedagogy, xiii
peer review, 163
peer support, 99, 181
peers, 5, 17, 98, 99
pelvis, 194
penicillin, 88
perceived control, 93, 144, 147, 148
perceived self-efficacy, 93, 140
percentile, 9
perception(s), 3, 16, 30, 80, 83, 91, 98, 100, 101, 102, 106, 123, 150, 160, 161, 166

perinatal, 7, 131, 137
permit, 66
perseverance, ix, 141, 144
personal accomplishment, 74
personal control, 33, 145
personal history, 33
personal qualities, 116
personal responsibility, 179
personality, 4, 16, 17, 18, 20, 35, 53, 75, 84, 106, 146, 151
personality characteristics, 20
personality traits, 4, 16, 17
persons with disabilities, xii, 165
pharmacokinetics, 128, 134
pharmacology, 87, 114
phenomenology, 54, 55, 58, 151
philosophers, 67, 196
phlebitis, 194
phobia, 93, 131
physical abuse, 6, 16, 102
physical activity, 102, 124, 127, 137
physical environment, 34, 79, 88, 99, 100
physical health, 145, 152
physical therapy, 131
physics, 85, 199
physiological factors, 79
physiology, 106, 118
pilot study, 129, 140, 166
pitch, 196
placebo, 93
placenta, 104
planets, 122
planning, viii, 1, 9, 10, 12, 13, 14, 16, 17, 31, 53, 98, 99, 120, 121, 129, 135, 137, 145, 155, 156, 157, 159, 165, 172, 175, 176
plants, 68, 111
plastic products, 122
pleasure, 32, 33, 116, 146, 149, 150
pneumothorax, 197
pollution, 67, 68, 133
polymorphisms, xiv
poor, 17, 21, 188
population, ix, xi, 7, 65, 66, 67, 69, 77, 82, 92, 97, 112, 117, 118, 120, 124, 126, 131, 154, 160, 164, 168, 169, 177, 179, 180, 183
population group, xi, 169, 177, 179, 180
positive emotions, ix, 141, 144, 147
positive interactions, 103
positivism, 48
postmodernism, 50
posttraumatic stress, 139
post-traumatic stress disorder, 91

poverty, xi, 3, 14, 17, 19, 21, 120, 125, 154, 165, 170, 171, 172, 177
power, 50, 51, 54, 56, 61, 102, 112, 113, 116, 139, 156, 164, 177, 178, 179, 180, 181, 188, 192, 198, 199
power plants, 113
practical knowledge, 179
praxis, 157, 164, 167
precipitation, 80
predictors, 17, 90, 139
preeclampsia, 104, 138
preference, 72, 192
pregnancy, 3, 80, 81, 99, 105, 126
premature infant, 7
preschoolers, 19, 127
president, xiii
pressure, x, 97, 138, 153, 179, 183
pressure sore, x, 153
prevention, x, xi, 81, 120, 121, 127, 143, 150, 153, 158, 159, 167, 170
private education, 171
private practice, 135
private sector, x, 169, 173, 175
problem-solving, 9, 15, 16, 31, 95, 131, 143, 180
problem-solving strategies, 15
production, 38, 52, 53, 59, 68, 83, 86, 90, 91, 112, 113, 115, 118, 128, 174
productivity, 79, 122
profession(s), ix, 47, 48, 54, 56, 126, 135
profit(s), x, 98, 108, 112, 114, 115, 116, 119, 120, 169
prognosis, 139
program, xii, xiii, 6, 36, 100, 127, 133, 134, 139, 155, 160, 161, 162, 163
programming, 80, 134, 158, 164
proliferation, 105
propane, 197
proposition, 128
prostate, 129
prostate cancer, 129
prostheses, 75
protective factors, 4, 5, 15, 16, 17, 106
proteins, 85
Prozac, 137
psychiatric disorders, 143
psychiatrist, 96
psychobiology, 19, 139
psychological distress, 128
psychological health, 7
psychological problems, 143
psychological resources, 145
psychological stress, 4
psychologist, 106

psychology, iv, vii, ix, xii, xiv, 9, 19, 36, 52, 55, 71, 78, 85, 93, 95, 105, 118, 124, 127, 132, 134, 137, 141, 144, 145, 146, 147, 148, 151, 152
psychometric properties, 8, 9
psychopathology, 130, 146, 151
psychosis, 128
psychosocial factors, 93
psychosomatic, 4
psychotherapy, ix, xiv, 106, 134, 141, 142, 144, 145, 146
public health, x, xii, 66, 85, 100, 118, 120, 123, 125, 132, 136, 169, 170, 172, 175
public schools, 159
public sector, 173, 175

Q

qualifications, 53
qualitative research, xiii
quality of life, viii, 23, 70, 71, 75, 79, 83, 99, 106, 118, 119, 121, 132, 142, 156, 163
questioning, x, 48, 52, 57, 141, 145
questionnaires, 6, 75

R

race, 84, 191, 198
racial minorities, 166
racism, 166
radiation, 131, 138
radiation therapy, 131
radio, 68
rain, 189
range, 23, 25, 32, 142, 148
rationality, 53, 57, 58, 59, 67, 174, 192, 195
reading, 116, 150, 189, 191, 192
realism, 193
reality, xii, xiii, 5, 32, 39, 52, 53, 56, 59, 81, 156, 175, 189, 191, 193, 195, 198
reasoning, 38, 39, 43, 44, 60, 116
recall, 8, 29, 96
recalling, 54
reciprocal interactions, 70
reciprocity, 97
recognition, xi, 8, 33, 52, 94, 100, 170, 183
reconstruction, 46, 125
recovery, 82, 130, 138
recreation, 140
recycling, 120, 121
redistribution, 181
reduction, 40, 74, 82, 92, 93, 107, 129
reflection, 25, 40, 74, 103, 157, 164

reflexes, 4
reflexivity, 56, 59
reforms, 75, 119
refugees, 85, 126
regeneration, 114
regulation(s), 20, 80, 81, 91, 95, 99, 104, 106, 111, 114, 117, 118, 122, 123, 128, 131, 132, 137, 139
rehabilitation, viii, xii, xiii, 38, 41, 47, 71, 74, 82, 93, 95, 106, 113, 124, 126, 127, 128, 132, 133, 135, 137, 140, 142, 155, 156, 160, 161, 162, 163, 165, 168
Rehabilitation Act, 156
rehabilitation program, 127
reinforcement, 101, 179
rejection, 39, 193
relationship(s), ix, x, 3, 6, 9, 30, 36, 49, 56, 59, 67, 69, 72, 77, 79, 80, 82, 85, 86, 90, 110, 106, 108, 120, 128, 130, 143, 161, 162, 163, 169, 170, 173, 176, 177, 178
relatives, 81, 94, 95, 98, 99, 105, 113, 119, 128
relaxation, 129, 149
relevance, 1, 92, 119, 121, 156, 195
reliability, 8, 9
religion, 50, 51, 55, 67, 129, 138, 193
renewable energy, 121
repair, 28, 68, 89, 91
replacement, 122
reprocessing, 106
resilience, viii, 1, 2, 3, 4, 5, 13, 15, 16, 17, 20, 82, 88, 91, 98, 103, 106, 125, 133, 134
resistance, 69, 171, 175
resolution, xi, 62
resources, vii, x, 32, 38, 39, 66, 68, 69, 72, 78, 79, 86, 89, 90, 91, 95, 97, 107, 108, 110, 111, 112, 113, 114, 117, 118, 119, 120, 139, 144, 145, 146, 152, 154, 156, 161, 162, 164, 169, 170, 173, 174, 177, 181, 183
respiratory, 133
responsiveness, 35
restructuring, 143
retention, 8
returns, 88
rheumatoid arthritis, 36
risk, xi, 3, 4, 14, 42, 51, 59, 69, 70, 75, 80, 81, 93, 98, 105, 107, 128, 129, 130, 133, 134, 154, 169, 178
risk factors, 69, 70, 75, 98, 128
routines, 30, 68, 78, 103, 131
rubber, 196
rural development, 174
rural population, 124

S

sadness, 116, 192, 197
sample, 26, 159, 166
satisfaction, ix, 24, 25, 32, 52, 79, 102, 130, 141, 144, 146, 147, 158, 161, 164
Scandinavia, 120
scarcity, 158
scheduling, 150
schizophrenia, 75, 128, 133
scholarship, xiv
school, xi, 4, 7, 9, 19, 21, 25, 71, 83, 85, 90, 97, 99, 101, 107, 109, 131, 136, 164, 199
school achievement, 21
scientific knowledge, 67, 85
scientific method, 114
scientific understanding, 96
scores, 1, 8, 9, 10, 11, 14
search, 48, 51, 52, 53, 56, 107, 116, 189
searching, 32, 38, 162
Second World, 74, 100
security, xi, 34, 98, 100, 109, 170, 174
segregation, 97
selecting, 34
selective attention, 8
self-concept, 73
self-confidence, 101, 102, 179
self-consciousness, 150
self-control, 92, 95, 117, 118, 121, 122
self-definition, 139
self-destruction, 193
self-efficacy, 74, 92, 93, 102, 118, 120, 124, 135
self-empowerment, 156
self-esteem, x, 5, 16, 73, 98, 101, 102, 162, 169, 174, 179, 183
self-image, 38, 101, 102
self-monitoring, 73, 148
self-observation, 73
self-reflection, 74, 95, 117
self-regulation, 9, 65, 74, 80, 81, 83, 92, 93, 95, 96, 104, 105, 106, 107, 114, 117, 119, 121, 124, 128, 129, 132, 134, 135, 136, 137, 140
self-worth, 102
sensations, 96, 116
sensory experience, 149
series, 8, 26, 48, 71, 87, 121, 133, 136, 151, 159
serum, 138
service provider, xi, xiv, 154, 155, 157, 159, 161, 164, 165
SES, 1, 2, 3, 5, 6, 7, 10, 11, 13, 14, 17
severity, 90, 142
sex, 78
sexual abuse, 6

sexual behaviour, 116
shamanism, 193
shape, 24, 26, 41, 44, 70, 73, 80, 104, 135, 139, 192, 199
shaping, 25, 80
sharing, 31, 42, 113, 120, 150, 160
sheep, 118
shelter, 157, 166, 181
shock, 137
short run, 90
side effects, 87
signs, 113
silk, 41
sites, 160
skills, 3, 6, 15, 72, 76, 84, 88, 92, 95, 101, 102, 103, 116, 117, 118, 121, 122, 143, 155, 162, 164, 171, 172, 178, 179, 181, 182, 183, 192
skin, 188, 194
slavery, 118
Slovakia, 130
smog, 68
smoke, 187
smoking, 69, 95, 100, 116, 124, 144
social behaviour, 73, 118, 130
social capital, 97, 120, 181
social change, 161, 164
social cohesion, 98, 184
social construct, 54
social control, 134
social costs, 119
social development, 134, 136, 177
social environment, 79, 84, 86, 88, 96, 97, 98, 100, 106, 109, 133
social events, 44
social exchange, 44
social exclusion, 182
social group, 120
social identity, 101
social inequalities, 110, 127
social integration, 75
social justice, 95, 167
social learning, 103
social life, 97
social network, 80, 136
social organization, 97
social participation, xii, 74, 75, 78, 79, 82, 83, 90, 97, 106, 107, 108, 127, 128
social perception, 134
social problems, 111, 170
social psychology, 78
social relations, 4, 42
social roles, 75, 77, 82, 87, 97
social rules, 87

social sciences, 71, 118
Social Security, 161
social services, xiii, 85
social skills, 16
social structure, 117
social support, xi, 16, 79, 97, 145, 158, 169
social support network, 16
social workers, 98
socialization, 101
society, 36, 71, 75, 95, 97, 102, 110, 112, 116, 121, 129, 139, 154, 163, 164, 172, 179, 194
socioeconomic status, viii, 1, 2, 3, 136
Socrates, 199
software, 10
solidarity, 121, 174
sounds, 173, 181
Spain, 167
specialization, xiii, 51
species, 67, 68, 70, 82, 84, 110, 111, 112, 113, 115, 116, 117, 118, 121, 122, 134
specificity, 114
spectrum, 137
speech, xiii, 18, 49, 58, 99, 120
speed, 8, 9, 191
spinal cord, x, 102, 128, 140, 153, 156, 160, 163, 165, 166
spinal cord injury, 102, 128, 140, 156, 165, 166
spine, 194
spirituality, vii, ix, xiii, 16, 47, 48, 49, 50, 51, 52, 53, 54, 55, 56, 57, 58, 59, 60, 61, 62, 63, 79, 112, 141, 144, 158, 196
spontaneity, 52, 61
spontaneous pneumothorax, 197
sports, 93, 101, 102, 113, 161
SPSS, 10
stability, 111, 144
stages, viii, 17, 23, 32, 34, 35, 70, 143, 146, 148, 171, 176
stakeholders, 158, 159
standards, 31, 32, 94, 97, 181
stars, 190, 192
steel, 201
stethoscope, 187
stigma, 131, 179, 180
stimulus, 115, 139
strategic planning, 172
strategies, ix, x, xi, 26, 31, 32, 34, 35, 72, 73, 81, 82, 86, 93, 100, 106, 113, 131, 139, 140, 141, 145, 148, 150, 153, 154, 155, 157, 164, 170, 172, 177, 183, 194
strength, vii, 72, 82, 198
stress, viii, 4, 15, 16, 80, 81, 91, 93, 96, 104, 114, 126, 130, 131, 134, 139, 144, 151

stressful events, 80, 81
stressors, 4, 80, 86, 104, 139, 147
strikes, 165, 190
stroke, 166
structural changes, 180
structuralism, xiv
structuring, 49, 50
students, 131, 199
subjective experience, ix, 86, 141, 144
subjectivity, 58
substance abuse, xi, 144, 158, 170, 172
suffering, xii, 25, 38, 99, 105, 122, 187, 188, 189, 190, 193, 194, 195, 196
sugar, 69, 83
suicide, xi, 170, 188, 191
summaries, x, 141, 145
summer, 187
supernatural, 50, 51
supervision, 161
supervisor(s), 9, 98, 109, 148, 161
supply, 111, 115, 161, 162
surprise, 150
surveillance, 109
survival, 68, 70, 74, 75, 82, 83, 88, 91, 113, 119, 125
survival rate, 74
survivors, 102, 126, 136
susceptibility, 93, 126, 130
suspense, 44
sustainability, 181
sustainable development, 66, 114, 118, 119, 120, 121
swallowing, 198
Sweden, xii, 37
symbols, 67, 73, 102
symptom(s), vii, 25, 40, 58, 76, 80, 96, 105, 142, 143, 144, 145, 146
syndrome, xiv, 20
synthesis, 66, 81
systems, x, 4, 36, 55, 66, 71, 72, 75, 76, 78, 80, 81, 84, 85, 87, 102, 104, 112, 113, 117, 119, 120, 122, 129, 153, 154, 155, 170, 175, 181, 182, 195

T

T lymphocyte(s), 93
talent, ix, 141, 144
tangles, 190
Tanzania, 118, 124
targets, 8, 79, 84, 88, 121
TBI, 16, 132
teachers, 97
teaching, xiii, 107, 148, 150
technical assistance, 172
technology, xii, 59, 68, 114, 119, 193, 197

Index

telephone, 68, 163
television, 68
temperament, 123
temperature, 149
tension, 197
tenure, xiii
territory, vii, 82, 89, 112, 113
textbooks, 194
theory, xii, 38, 47, 49, 51, 58, 67, 71, 73, 74, 78, 82, 93, 94, 95, 100, 106, 110, 117, 122, 123, 124, 127, 128, 129, 131, 132, 135, 136, 137, 138, 145, 146, 147, 148, 151, 152, 167, 168
therapeutic goal, 30
therapeutic interventions, 60
therapeutic practice, 147
therapeutic relationship, 59
therapists, x, 41, 45, 47, 48, 50, 51, 54, 60, 61, 71, 78, 79, 86, 94, 95, 98, 101, 109, 125, 141, 145, 146, 147, 148, 160
therapy, x, xiii, 25, 26, 30, 31, 37, 45, 48, 50, 54, 56, 60, 61, 62, 94, 96, 99, 107, 124, 125, 130, 141, 142, 143, 144, 145, 146, 147, 148, 149, 150, 151, 152, 161, 163
thinking, vii, viii, ix, 15, 25, 30, 38, 49, 57, 59, 66, 67, 74, 119, 121, 122, 141, 142, 143, 144, 145, 148, 149, 150, 188, 192, 197
Third World, 125
threat, 195
time, x, xiv, 4, 6, 7, 8, 29, 30, 35, 38, 39, 40, 42, 43, 49, 56, 58, 67, 69, 73, 79, 82, 83, 84, 86, 90, 91, 96, 97, 98, 100, 108, 109, 112, 113, 114, 119, 122, 131, 133, 136, 138, 146, 148, 150, 156, 157, 160, 164, 169, 173, 177, 179, 189, 190, 192, 193, 194, 195, 196, 197, 198, 199, 200
time frame, 177
time use, 30
timing, 138, 148
tissue, 24
tobacco, 158
torture, 199
toxic products, 69, 96, 113, 114, 120
toxicology, 98
toys, 42
trachea, 196
tracking, 161, 162
trade, 69, 173
tradition, 38, 39, 41, 76, 146
training, xiv, 9, 48, 66, 94, 109, 120, 130, 134, 136, 159, 160, 171, 172, 182
traits, ix, 4, 17, 141, 144, 146
transcendence, 50, 55
transference, 4
transformation(s), 17, 54, 91, 106, 122, 133, 179

transition(s), xi, xii, 69, 84, 85, 103, 124, 181
transmission, 69, 80, 104, 115, 117
transparency, 181
transport, 71, 107
transportation, 66, 68, 86, 97, 100, 107, 112, 114, 140, 154, 157, 161, 162, 171, 181
trauma, 4, 5, 15, 16, 20, 75, 76, 90, 96, 102, 107, 113, 130, 133, 134, 137, 139
traumatic brain injury, xii, xiii, 7, 16, 20, 90, 94, 95, 103, 108, 126, 127, 130, 131, 136, 139, 140, 165
traumatic events, 16, 81, 88, 96
trees, 197
trend, 38, 49, 55, 197
trial, 20, 50, 112, 167
trial and error, 112
tribes, 113
triggers, 143
trust, ix, 5, 16, 141, 144, 174, 181
tundra, 189, 194, 196, 199, 200
type 1 diabetes, 83, 134, 137
type 2 diabetes, 69, 104, 129

U

UK, 61
umbilical cord, 7
underlying mechanisms, 104
unemployment, 170, 171, 172
unemployment rate, 172
unions, 173
United Nations, 129
United States, 19, 129, 130, 166, 168, 174
universe, 50, 67, 85, 122, 188, 189, 192, 197, 199
universities, 121
urbanization, 118
users, 97, 139

V

validation, 35, 152, 167
validity, 8, 9, 53, 143
values, 24, 26, 30, 31, 32, 33, 34, 35, 52, 53, 59, 73, 78, 79, 84, 86, 101, 102, 110, 121, 157, 158, 174, 175, 181, 188
variable(s), x, 10, 13, 15, 34, 90, 153, 179
variance, 12
variation, 80, 150
Venus, 122
verbal fluency, 10
vertebrates, 115
victims, 5, 15, 16, 20, 100, 113, 160, 163, 164, 182
village, 97, 174, 196, 197

violence, x, 20, 96, 100, 111, 151, 153, 160, 163, 164
violent crime, 160
vision, xi, 42, 54, 65, 76, 82, 119, 125, 176, 179, 181, 191
visual stimulus, 9
vocabulary, 3, 125
vocational rehabilitation, xi, 132
voice, 26, 164, 167, 190
vomiting, 193
vulnerability, 6, 40, 68, 74, 125, 137

W

walking, 77, 94, 140
war, 69, 74, 96, 113, 190
weakness, 191
wealth, 97, 100, 120
wealth distribution, 97, 120
weapons, 118
web, 166, 174
Wechsler Intelligence Scale, 21
welfare, 21, 140, 167
welfare system, 140, 167
well-being, ix, x, 25, 45, 50, 52, 72, 74, 79, 100, 101, 109, 116, 117, 122, 125, 136, 138, 141, 144, 162, 169, 170, 172, 173, 184
wellness, 23, 142
wells, 67

wheat, 137, 187
William James, 138
wind, 187, 189
winter, 197
witchcraft, 67
women, 43, 100, 102, 105, 112, 120, 131, 132, 136, 139, 151, 158, 173, 177, 188, 197, 201
wood, 42
work environment, 98, 109
work roles, 30
workers, 6, 16, 127, 138, 142
working conditions, 172
workplace, 83, 86, 91, 97, 101, 109, 154
workstation, 88, 109
World Health Organisation, 69, 135, 140
worry, 25, 142
writing, 92, 190, 191, 194, 199

Y

young adults, 112
young men, 160

Z

Zimbabwe, 124